Design for Pediatric and Neonatal Critical Care

Design for Pediatric and Neonatal Critical Care provides an overview of the design and research issues associated with the development of environments for pediatric and neonatal intensive care. This is the first and only book dedicated to this topic and was created to support individuals interested in developing and studying critical care environments for children and their families.

In addition to a detailed analysis of the literature from research and practice, the author provides a summary of the historical development of critical care for infants and children, and information regarding the role of PICUs and NICUs in the critical care system. A discussion of current codes and future trends is also provided.

Design for Pediatric and Neonatal Critical Care includes essays from prominent voices in the field ranging from inspired young architects and researchers to world-renowned healthcare design and research icons. Illustrations of work that has been identified as exemplary or representative of recent directions are included, which will help those planning new or remodeled projects to identify and examine precedents.

This book is intended to help designers and researchers enhance healing environments for young patients in critical care settings and provide information in support of the families and staff who provide care for these children and infants.

Mardelle McCuskey Shepley is a Professor of Architecture and Director of the Center for Health Systems & Design at Texas A&M University. A registered architect with 25 years of experience in practice, her books include *Design for Critical Care* and *Health Facility Evaluation for Design Practitioners.*

Planning for a new pediatric or neonatal ICU is daunting for most clinicians. Few have prior experience, and the skills needed are far different from those they use on a regular basis. Until now, the accumulated wisdom available to them from others who have gone through the planning process has been incomplete, inconsistent, and at times even inaccurate. With the publication of Mardelle Shepley's *Design for Pediatric and Neonatal Critical Care*, this void has been filled in remarkable fashion.

A first attempt to address such a complex issue tends to be rudimentary in areas where the author(s) may not have expertise. But *Design for Pediatric and Neonatal Critical Care* excels in every area. Form and function, design as well as operational issues which might impact design are considered by experts from every relevant discipline, with an international perspective.

Clinicians now have a superb resource to guide them through the planning process for a new ICU, and many babies, families, and caregivers will benefit as a result.

Bob White, Director, Regional Newborn Program, Memorial Hospital, South Bend, IN.

Design for Pediatric and Neonatal Critical Care

Mardelle McCuskey Shepley

Routledge
Taylor & Francis Group
LONDON AND NEW YORK

First edition published 2014
by Routledge
2 Park Square, Milton Park, Abingdon, Oxon OX14 4RN

and by Routledge
711 Third Avenue, New York, NY 10017

Routledge is an imprint of the Taylor & Francis Group, an informa business

British Library Cataloguing in Publication Data
A catalogue record for this book is available from the British Library

Library of Congress Cataloging in Publication Data
Shepley, Mardelle McCuskey.
Design for pediatric and neonatal critical care / Mardelle McCuskey Shepley. -- First edition.
pages cm
Includes bibliographical references and index.
1. Health facilities--Design and construction. 2. Pediatrics. 3. Neonatal intensive care. I. Title.
RA967.S54 2014
725'.57--dc23
2013030252

ISBN: 978-0-415-63922-4 (hbk)
ISBN: 978-1-315-81935-8 (ebk)

Typeset in 10/12pt Syntax
by Fakenham Prepress Solutions, Fakenham, Norfolk NR21 8NN

Printed and bound in India by Replika Press Pvt. Ltd.

Contents

List of figures

Foreword

D. Kirk Hamilton

There is a significant difference between the patients of adult intensive care units, and those of pediatric and neonatal ICUs. These neonates, infants, children, and adolescents are not simply smaller versions of an adult. Providing for their care is not the same as providing care for adults. The patients, diagnoses, treatments, equipment, social support systems, and outcomes are quite different, and so the design of pediatric and neonatal critical care environments inevitably must also be distinctly different. Design of these settings has profound consequences for the patients, families, and caregivers who must experience them. I believe those who design and build them well are doing sacred work.

It is a pleasure for me to recommend the latest work on the part of Mardelle Shepley, a dear friend and valued colleague at Texas A&M University. Dr. Shepley is a superb scholar, widely recognized for her world-class expertise in the realms of design for pediatric and neonatal care, as well as adult critical care. She co-authored *Design for Critical Care: An Evidence-based Approach* (2010), and was the lead author for *Healthcare Environments for Children and their Families* (1988). She has numerous scholarly publications in the areas of evidence-based healthcare design, pediatric and neonatal design, and post-occupancy evaluation. She has long participated in the annual Gravens Conference on the Physical and Developmental Environment of the High Risk Infant, and is a co-author of the current principal guidelines for NICU design, *Recommended Standards for Newborn Intensive Care* (2013).

Dr. Shepley is joined by a distinguished list of contributors from the clinical and design communities, who provide meaningful additional perspectives on this important topic. These noted experts offer a range of facts and opinions that enhance the value of the contents. Their multiple contributions enrich the text.

I am impressed by the comprehensive nature of the volume. It begins with history and definitions. It deals separately with the pediatric ICU and the neonatal ICU. It has sections to examine the physical setting, and the interaction of persons with the environment. Shepley grounds her material in the assumption that improved design decisions, based on reference to findings from research and experience, will contribute to improved outcomes, and will therefore contribute to the environment itself playing a therapeutic role in the course of care. I find her arguments to be completely convincing.

This volume is especially timely in offering research-informed assistance to designers and their clinician clients at a time when there are trends in the air that may profoundly change the character of pediatric and neonatal ICU designs, as in the case of transitions to new technologies, the increasing use of private rooms, or new models for enriched family involvement. Shepley provides us with an exhaustive set of references for the evidence that might influence design. It is comprehensive, and includes substantial international content. There is a consistent orientation to the future.

I recommend this book to anyone involved in the care of very sick children and infants, and especially to the architects, engineers, interior designers, and industrial designers who are involved with creating pediatric and neonatal intensive care environments. Shepley has created a valuable resource and companion for anyone involved in an evidence-based design process, intending to create these important critical care settings for children and their families. It needs to be on the bookshelf of everyone who cares.

D. Kirk Hamilton is a Professor of Architecture and Fellow of the Center for Health Systems & Design at Texas A&M University where he researches the relationship between evidence-based design of healthcare facilities and measurable organizational performance. He holds a professional degree in architecture, a Master's degree in organization development, and is currently working towards a doctorate in nursing and healthcare innovation. He is a long-time member of the Society of Critical Care Medicine and co-editor of the quarterly, peer-reviewed Health Environments Research and Design *journal.*

Acknowledgments

I would like to thank Yilin Song, who served as my graduate research assistant while this book was being produced and is conducting her doctoral research on light in neonatal intensive care units; Genoa Shepley, who reviewed the book for editorial content; Judy Pruitt, who provided administrative assistance; Nidhi Setya, who helped with the plan analysis, and the various design firms who contributed images for the book.

I would also like to thank the various guest authors for their contributions. Their biographies follow.

Samuel Alan Black, AIA, ACHA, LEED AP

FKP Architects, Houston, TX

Alan Black is a Senior Vice President and Pediatric Practice Leader at FKP Architects. A healthcare programmer, designer, and planner with 20 years of experience, he works with top-tier children's hospitals to create results-driven patient care environments. Alan has helped bring millions of square feet of care spaces to reality for clients such as Texas Children's Hospital, Cook Children's Health Care System, Children's Hospital Colorado, and Le Bonheur Children's Hospital.

Annie Coull, AIA, ACHA, EDAC

Stantec, San Francisco, CA

Annie Coull has pursued a special interest in the programming, conceptual planning, and detailed design of healthcare facilities for children. With her education in psychology, child development, and architecture, including a Master of Architecture from the Southern California Institute of Architecture, a Master of Education in Child Development from Tufts University, and a BS in Psychology from the University of Pittsburgh, she brings a unique sensitivity to the special needs of children, families, and staff in the healthcare setting. She strives to create environments that respect and dignify patients through the continuum of human development, that support families in stress, and that enhance the ability of staff to provide care. Her involvement in planning one of the first private room neonatal intensive care units in the US led her to pursue a special interest in design for critical care of newborns that is informed by the latest research on environmental and developmental issues.

Thomas K. Ferris, PhD

Texas A&M University, College Station, TX

Dr. Ferris is an Assistant Professor of Industrial and Systems Engineering at Texas A&M, specializing in the fields of Human Factors and Cognitive Systems Engineering. His research focuses on the design of tools and technologies to support human operators in complex work domains, such as military operations, aviation, ground transportation, and, most notably, in healthcare.

Peter Fröst, Architect, PhD, Professor

Sweco Architects AB, Chalmers University of Technology

Peter Fröst has 30 years of experience as a practicing architect and a PhD in Architecture. Since 2007, he has held an adjunct professorship in Healthcare Architecture at Chalmers University of Technology in Gothenburg, Sweden in combination with his architectural practice. In his doctoral thesis (2004) he developed a protocol for a dialogue-based collaborative design method for the early stages of building projects – Design Dialogues. This method has been met with extensive interest, especially in the healthcare sector, and healthcare is a predominant part of his architectural practice. Dr. Fröst is also Director of the Center for Healthcare Architecture at Chalmers University, where he is responsible for research and development projects as well as undergraduate and graduate programs in the healthcare architecture area.

Breeze Glazer, LEED AP BD+C

Perkins+Will, New York, NY

Breeze Glazer is a designer who has focused his career on sustainability in architecture. He is passionate about redefining the role and impacts of the built environment on human and ecological health. He has applied this passion and his expertise to a broad variety of projects across a multitude of scales, including acute care hospitals, academic medical centers and health clinics, to corporate office renovations and transitional homeless shelters, among others. His research into sustainability covers topics as diverse as alternative energy systems, climate change mitigation, the business case, and material health and toxicity, often in collaboration with academic institutions and non-profit organizations.

Boubou Hallberg MD, PhD

Clinical Director, Neonatal Department, Huddinge, Karolinska Institutet and University Hospital

Boubou Hallberg is Clinical Director and Senior Consultant in the Neonatal Department at Karolinska Institutet and Karolinska University Hospital. His main research focuses on new strategies for preventing neonatal brain injury. He wrote his PhD on neonatal brain injury, hypothermia treatment and outcome following birth asphyxia. He is also involved in family-centered and couplet care in neonatal medicine and has, for the past several years, directed his attention toward parental and staff interaction and the process of designing a new NICU to find ways for supporting this process.

Debra Harris, CEO, PhD

RAD Consultants, Austin, TX

Dr. Debra Harris is the CEO of RAD Consultants, a planning and research consulting firm located in Austin, Texas. She is internationally recognized for research in building performance and occupant outcomes for healthcare, education, and government organizations. She has written over 40 peer-reviewed and trade publications, books, and book chapters; and has presented to thousands of industry professionals on issues significant to the quality of the indoor environment. Her most recent published book is *Design Details for Health: Making the Most of Design's Healing Potential*, 2nd Edition, a reference work which draws upon a rich source of evidence that supports the application of specific research-based design for acute care, ambulatory care, and long-term care facilities. In practice since 1985, she specializes in assimilating research into evidence-based strategies for facility design. Her research focuses on factors affecting user experience and outcomes, especially related to health, productivity, safety, and cost implications of the physical environment.

Dominique Haumont, MD

Neonatal Unit CHU Saint-Pierre, Brussels, Belgium

Professor Haumont is Head of the NICU in Saint-Pierre University Hospital of the Free University of Brussels, Belgium. She has been very active and among the pioneers in moving away from the traditional stressful NICU toward developmentally supportive and family-centered neonatal units. She is President of the educational committee of the EAPM (European Association of Perinatal Medicine), President of the Belgian College of Physicians in Neonatology, and a faculty member at the ECPN (European Chinese Perinatal Network). Besides developmental care, her research fields of interest are intravenous lipids, DNA damage and oxidative stress, and perinatal ethics).

Yamile C. Jackson, CEO, PhD, PE, PMP

Nurtured by Design, Houston, TX

A native of Bogotá, Colombia, Yamile Jackson has a PhD in industrial engineering with concentration in ergonomics and human factors. Since 2001 when her son Zachary was born prematurely weighing less than 2lb., she has applied ergonomics, engineering and technology, and parental intervention to prevent deficiencies commonly attributed to prematurity. Her designs provide each NICU patient with a constant level of individualized developmental care, support for brain maturation, and the best possible quality of life. She is a global leader of kangaroo care, and a strong advocate for humanizing the care of preemies with evidence-based developmentally supportive care that is centered in the family.

Lauren Johnson, MS, RN, CNS-BC

University of Minnesota Amplatz Children's Hospital, Minneapolis, MN

Lauren Johnson's career spans more than 30 years of patient care and roles in nursing education. She earned her BSN from the University of Wisconsin – Eau Claire and master's degree in nursing from the University of Minnesota. She was clinical planning lead for the University of Minnesota Amplatz Children's Hospital building project from 2006 to 2011.

Gregory C. Mare, AIA, EDAC

Stantec, San Francisco, CA

Greg Mare has over three decades of experience as an innovator and expert in healthcare planning and design. As lead medical planner and designer for new free-standing children's hospitals, hospital additions and alterations, for academic healthcare systems and children's hospitals within a hospital, Mr. Mare brings significant knowledge to children's hospitals across the country. He is an industry leader in evidence-based design and patient quality/safety environments, and a prolific national speaker on pediatric healthcare design issues. He has been named in *Healthcare Design Magazine*'s "Twenty Who Are Making a Difference," published in the December 2008 issue.

Michele Moss, MD

Arkansas Children's Hospital, Little Rock, AK

Dr. Moss grew up in Dallas, Texas, and received her BS in Zoology from Texas A&M University. She attended the University of Texas Southwestern Medical School, receiving her MD in 1979. She performed her residency in Pediatrics at the Children's Hospital of Alabama in Birmingham, Alabama, and her dual fellowships in Pediatric Critical Care and Cardiology at Yale University School of Medicine in New Haven, Connecticut. She is currently a Professor and Vice Chairman of Pediatrics in Critical Care and Cardiology at the University of Arkansas for Medical Sciences. She is an attending intensivist in the Pediatric ICU and the Pediatric Cardiovascular ICU at Arkansas Children's Hospital. In addition, she serves as Medical Director for Angel One, the pediatric transport service for Arkansas Children's Hospital.

Diane R.K. Osan, FAIA, ACHA

FKP Architects, Houston, Texas

A Fellow in the American Institute of Architects and founding member of the American College of Healthcare Architects, Diane Osan is Chairman of the Board and Chief Visionary Officer at FKP Architects. An award-winning designer, her work with many of the world's leading healthcare organizations over her 30-year career has led to breakthrough deliveries of transformative design and smart operations improvement programs. Her work spans the country and the globe, from California to Philadelphia and beyond, including Canada, China, and Australia.

M. Kathleen Philbin, RN, PhD

Member: Committee to Establish Recommended Standards for Newborn ICU Design, Pragmatix: consultation, Moorestown, NJ

Dr. Philbin consults with newborn intensive care units in staff education for infant handling (Six Lessons for Hands) and feeding preterm infants (SOFFI method). She has long experience in acoustic planning and remediation for newborn intensive care and publishes professionally in each of these areas. She was awarded a doctorate in child development psychology (infancy studies) by Boston University with training in child development with T. Berry Brazelton and dissertation supervision by Heidelise Als.

Laura Poltronieri, Principal, AIA

Poltronieri Tang & Associates, Swarthmore, PA

Laura Poltronieri founded Poltronieri Tang & Associates, a firm dedicated exclusively to the planning and design of children's healthcare facilities, in 2000. Her firm's mission is to design functional, humane, and inspiring pediatric environments. PTA's current clients include Morgan Stanley Children's Hospital of New York, St. Louis Children's Hospital, Children's Hospital of Wisconsin, Miami Children's Hospital, Penn State Hershey Children's Hospital, and the Children's Inn at NIH. Laura speaks frequently at national and international conferences. She has also written extensively on the subject and her firm has sponsored numerous pediatric specific evidence-based design research projects.

Uma Ramanathan, AIA

Shepley Bulfinch Architects, Boston, MA

Uma Ramananthan is a principal with the architecture firm of Shepley Bulfinch and a leader of the firm's pediatric healthcare practice. Her current and recent clients include Women's and Children's Hospital of Buffalo; DMC Children's Hospital of Michigan; Children's Hospital Boston; East Tennessee Children's Hospital; Lahey Clinic, and Hartford Hospital. Her understanding of the rigorous demands of medical staff is complemented by her ability to work effectively with high-level medical faculty and administrators to build consensus among diverse viewpoints. Uma holds a Master's degree in Architecture from the University of Michigan, where she serves on the alumni board of the College of Architecture.

Martha Rothman, FAIA, LEED AP

Shepley Bulfinch Architects, Boston, MA

Martha Rothman is a consulting principal with Shepley Bulfinch, and a national voice in the planning and design of healthcare and academic science facilities. She co-founded Rothman Partners in 1969, where she grew a thriving institutional practice. In 2005 Rothman Partners merged with Anshen+Allen, where she became a principal. She joined Shepley Bulfinch in 2010. At Shepley Bulfinch, Martha has served as consulting principal for projects at Harvard Medical School and Women's and Children's Hospital of Buffalo. Prior to joining Shepley Bulfinch, her work included the LEED Gold South Pavilion at Women and Infants Hospital (Providence, RI) and Beth Israel Deaconess Medical Center's award-winning Shapiro Clinical Center (Boston). She was a founding member and Fellow of the American College of Healthcare Architects and served on the editorial board of the *Journal of the International Academy for Design and Health*.

Zofia K. Rybkowski, PhD, LEED AP

Texas A&M University, College Station, TX

Zofia Rybkowski is an Assistant Professor in the Department of Construction Science of the College of Architecture and Fellow of the Center for Health Systems and Design at Texas A&M University. Dr. Rybkowski's research experience includes environmentally sustainable architecture and construction, life cycle cost analysis, evidence-based design, and lean construction. She researched with Lean Construction Institute founders Dr. Glenn Ballard and Dr. Iris Tommelein while at the University of California, Berkeley. She has extensive experience as a biologist, as well as in architectural and engineering research and as a design consultant. She has consulted for firms in Boston, San Francisco, Tokyo, and Hong Kong. Dr. Rybkowski holds degrees from Stanford, Brown, Harvard, and HKUST. She earned her MArch degree from the Harvard Graduate School of Design and her PhD in civil and environmental engineering from the University of California, Berkeley.

Blair L. Sadler, JD

Institute for Healthcare Improvement, Cambridge, MA

Blair L. Sadler is a Senior Fellow at the Institute for Healthcare Improvement (IHI), and a member of the faculty at the UCSD School of Medicine and Rady School of Management. He served as President and CEO of the Rady Children's Hospital in San Diego from July 1980 until July 2006 and was a member the Board of the Center for Health Design. He is a founder of the Blair L. Sadler International Healing Arts Awards Competition in partnership with the Society of the Arts in Health Care and co-author of *Transforming the Healthcare Experience through the Arts*. Mr. Sadler is a strategic advisor to Health Care without Harm and their Healthy Hospitals Initiative. He is a Founding Fellow of the Hastings Center and serves on its Board of Directors. He is the co-author of leading articles relating to organ and tissue donation as well as two additional books: *The Physician's Assistant Today and Tomorrow* and *Emergency Medical Care: The Neglected Public Service*.

Yilin Song, M.Arch., Doctoral Candidate

Texas A&M University, College Station, TX

Yilin Song, B.Arch., M.Arch, is a doctoral student and graduate assistant in the College of Architecture at Texas A&M University. She received a Bachelor of Architecture degree from Tianjin University, China. While matriculated at Texas A&M University, she was the recipient of multiple scholarships, a Master of Architecture degree, Certificate in Health Systems and Design, and a Certificate in Applied Statistics. She has worked as an intern in several design firms. Her dissertation research focuses on the presence of windows and natural light in neonatal intensive care unit design.

Peter Syrett, AIA, LEED AP BD+C

Perkins+Will, New York

Peter Syrett's experience in sustainability and living built environments has made him one of the firm's leading experts in green design. He heads the sustainability efforts in Perkins+Will's New York office as well as being the northeast region leader of Perkins+Will's Sustainable Advisory Services, which help clients to build a more sustainable future for their organizations. His projects range in scale from large urban planning studies down to critical analysis of the substances we use to build. He led the effort in 2009 to develop the Precautionary List, the architectural industry's first major list of substances to avoid using in building design as well as the development of the 2011 Transparency website on material health and the built environment.

Robert White, MD

Memorial Hospital of South Bend, South Bend, IN

Dr. Robert White is a neonatologist and Director of the Regional Newborn Program at Memorial Hospital of South Bend, Indiana. He has co-chaired the annual Gravens Conference on the Physical and Developmental Environment of the High-Risk Newborn and chaired the Consensus Committee to Establish Recommended Standards for Newborn ICU Design. He also chairs an annual conference on brain monitoring and neuroprotection in the newborn, and has appointments at the University of Notre Dame and the Indiana University School of Medicine. Dr. White is a member of the American Institute of Architects Guidelines Revision Committee, the American Academy of Pediatrics representative to the AAMI Committee on Incubators, and the US representative to the International Electrotechnical Equipment Working Group for Pediatric Equipment.

Introduction

> I could see all these babies laying on these tables and all these monitors and respirators, and God knows what, all hooked up to these things. And I knew my baby was coming into here... and that was pretty scary for me...that took me by surprise. I wasn't prepared for that.
>
> (NICU parent: Huber, 1998, p. 48)

> A monster wanted to eat me – to eat me to bits.
>
> (PICU, hallucination of a boy, aged 7: Colville *et al.*, 2008, p. 978)

The voices of the children and families who have experienced pediatric and neonatal intensive care units provide the most articulate justification for the creation of quality environments. Designing these environments is challenging, however. While a vast amount of data and experience on pediatric and neonatal environments exists, the appropriate mechanisms for accessing, analyzing, and synthesizing this information and experience do not.

Gathering the literature and information on this topic involves a five-point offensive. First, I place pediatric intensive care units (PICUs) and neonatal intensive care units (NICUs) in the context of the overall medical system (Chapter 1). This information sets the context for a discussion of design and research issues.

Chapters 2 and 3 offer definitions of PICUs and NICUs and analyze their development from a historical perspective. Comprehension of organizational and environmental developments in these settings enables us to better understand the current state-of-the-art of their design.

Chapter 4 addresses design recommendations as supported by the general knowledge shared by architects and designers. In this chapter, commonly held opinions are integrated with data to provide justification for design strategies to identify congruencies. Chapter 4 concludes with a summary of recent or well-thought-of PICU and NICU prototypes.

Chapter 5 directs attention toward the science of this knowledge-gathering mission by conducting an in-depth literature review of studies relating to the design of PICUs and NICUs. In addition, literature analyses address the needs of the patients, families and staff who occupy these spaces. While some of these studies are more focused on organization issues than the physical environment, the design of the environment supports the successful execution of the organizational, psychological and sociological objectives.

Chapter 6 informs the reader of the various standards regarding PICUs and NICUs from an international perspective. Much of the literature summarized elsewhere in the book is focused on research and experience in North America, and this section provides the opportunity for some exposure to other perspectives on design objectives.

Chapters 1 through 6 serve as a history of PICU and NICU design, and as a snapshot of the present. Chapter 7 looks toward the future and raises issues regarding potential trends.

This book was conceived to be a companion piece with *Design for Critical Care* (Hamilton and Shepley, 2010), and is organized in a similar fashion. *Design for Critical Care* explicitly focused on facilities for adults. This volume, *Design for Pediatric and Neonatal Critical Care*, completes the coverage of intensive care facilities by extending the subject to children, their families, and the staff who support them.

References

Colville, G., Kerry, S., and Pierce, C. (2008). Children's factual and delusional memories of intensive care. *American Journal of Respiratory and Critical Care Medicine*, *177*(9), 976–982.

Hamilton, D. K., and Shepley, M. (2010). *Design for Critical Care: An Evidence-based Approach*. New York: Architectural Press.

Huber, D.T. (1998). *Parents' lived-experience with the admission of their newborn into a newborn intensive care unit: A phenomenological study*. (Doctoral dissertation). Retrieved from ProQuest Dissertations and Theses. http://search.proquest.com.lib-ezproxy.tamu.edu:2048/docview/304455409/fulltextPDF?accountid=7082

Part One: PICU and NICU background and history

The role of pediatric and neonatal intensive care in healthcare delivery

1

Prior to describing the activities of pediatric and neonatal intensive care units, it is helpful to provide the historical and functional context of these health services. This chapter summarizes the history of critical care, the relationship between different types of critical care units, the need for specialized critical care for children, and basic information regarding pediatric and neonatal intensive care services.

1.1 The history of critical care

The role of pediatric and neonatal intensive care is linked to overall developments in the general field of critical care. Although contemporary critical care traces back to the growth of scientific medicine in the early 1800s, it crystalized around the treatment of patients suffering from shock and trauma during wartime. The Crimean War (1853–1856) provided the knowledge base for the intensive care protocols employed in the US Civil War, which in turn served as the basis for care procedures used in the Franco-Prussian War (Hamilton and Shepley, 2010). Critical care has also been directly connected to the development of anesthesia science and the discovery of X-rays. The recommendation by Florence Nightingale that the sickest patients be located near supervision points is a core notion in critical care environments.

The first contemporary ICU is thought to have been founded by anesthesiologist Björn Ibsen at the Municipal Hospital (*Kommunehospitalet*) (Berthelsen and Cronqvist, 2003) in Copenhagen in 1952/1953 during a polio epidemic (Reisner-Sénélar, 2011). Ibsen's innovative design recognized that the source of the disease was less important than the efficacy of the treatment facility in terms of responding to common symptoms. In these cases the structure thus necessitated the same attributes, regardless of cause. According to Reisner-Sénélar,

> Ibsen's great achievement was to understand that, in terms of treatment, it was rather irrelevant which disease caused the respiratory failure; the treatment should remain fundamentally the same: secure proper ventilation. Today this seems evident, but at that time the idea was quite revolutionary. Starting from this conclusion he understood that patients could only be dealt with adequately if the hospital was reorganised to treat respiratory failures in a multidisciplinary centralised unit.
>
> (Reisner-Sénélar, 2011, p. 1086)

The debate as to which unit was the first is complicated by the activities taking place in various hospitals; these activities entailed multiple intensive care-related interventions, but they were not necessarily conducted in a dedicated unit. However, the first ICU in the United States was likely located at the Dartmouth-Hitchcock Medical Center opened in 1955 (D.C.G., 2013). Shortly thereafter, in 1958, Baltimore City Hospitals (Johns Hopkins Bayview Medical Center) announced the creation of an ICU as well (Safar et al., 1961). Dr. Safar was the physician behind the development of this unit, and while the Baltimore facility may not have been the first ICU, Safar has been credited with establishing methods of modern cardiopulmonary resuscitation (Acierno and Worrell, 2007), and was conducting procedures associated with critical care settings in anticipation of the unit. The ICU at the Baltimore City Hospitals was an outgrowth of the progressive care model, which assumes a distribution of patients by intensity of care needs rather than by disease (Safar et al., 1961), an approach that has characterized inpatient distribution since that time. The costs, including physicians' services, relative to the various levels of progressive care at the Baltimore City Hospitals at the time of the 1958 ICU, are summarized in Figure 1.1.

Figure 1.1: *Costs associated with units at Baltimore City Hospitals (Source: Safar et al., 1961)*

	Beds	*Avg. cost per patient/day*
ICU/recovery room	17–20	$50–80
Acute unit	375	$27
Chronic unit	431	$13
Tuberculosis unit	337	$9
Infirmary and self-care unit	920	$4
Total	2,083	$25 (average)

Another early ICU was located at the Baylor Hospital in Texas which was opened in 1960 (N.A., 2013). In response to the growth of this specialization, the Society of Critical Care Medicine was founded in 1971 (Weil, 1973). The first pediatric and neonatal organizations and units followed suit shortly after the adult units. A discussion of the history of PICUs and NICUs follows in Chapters 2 and 3.

1.2 Current critical care pediatric services and specializations

In 2009, the United States had 5,795 hospitals serving a total of 944,277 beds (AHA, 2012). Within the total patient population, approximately 55,000 critical care patients are admitted each day (SCCM, 2012). According to the Society of Critical Care Medicine (SCCM, 2012), there were approximately 337 pediatric ICUs (4,044 beds) and 1,500 NICUs (20,000 beds) in 2009. Estimates of these totals (see Chapters 2 and 3) vary depending on the source, but the role of these specializations within critical care services is significant. Halpern and Pastores (2010) note that critical care medicine continues to expand within a diminishing US hospital system.

There are 19 pediatric subspecialties (see Figure 1.2). Pediatric intensivists are certified by the American Board of Pediatrics Sub-board of Critical Care Medicine and neonatologists are certified by the American Board of Pediatrics Sub-board of Neonatal Perinatal Medicine (COPS, 2012).

Many of the subspecialties overlap; for example, cardiology and critical care, and behavior/developmental and neonatology.

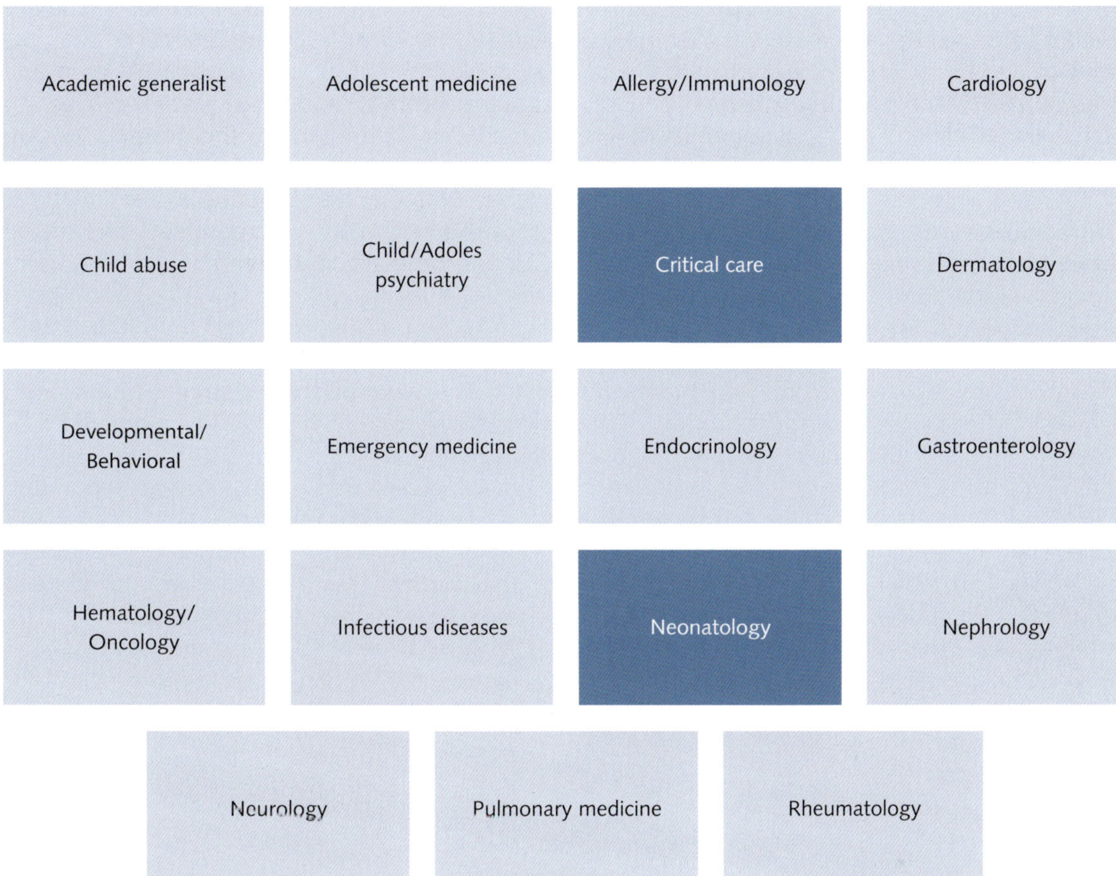
Academic generalist
Adolescent medicine
Allergy/Immunology
Cardiology
Child abuse
Child/Adoles psychiatry
Critical care
Dermatology
Developmental/ Behavioral
Emergency medicine
Endocrinology
Gastroenterology
Hematology/ Oncology
Infectious diseases
Neonatology
Nephrology
Neurology
Pulmonary medicine
Rheumatology

Figure 1.2: *Pediatric subspecialties (Source: COPS, 2012)*

1.3 The relationship between inpatient and critical care units

In addition to the role of pediatric critical care in the context of a range of specializations, the units serve as a key component in the spectrum of inpatient functions. Inpatient facilities in hospitals incorporate a variety of settings, including acute care beds of various specializations (e.g. maternity, oncology, orthopedic, medical surgery), and various levels of care (acute, step-down, intensive). Intensive care beds typically fall into one of three categories based on age of the patient: adult intensive care, pediatric intensive care, and neonatal intensive care. Within these categories are subcategories relating to specialized care, such as cardiac intensive care, or psychiatric intensive care.

The infant intensive care, sometimes referred to as an infant care center (ICC), and NICU provide care for infants who are premature, have congenital anomalies, are impacted by maternal drug dependency, low birth weight, have suffered the negative impacts of the birthing process, or other complex diagnoses. The ICC focuses on babies up to one year of age who are in need of a higher level of care than the standard pediatric patient (Smith, 2012). The PICU serves patients up to 18 years of age for emergency and continuing care needs (Smith, 2012). Some older PICU patients may be treated on the unit when their diagnoses are related to traditional pediatric diseases. Pediatric medical and surgical inpatient units support children with less critical conditions (Smith, 2012).

Contemporary acute care pediatric inpatient units are similar in some ways to contemporary critical care units, for example, with regard to the provision of private rooms, but are dissimilar in a variety of ways in addition to the level of supervision. A literature review on the similarities and differences between these units, however, reveals few studies. Among the most recent, Smith (2012) examined the differences in staff activities in several pediatric inpatient settings. The purpose of this research was to analyze the way in which staff activities were performed prior to a proposed conversion from shared to private rooms in one children's hospital. Smith (2012) compared four types of inpatient units in the hospital. Those units included an ICC, a medical/surgical unit, a NICU, and a PICU – each of which included both private and shared rooms. Researchers noted ergonomic design features, task activity analyses of staff, and surveys of perceptions of nurse and house staff regarding the environment. The ICC and NICU received the highest ratings regarding job satisfaction, quality of patient care, job, work environment, team interaction, and general occupancy. Regarding the physical environment, noise and equipment problems surfaced. The authors drew three conclusions from their data: (1) the most common tasks were interactions with patients, families and the care team members, charting and working with equipment, (2) for these activities, no unit was consistently different, and (3) NICU staff stand for significantly longer periods than staff in other units (see Figure 1.3).

1.4 The need for specialized critical care units for children

Some of the differences between adult and pediatric critical care units are based on the specialized needs of children. According to Downes et al. (1972) per Crone (1988), the primary objective of pediatric critical care is to maximize surveillance and support of organ systems during life-threatening but reversible illness. Fewer children than adults are admitted to critical care units who have been diagnosed with chronic or degenerative organ system complications (Crone, 1988). These children must be cohorted to units dedicated to pediatric issues, which are unique to young patients and require specialized staff and equipment.

1.4.1 Pediatric critical care

While the spatial requirements of PICUs are similar in some ways to adult ICUs, the children in these facilities have unique needs (see Chapter 4), and a range of diagnoses particular to the young age of the patients. In a study of 20 PICUs, Gregory et al. (2008) found that trauma, pneumonia/bronchiolitis, seizures and asthma are the primary admission diagnoses (see Figure 1.4).

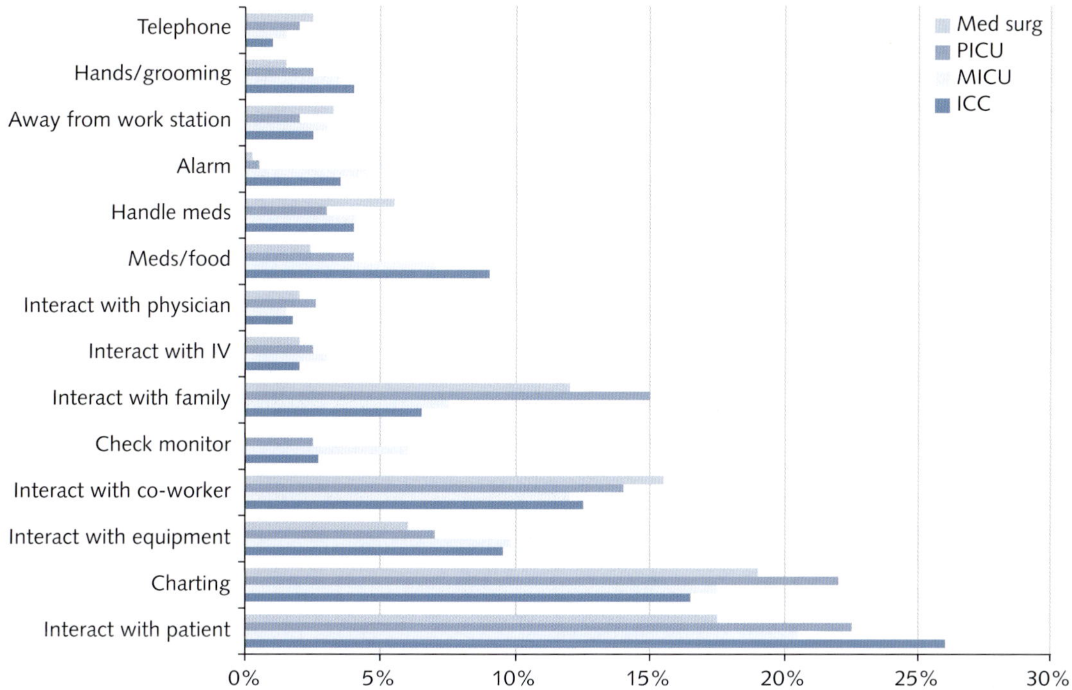

Figure 1.3: *Percent of task activities on ICC, NICU, PICU, and medical surgery units in a pediatric hospital (Source: Smith, 2012)*

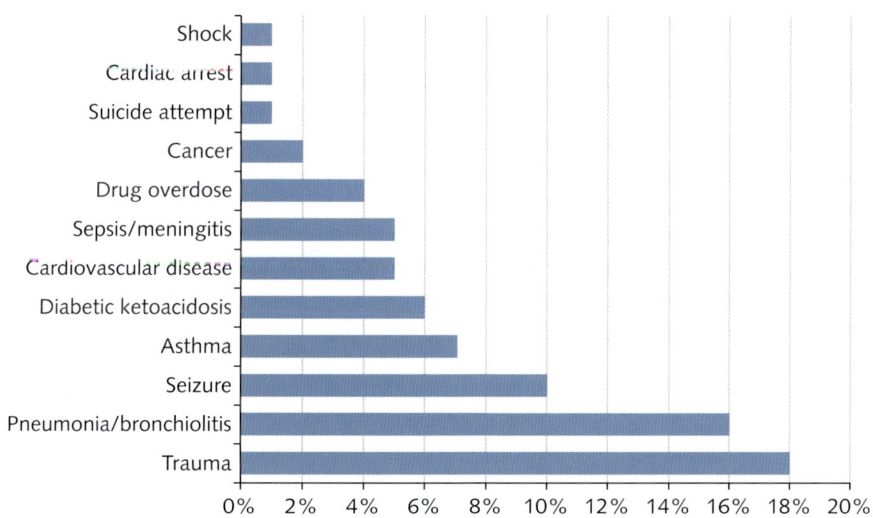

Figure 1.4: *Primary PICU admissions by diagnosis (Source: Gregory et al., 2008)*

Data provided by Rosenberg et al. (2000), regarding the 15 most frequent diagnoses of non-operative adult admissions to adult ICUs, provide a framework for comparison to PICU and NICU admissions, noting myocardial infarction and congestive heart failure to be the primary reasons for admission (See Figure 1.5).

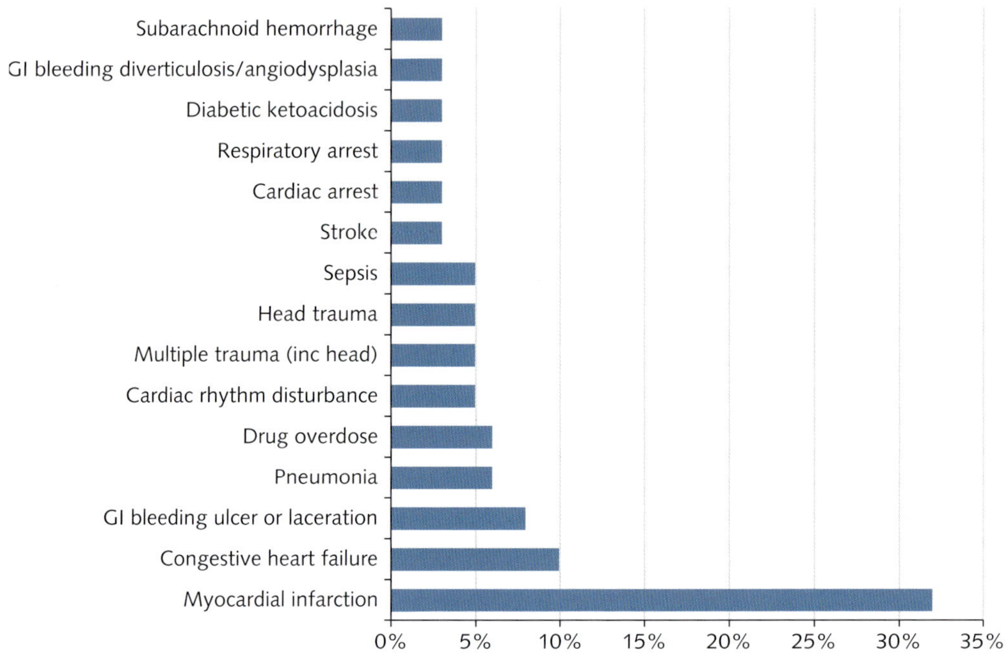

Figure 1.5: *Top 15 non-operative adult ICU diagnoses (as % of top 15) (Source: Rosenberg et al., 2000)*

1.4.2 Neonatal critical care

Neonatal critical care is provided to all newborns whose health status is of concern, but almost half of NICU babies are premature (March of Dimes, 2011). Premature birth has been a significant problem in the United States. Approximately 11.9 percent of babies were born prematurely in 2010 (less than 37 weeks' gestation) and 1.96 percent were born at 32 weeks or less (U.S. Department of Health and Human Services (USDHHS), 2012). While U.S. hospitals have an excellent record for the survival of these infants, the statistics for premature birth are comparable to those in developing countries and below all Western European and Scandinavian countries (McNeil, 2012). Risk factors for preterm birth include previous preterm delivery, smoking, infection, substance abuse, and advanced maternal age. However, the reasons for half of all preterm births are not known (Nelson, 2004).

Premature birth is also race/ethnicity related. In 2010, 17.12 percent of babies born to non-Hispanic Black women were premature, while 10.77 percent of babies born to White women were premature (USDHHS, 2012). American women are at high risk for high blood pressure, obesity, diabetes and smoking; the negative outcomes of lack of prenatal care due to lack of insurance (McNeil, 2012). The percentage of live preterm births by gestational age is reported in Figure 1.6.

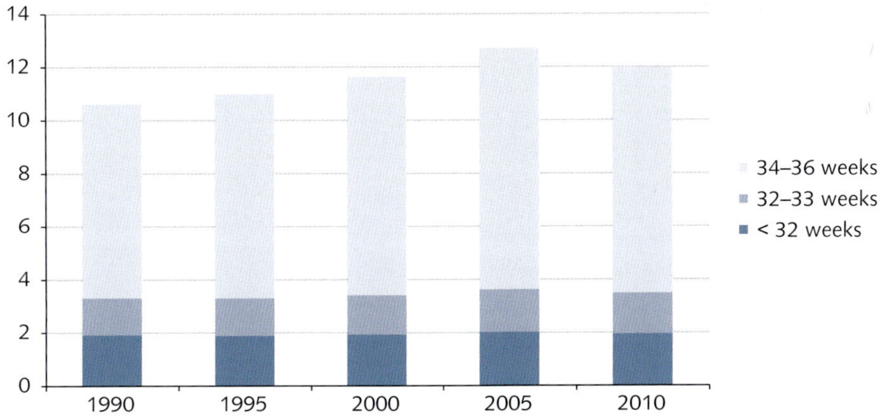

Figure 1.6: *Percent of live preterm births by weeks of gestation (Source: Martin et al., 2010; Centers for Disease Control and Prevention, 2013)*

In the one-year study from July 2009 to June 2010 by the March of Dimes and the National Perinatal Information Center/Quality Analytic Services (NPIC/QAS) (2011), premature babies accounted for 49.1 percent of admissions, and 50.9 percent were term or post-term. Some 14.4 percent of all infants delivered at or transferred to a NPIC/QAS member hospital were admitted to a special care nursery (March of Dimes, 2011). The five most common diagnoses in this study are shown in Figure 1.7.

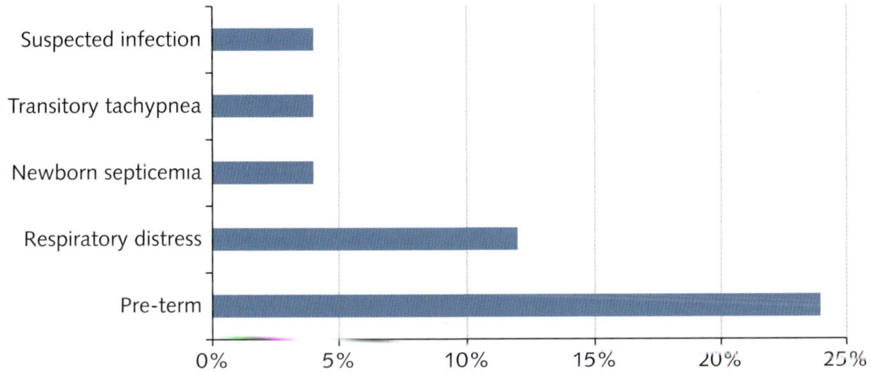

Figure 1.7: *Five most common diagnoses for neonatal special care admissions (Source: March of Dimes, 2011)*

Addressing the suffering and stress experienced by premature babies and their families is the primary reason for providing the best specialized care and finding means to reduce the number of premature births. The medical cost of this care, which is currently being provided, has been acknowledged by policy makers (Almond et al., 2010). One of the factors influencing medical costs for premature babies is gestational age. The relationship between length of stay and hospital charges as found in the March of Dimes study is reported in Figure 1.8.

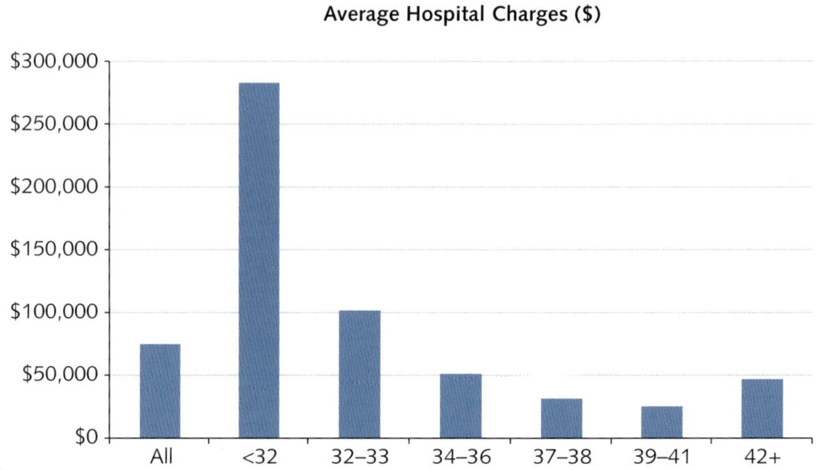

Figure 1.8: *Special care nursery admissions hospital charges by gestational age of infant (Source: March of Dimes, 2011)*

The content of this chapter has focused on the role of pediatric and neonatal critical care in the context of the broader inpatient healthcare system. The following two chapters discuss the developments within PICUs and NICUs over time.

References

Acierno, L.J., and Worrell, L.T. (2007). Peter Safar: Father of modern cardiopulmonary resuscitation. *Clinical Cardiology*, *30*(1), 52–54.

Almond, D., Doyle, J., Kowalski, A., and Williams, H. (2010). Estimating marginal returns to medical care: Evidence from at-risk newborns. *Quarterly Journal of Economics, 125*(2), 591–634.

American Hospital Association (AHA). (2012). *Fast Facts on Hospitals*. Chicago, IL: American Hospital Association.

Berthelsen, P. G., and Cronqvist, M. (2003). The first intensive care unit in the world: Copenhagen 1953. *Acta Anaesthesiologica Scandinavica*, *47*(10), 1190–1195.

Centers for Disease Control and Prevention. National Center for Health Statistics. (2013). *VitalStats*[data file]. Retrieved from http://www.cdc.gov/nchs/vitalstats.htm

Council of Pediatric Subspecialties (COPS). (2012). Descriptions of pediatric subspecialties. Retrieved from http://pedsubs.org/SubDes/index.cfm

Crone, R.K. (1988). Paediatric and neonatal intensive care. *Canadian Journal of Anesthesia/Journal Canadien d'Anesthésie*, *35*(3), S30–S33.

D.C.G. (2013). Vital signs: Remembering Dr. William Mosenthal: A simple idea from a special surgeon. *Dartmouth Medicine, 28*(3). Retrieved from http://dartmed.dartmouth.edu/spring04/html/vs_mosenthal.shtml

Downes, J.J., Fulgencio, T., and Raphaely, R.C. (1972). Acute respiratory failure in infants and children. *Pediatric Clinics of North America, 19*(2), 423–440.

Gregory, C.J., Nasrollahzadeh, F., Dharmar, M., Parsapour, K., and Marcin, J.P. (2008). Comparison of critically ill and injured children transferred from referring hospitals versus in-house admissions. *Pediatrics*, *121*(4), e906–e911.

Halpern, N.A., and Pastores, S.M. (2010). Critical care medicine in the United States 2000–2005: An analysis of bed numbers, occupancy rates, payer mix, and costs. *Critical Care Medicine*, *38*(1), 65–71.

Hamilton, D.K., and Shepley, M. (2010). *Design for Critical Care: An Evidence-based Approach*. Oxford, UK, and Burlington, MA: Elsevier/Architectural Press.

March of Dimes. (2011). Special care nursery admissions. Retrieved from http://www.marchofdimes.com/peristats/pdfdocs/nicu_summary_final.pdf

Martin, J.A., Hamilton, B.E., Ventural, S.J., Osterman, M.K., Wilson, E.C., and Mathews, T.J. (2010). *Births: Final Data for 2010*. National vital statistics reports, 61(1). Hyattsville, MD: National Center for Health Statistics 2012.

McNeil, D.G. (2012, May 2). U.S. lags in global measure of premature births. *The New York Times*. Retrieved from http://www.nytimes.com/2012/05/03/health/us-lags-in-global-measure-of-preterm-births.html?_r=0

N.A. (2013). 1960 – First intensive care unit (ICU) opens at Baylor. Baylor Online Newsroom. Retrieved from http://media.baylorhealth.com/channels/Historical/photos?page=3

Nelson, R. (2004). Premature births on the rise: The March of Dimes and AWHONN educate providers and patients. *AJN The American Journal of Nursing*, *104*(6), 23–25.

Reisner-Sénélar, L. (2011). The birth of intensive care: Björn Ibsen's records. *Intensive Care Medicine*, *37*(7), 1084–1086. doi:10.1007/s00134-011-2235

Rosenberg, A.L., Zimmerman, J.E., Alzola, C., Draper, E.A., and Knaus, W.A. (2000). Intensive care unit length of stay: Recent changes and future challenges. *Critical Care Medicine*, *28*(10), 3465–3473.

Russell, R.B., Green, N.S., Steiner, C.A., Meikle, S., Howse, J.L., Poschman, K., and Petrini, J.R. (2007). Cost of hospitalization for preterm and low birth weight infants in the United States. *Pediatrics*, *120*(1), e1–e9.

Safar, P., DeKornfeld, T.J., Pearson, J.W., and Redding, J.S. (1961). The intensive care unit. *Anaesthesia*, *16*(3), 275–284.

Smith, T. (2012). A comparative study of occupancy and patient care quality on four different types of intensive care units in a children's hospital. *Work*, *41*, 1961–1968. doi:10.3233/WOR-2012-0415-1961

Society of Critical Care Medicine (SCCM). (2012). Critical care statistics in the United States. Retrieved from http://www.sccm.org/SiteCollectionDocuments/StatisticsBroch_d4.pdf

U.S. Department of Health and Human Services (USDHHS), Health Resources and Services Administration, Maternal and Child Health Bureau. (2012). *Child Health USA 2012*. Rockville, MD: U.S. Department of Health and Human Services.

Weil, M.H. (1973). The Society of Critical Care Medicine, its history and its destiny. *Critical Care Medicine*, *1*(1), 1–4.

Definition and history of pediatric intensive care environments

2

This chapter will describe the events that led to the development of pediatric intensive care. The origins of pediatric intensive care are linked to pediatric surgery, respiratory medicine, and pediatric anesthesiology (Epstein and Brill, 2005). The formulation of these specializations grew in tandem with the pediatric intensive care unit (PICU).

Apart from definitions and a discussion of the milestones regarding the development of pediatric intensive care, this chapter describes the evolution of characteristics of the levels of care. The role of subspecialty units is also addressed. By addressing the history and components of PICUs it is easier to understand programmatic needs.

2.1 Definition of the pediatric intensive care unit

Since the 1960s, the intention of pediatric critical care medicine, a subspecialty of intensive care and pediatric care medicine, has been the "surveillance and support of vital system functions in critically ill or injured infants, children, and adolescents, and their eventual restoration to health" (Downes, 1992, p. 1). An intensive care unit is an inpatient unit that provides medical care to patients with severe or life-threatening illnesses. The equipment and intensity of supervision are at a level of sophistication that addresses potential medical crises and the frailty of the patient. In the case of pediatric intensive care, the patient population is typically children who are 18 years and younger. Although there will be some infants in the PICU, newborn infants will be admitted to the neonatal intensive care unit.

A central issue in pediatric healthcare has been the need for specialized environments for children. Apart from addressing the unique medical needs of pediatric patients, we must address their psychosocial needs. The need for specialized units for intensive care has been clearly articulated by the Committee on Hospital Care of the American Academy of Pediatrics (CHCAAP) and Pediatric Section of the Society of Critical Care Medicine. In *Guidelines for Pediatric Units*, the CHCAAP states, "Children have special medical needs, and it is appropriate, therefore, to provide their critical care in units of excellence dedicated exclusively to children, where care is provided by pediatric specialists" (CHCPS, 1983, p. 364). In addition to specific diagnoses common to pediatric patients, because a child's physiology is different from that of an adult, routine treatments for adults may not be appropriate for a developing child. Additionally, the interaction between a caregiver and a pediatric patient requires specialized experience on the part of the practitioner due to the varying communication styles of children of differing ages.

2.2 Evolution of pediatric intensive care

According to Downes (1992), pediatric critical care medicine originated from five fields in the 1950s in Europe and the United States: adult respiratory care, neonatal critical care, pediatric anesthesiology, pediatric general surgery, and pediatric cardiac surgery. As a precursor to pediatric critical care, Downes traces the origins of adult intensive care to the period between 1890 and 1910 in the US and Germany, represented primarily in the work of thoracic surgeons addressing lung neoplasms and tuberculosis. In 1929 Philip Drinker invented the first viable ventilator, also referred to as an iron lung (Downes, 1992). Several units were established throughout the US using tracheostomy and ventilators to address the needs of polio patients. These served as the first respiratory intensive care units, as they were staffed 24 hours per day.

Although adult/general intensive care preceded pediatric intensive care, much of the impetus surrounding the development of all levels of critical care was spurred by experiences providing intensive care to children. The activities of Dr. Björn Ibsen are an example of the precedents involving pediatric patients. Dr. Ibsen, who is credited by Reisner-Sénélar as fathering the birth of intensive care, used the respiratory technology that commonly characterizes critical care settings. The example given by Reisner-Sénélar (2011) regarding the first use of intensive care focuses on an experience Dr. Ibsen had while treating a young girl with polio.

> On 27 August 1952, Ibsen demonstrated his anesthetic skills on a 12-year-old girl named Vivi E., who was in a state of severe respiratory failure. Ibsen ventilated the tracheotomised girl with a to-and-fro system, sucking the mucus from her lungs and narcotising her in order to release her bronchospasm. As it became clear that the available cuirass respirator could not provide sufficient ventilation, Ibsen continued to ventilate the girl manually and eventually saved her life. Within 8 days, the method of manual ventilation via tracheostomy was conducted on every patient with respiratory failure from poliomyelitis within Blegdam Hospital.
>
> (Reisner-Sénélar, 2011, p. 1086)

The poliomyelitis epidemic in the 1950s resulted in a high level of care outside of surgery venues. Later that year, when a newborn presented with congenital tetanus, Dr. Ibsen tracheotomized the child and applied artificial ventilation on a rocking bed. A third event occurred in 1953 when Ibsen treated a young patient with tetanus by using narcosis and curare.

The effectiveness of pre-set ventilators and the professed need to co-locate patients with respiratory failure were the impetus for respiratory and general medical-surgical units in the UK, Denmark, and Sweden (Downes, 1992). As Downes notes, although there were post-anesthesia recovery rooms in North America in the late 1950s, the first adult units were not established until 1958. These units were located at the Baltimore City Hospital and the Toronto General Hospital. Children rarely received care in these facilities with the exception of one dedicated unit in Sweden, although support was growing for this specialized care. C. Everett Koop was one of the earliest and strongest advocates for providing neonatal and pediatric intensive care for all critically ill children (Downes, 1992).

Subsequent to these early steps in adult care, pediatric critical care medicine began to take root (CHCPS, 1993; Epstein and Brill, 2005) due to advancements in pathophysiology and technology

(CHCPS, 1993). In 1981 the Section on Pediatric Critical Care in the Society of Critical Care Medicine was created (Downes, 1992). Other events have also contributed to the founding and maturing of pediatric critical care, as demonstrated in the timeline shown in Figure 2.1. Regarding standards, the first set of guidelines for facility requirements was published in 1983. Recognition was formally achieved when pediatric critical care was designated as a subspecialty in 1985 by the American Board of Pediatrics (ABP), the American Board of Medicine (ABM), the American Board of Surgery (ABS), and the American Board of Anesthesiology (ABA) (Committee on Hospital Care (CHC) and Pediatric Section of the Society for Critical Care Medicine (SCCM), (SCCM, 1993). The guidelines were revised in 1993 and 2004, reaffirmed in 2008, and are likely subject to revision in 2014.

One indication of the substantiation of a specialty is the development of germane training and certification programs, and the formulation of professional organizations. In 1986, the American Association of Critical Care Nurses certification program was established, and in 1990 the Residency Review Committee of the Accreditation Council for Graduate Medical Education held the first accreditation of pediatric critical care medical training programs. In 1999 the certification program for clinical nurse specialist in pediatric critical care was initiated.

Significant steps were made on the international front when, in 1997, the World Federation of Pediatric Intensive and Critical Care Societies was established and in 2002 the first World Conference on Pediatric Intensive Care was held. This educational forum has retained its momentum. The seventh world conference will be held in Turkey in 2014.

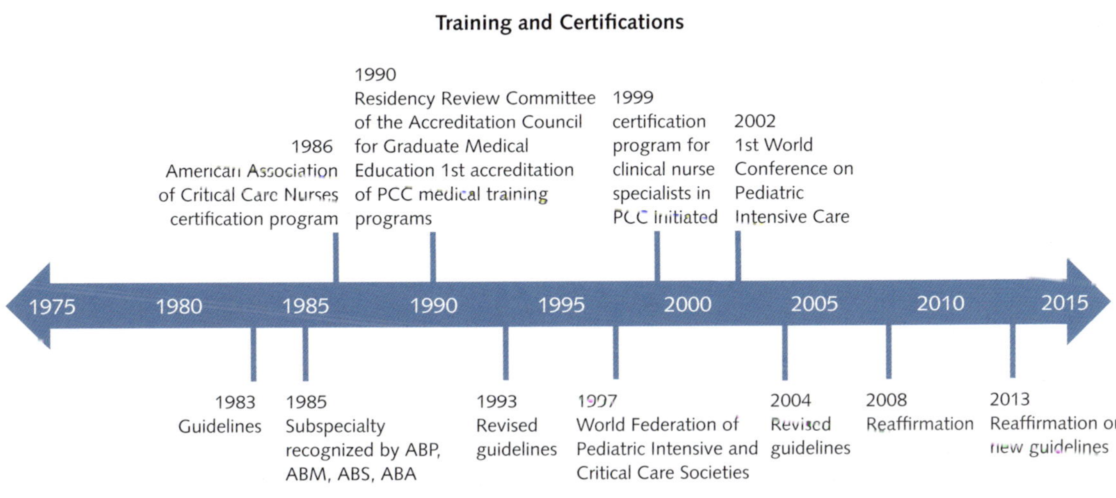

Figure 2.1: *Timeline of events in the history of pediatric intensive care*

2.3 The first PICUs

While the first modern hospital for children was created in Paris in 1802, the first pediatric intensive care unit is attributed to Goran Haglund in 1955 (Costarino and Downes, 2005) (see

Figure 2.2: *The first PICUs (Source: Derived from Downes, 1992)*

Year	*Institution*	*City, Country*	*Director*
1955	Children's Hospital of Goteburg	Goteburg, Sweden	G. Haglund
1961	Stockholm	Stockholm, Sweden	H. Feychting
1963	Hôpital St. Vincent de Paul	France	J.G. Jolu, G. H'ualt
1963	Royal Children's Hospital	Melbourne, Australia	I.M. McDonald, J.G. Stocks
1964	Alder Hey Children's Hospital	Liverpool, UK	G. Jackson Rees
1967	Children's Hospital of Philadelphia	Philadelphia, US	J.J. Downes
1969	Children's Hospital of Pittsburg	Pittsburg, US	S. Kampschulte
1969	Yale-New Haven Medical Center	New Haven, US	J. Gilman, N. Talner
1971	Hospital for Sick Children	Toronto, Canada	A. Conn
1971	Massachusetts General Hospital	Boston, US	D. Todres, D. Shannon

Figure 2.2). This facility, located at the Children's Hospital in Goteburg, Sweden was a 12-bed unit. During the early to mid-1960s similar facilities were set up in Stockholm, Liverpool, and Melbourne (Downes, 1992). The first PICU in the UK included 13 beds, a laboratory, and a resuscitation/procedures room.

The first multidisciplinary PICU in North America was created in 1967 at the Children's Hospital of Philadelphia, which was a seven-bed unit with a full-time nursing staff (Bachman et al., 1967). Shortly thereafter PICUs were established at the Children's Hospital of Pittsburgh (10 beds), the Massachusetts General Hospital, The Hospital for Sick Children in Toronto, and the Yale-New Haven Medical Center (Costarino and Downes, 2005). Downes credits the 20-bed 1971 PICU, at the Hospital for Sick Children in Toronto, as the forerunner for PICUs for the next 10 years.

2.4 Pediatric intensive care subspecialties

There are several subspecialties of PICU, including infant care centers (ICCs) for children up to a year old who require a higher level of care than those admitted to pediatric care (Smith, 2012). Others are pediatric cardiac intensive care (PCIC), and pediatric burn care units (PBCUs). Concerning PCIC, data suggest that cardiac disease is the most common birth defect and accounts for the largest percentage of children in critical care settings. In a study of a cardiac surgery program that introduced a cardiac pediatric intensive care unit, researchers found that wound infection, chest re-exploration, mortality, and frequency of resuscitation decreased (Eldadah et al., 2011). Depending on the severity of the injury, burn units may serve as intensive care units. They share similarities to standard PICUs in terms of painful medical procedures, patient observation of other ill patients, and reduced sensory stimulation (Tarnowski et al., 1989). They are different from standard PICUs in that patients typically have a longer length of stay and are less confined to their beds. Another way in which PBCUs are different from PICUs is that patients are more likely to experience daily intrusive procedures, while PICU patients tend to need fewer procedures after surgery (Tarnowski et al., 1989).

2.5 Guidelines for pediatric intensive care

Guidelines describing the levels of pediatric intensive care were produced in 1983, 1993, and 2004. The next iteration is likely to be available in 2014. A history of the Guidelines is useful as a demonstration of the trends in the requirements for these settings and suggests future needs. All the Guidelines cover a range of topics, including organizational structure, physician staff, nursing staff, other team members, support services, external and internal physical facility features, and equipment. The most recent iterations include guidelines for transport, for quality assessment, and for training features.

2.5.1 *Guidelines of 1983*

The first Guidelines for pediatric intensive care were published in 1983. This took place shortly after the acceptance by the American Board of Medical Specialists of the submission for a Certificate of Special Competency in Critical Care Medicine by the American Boards of Internal Medicine, Pediatrics, Anesthesiology, and Surgery. The authors of the 1983 Guidelines for Pediatric Intensive Care define a PICU as "a hospital unit that provides treatment to children with a wide variety of illnesses of a life-threatening nature, including children with highly unstable conditions and those requiring sophisticated medical and surgical intervention" (CHCPS, 1983, p. 364). According to the parameters described in this document, all critically ill children up to 16 years of age (except premature infants) were to be treated in units dedicated to pediatrics.

Only one level of care is described in the 1983 Guidelines, and this level is associated with a series of qualities described as important, desirable, or optional. The PICU Guidelines described in this document include the need for an organization committee, a medical director with a specialization in pediatrics, and physician and nurse pediatric specialists. A minimum of one registered nurse for every three patients is required along with 24-hour laboratory services, and extensive physiological monitoring. Regarding unit size, the authors of the 1983 Guidelines point out that fewer than six is inefficient and more than 16 is difficult to manage. Room size is not mentioned.

Figure 2.3 lists the internal and external physical environmental features from the minimum Guidelines of 1983. The evaluation of individual components is done using the terms "important," "desirable," and "optimal". The details of the 1983 Guidelines are published in volume 72 of *Pediatrics* (1983).

The document concludes with an appendix of technical considerations related to local building and state codes, "Minimum Requirements of Construction and Equipment for Hospitals and Medical Facilities" (U.S. Department of Health and Human Services) and the "Accreditation Manual for Hospitals" (Joint Commission on the Accreditation of Hospitals). Also included are specific requirements for electrical equipment; heating, ventilating, and air conditioning (HVAC); materials and finishes; plumbing; compressed air; and vacuum. The Guidelines make reference to the building codes. The codes for 1983 are summarized in Figure 2.4.

2.5.2 *Guidelines of 1993*

The next significant publication regarding pediatric intensive care guidelines was produced in 1993, shortly after the first accreditation for a pediatric critical care medicine training program in

Figure 2.3: *Physical environment of pediatric intensive care 1993 (Source: CHCPS, 1993)*

External feature	*Internal feature*	*Reqmt*
Distinct unit		
Controlled access		★★★
Adjacent to elevators		★★
Adjacent to OR		★★
Adjacent to ER		★★
Adjacent to recovery		★★
Adjacent to MD on-call		★★★
Adjacent to nurse manager's office		★
Adjacent to medical director's office		★
Adjacent to head nurse's office		★
No through-traffic		★★★
Key controlled elevators		★★★
Alarm to central hospital		★★★
Waiting room		★★
Family sleep		★★
Family counseling		★★★
Staff lounge		★★
Staff locker		★★
Janitor closet		★★★
Clean linen or	Clean linen	★★★
Nourishment station or	Nourishment station	★★★
Patients' effects or	Patients' effects	★★★
Clean workroom or	Clean workroom	★★★
Soiled workroom or	Soiled workroom	★★★
Intermediate care area		★★
	Patient isolation	★★★
	Patient privacy provisions	★★★
	Central station; direct visualize	★★★
	Med station + refrigerator/narcotics cabinet	★★★
	Separate charting area	★
	Conference area	★★
	Staff toilet	★★★
	Bedpan washing	★★★
	Emergency equip storage	★★★
	Hand washing facilities	★★★
	Patient toilet	★★
	Counter & cabinet space	★★★
	Bedside alarm	★★★
	Clocks, tvs, radios, windows	★★

External feature	*Internal feature*	*Reqmt*
	Access to patient head/neck	★★★
	11 electrical outlets/bed	★★★
	14 electrical outlets/bed	★★
	2 oxygen outlets/bed	★★★
	1 compressed air/bed	★★★
	2 or more compressed air/bed	★★
	2 vacuum outlets/bed	★★★
	3 or more vacuum outlets/bed	★★
	Building/Federal code conforming: HVAC, etc.	★★★
	Computer/microprocessor	★★

* I=Important ★★★, D=Desirable ★★, O=Optional ★

Figure 2.4: *Codes and Standards, 1983 (Source: CHCPS, 1983)*

Organization	*Code*
US Department of Health & Human Services	Minimum Requirements of Construction and Equipment for Hospitals and Medical Facilities
Joint Commission	Accreditation Manual for Hospitals
State and Municipal Organizations	Building codes
	Public health codes
National Fire Protection Association	Inhalation Anesthetics 56A
	Respiratory Therapy 56B
	Laboratories in Health Related Institutions 56C
	Standard for Nonflammable Medical Gas Systems 56F
	National Electric Code 70
	Essential Electric Systems 76A
	Air Conditioning and Ventilating Systems 90A
	Safe Use of Electricity in Hospitals, Code 76B
American Standards Institute	Code for Elevators A17.1
	Making Buildings and Facilities Accessible to the Physically Handicapped A117.1
American Society of Heating, Refrigeration and Air Conditioning Engineers	Energy Conservation in New Building Design 90-75
	Methods of Testing Air Cleaning Devices, Standard 52
	Standard for Air Filter Equipment, Standard 680
Compressed Gas Association	Standard for Medical-Surgical Vacuum Systems in Hospitals, Pamphlet P-2.1
American Society for Testing Materials	Laboratory Measurements of Airborne Sound Transmission, E90
	Classification for Determination of Sound Transmission Class, E 413
National Association of Plumbing-Heating-Cooling Contractors	National Standard Plumbing Code

1990 (Committee on Hospital Care and Pediatric Section of the Society of Critical Care Medicine, 1993). As with the previous Guidelines document, the list of requirements was not believed to be final, but rather a baseline for continuous improvement.

The 1993 Guidelines stand out as the first formal acknowledgment of the need for levels of care. The authors recognized this need in response to the impact on healthcare delivery of geographically isolated portions of the country with low populations (Committee on Hospital Care and Pediatric Section of the Society of Critical Care Medicine, 1993). Having multiple high-level care units in remote areas is likely infeasible due to the high capital costs of these facilities, the difficulty of recruiting sufficient qualified staff, and the inefficiency of small units. The function of the more remote locations, therefore, would be the stabilization of patients prior to relocation to facilities with higher levels of care, normally located in more densely populated portions of the country.

The primary differences between Level I and Level II were staffing and facilities requirements. Level I, which provides a higher level of care, addresses "a wide range of complex, progressive, rapidly changing, medical, surgical, and traumatic disorders, often requiring a multidisciplinary approach. ... Patients in Level II units will have less complex and more stable disorders whose course is more predictable" (Committee on Hospital Care and Pediatric Section of the Society of Critical Care Medicine, 1993, p. 166). The former was identified as having a full staff of subspecialists, including intensivists, but Level II must have a communications system that allows for timely referral. Contrary to the NICU levels, the higher the number designation of the PICU, the lower the intensity of care.

As with the 1983 Guidelines, on which the 1993 Guidelines were founded, the 1993 document addresses the organization and administrative structure of the PICUs, physical design, personnel, drugs, and equipment. Additional categories are quality assessment, training and education, and pre-hospital care. Unlike the 1983 version unit size is not addressed. Regarding staffing, the requirements are significantly more detailed than the 1983 iteration. The medical director must be board-certified in pediatric critical care, anesthesiology, or surgery. Level I must include a pediatric anesthesiologist, a pediatric surgeon, a neurosurgeon, a thoracic surgeon, a pediatric intensivist, a pediatric cardiologist, a pediatric neurologist, a radiologist, a pathologist, and a psychologist or psychiatrist. Regarding nursing staff the ratios range from two staff for one patient to one staff member for three patients, depending on the child's acuity.

Recognition of the role of child life and family is a hallmark of these Guidelines and the document speaks to providing a pleasant atmosphere, considering the health of parents, providing a proper location for the waiting area, and recognizing the psychosocial needs of families.

The following physical environmental features were listed in the minimum Guidelines of 1993, which include a two-tiered evaluation system of "required" and "desirable, but optional." A detailed summary may be found in Volume 92 of *Pediatrics* (1993) (see Figure 2.5).

As previously, the 1993 Guidelines were linked to building codes. In 1993, however, individual codes were not listed. The summary chart simply says that HVAC, fire safety, electrical grounding, plumbing, and illumination must conform to building code or federal code in both levels of PICU.

2.5.3 Guidelines of 2004

As with its predecessor, the 2004 Guidelines document was built on prior Guidelines. One of the distinct differences between 2004 and 1993 is the return to the three-tiered system of evaluation similar to that used in 1983. In lieu of "required" and "desirable but optional," from 1993, the 2004 document includes "essential," "desired," and "optional." Level II PICUs have fewer spatial adjacency requirements than Level I, and do not require an independent unit, among other differences (Rosenberg et al., 2004). The authors of the 2004 Guidelines point out that the standards of quality of care are equivalent for both levels. The primary difference is the proximity of specialized medical staff to the PICU site and resources.

The 2004 Guidelines reaffirmed much of the 1993 Guidelines, which is to be expected as the Guideline authors used the first two decades between 1983 and 2003 to iron out many of the primary issues. However, there are four changes/modifications with regard to the physical facility program:

1. The addition of the family sleep and shower area to be provided as an external feature (essential for Level 1, and desired for Level II) (external features are features outside of the immediate environment of the PICU).
2. The addition of the satellite pharmacy to be provided as an internal feature (desired for Level 1 and optional for Level II) (internal features are spaces located within the PICU).
3. The addition of toys in the internal environment (essential for both levels).
4. The specification of infrastructure. No electrical outlets were explicitly specified in 1993 (perhaps due to the link to the electrical code). Twelve or more were required for both levels in 2004, and the number of oxygen outlets increased from two in 1993 to two or more in 2004 (essential for both levels).

The 2004 Guidelines require at least 250 square feet per patient in a private room, and 225 per patient in a shared space. This was the first time room areas were indicated in the Guideline documents. Unlike the 1983 code, however, no mention was made of the number of beds.

As previously, the 2004 Guidelines are linked to building codes, and specific codes are not mentioned. However, the document states that the unit must conform to building or federal codes with respect to heating, ventilation and air conditioning; fire safety; electrical grounding; plumbing; and illumination.

Figure 2.6 lists the physical environmental features addressed in the minimum Guidelines of 2004. A detailed summary that includes all the other requirements (e.g. staff) may be found in Rosenberg et al. (2004).

Figure 2.5: *Physical environment of pediatric intensive care, 1993 (Source: Committee on Hospital Care and Pediatric Section of the Society of Critical Care Medicine, 1993) (items in* **bold** *are additions)*

External feature	*Internal feature*	*Lev I*	*Lev II*
Distinct unit		★★★	★★★
Controlled access (No through-traffic)		★★★	★★★
Proximity to elevators		★★★	★★
Proximity to OR		★★	★★
Proximity to ER		★★	★★
Proximity to recovery		★★	★★
Proximity to MD on-call		★★★	★★
Proximity to nurse manager's office		★★	★★
Proximity to med director's office		★★	★★
Proximity to waiting room			
Family counseling		★★★	★★★
Staff lounge		★★	★★
Staff locker		★★	★★
	Nourishment station	★★★	★★★
Patients' effects or	Patients' effects	★★★	★★★
	Clean **utility/linen**	★★★	★★★
	Soiled **utility/linen**	★★★	★★★
	Patient isolation	★★★	★★★
	Patient privacy provisions	★★★	★★★
	Med station+refrigerator/narcotics cabinet	★★★	★★★
Conference area		★★	★★
	Staff toilet	★★★	★★★
	Emergency equip storage	★★★	★★★
	Hand washing facilities	★★★	★★★
	Patient toilet	★★★	★★★
	Counter & cabinet space	★★★	★★★
	Clocks	★★★	★★★
	Television, radios	★★★	★★
	Access to patient head/neck	★★★	★★★
	2 oxygen outlets/bed	★★★	★★★
	2 or more compressed air/bed	★★★	★★★
	2 vacuum outlets/bed	★★★	★★★
	Building/Federal code conforming	★★★	★★★
	Computerized lab report	★★★	★★

R=Required ★★★, O=Optional but desirable ★★

Figure 2.6: *Physical environment of pediatric intensive care, 2004 (Source: Rosenberg et al., 2004)*

External Feature	*Internal Feature*	*Lev I*	*Lev II*
Distinct unit		★★★	★★
Controlled access (No through-traffic)		★★★	★★★
Located near elevators		★★★	★★★
Located near OR		★★★	★★
Located near ER		★★	★★
Located near recovery		★★	★★
Located near MD on-call		★★	★★
Located near nurse manager's office		★★★	★★
Located near med director's office		★★	★★
Located near waiting room		★★★	★★
Family counseling		★★★	★★
Staff lounge		★★	★★
Staff locker		★★	★★
Family sleep and shower area		★★★	★★
	Nourishment station	★★★	★★★
Patients' effects	Patients' effects	★★★	★★★
	Clean utility/linen	★★★	★★★
	Soiled utility/linen	★★★	★★★
	Patient isolation	★★★	★★★
	Patient privacy provisions	★★★	★★★
	Satellite pharmacy	★★	★
	Med station+refrigerator/narcotics cabinet	★★★	★★★
Conference area		★★	★★
	Staff toilet	★★★	★★★
	Emergency equip storage	★★★	★★★
	Hand washing facilities	★★★	★★★
	Patient toilet	★★★	★★★
	Counter & cabinet space	★★★	★★★
	Clocks	★★★	★★★
	Television, radios, **toys**	★★★	★★★
	Access to patient head/neck	★★★	★★★
	12 or more electrical outlets/bed	★★★	★★★
	2 **or more** oxygen outlets/bed	★★★	★★★
	2 or more compressed air/bed	★★★	★★★
	2 vacuum outlets/bed	★★★	★★★
	Building/Federal code conforming	★★★	★★★
	Computerized lab report	★★★	★★

E=Essential ★★★, D=Desired ★★, O=Optional ★

Thoughts on the design of pediatric intensive care units

Michele Moss, MD

The process of designing a pediatric intensive care unit is a complex one. As a rather senior pediatric intensivist, I have witnessed and participated in the process several times over the years both with a general pediatric intensive care unit and a dedicated pediatric cardiac intensive care unit. I am sure my observations are not new to architects skilled in ICU design but I am sharing thoughts on some recent processes I have experienced. As those who do the actual designing know, there must be a balance of creating a functional yet aesthetically pleasing space with the realities of overwhelming regulations and fiscal restraints.

The process should start with an assessment of why the new space is needed. Sometimes the design involves just the expansion or redesign of existing space but the most exciting but also challenging is designing all-new space. Is the new space because of the need for new beds and expanded capacity only? Is it because the current space needs a few more beds but the compelling reason is the need for better space – perhaps the current ICU is still an open-bed unit and antiquated in its design? Examining "why the new space" will help guide discussions and often create a matrix for decisions as the design is being developed.

Input from the end users is crucial. Often times just selected caregivers are included and sometimes not even all of them. It is imperative that there is representation from all the caregivers in the ICU – nurses, patient care techs, pharmacy, respiratory therapy, child life, social work, physicians, etc., but most importantly there needs to be a forum for input from all the frontline users. Can you really adequately design a reception desk without getting input from the unit secretary who has to man that desk? Thus, early on in the process the leaders and end users should be allowed to develop a "wish list" and dream big – write down everything that is needed and wanted in the new space. Of course, all the dreams are rarely accomplished but often themes develop that are important to almost everyone and these should be prioritized very highly. In addition, they can offer valuable input regarding the workflow patterns outside the patient room that may allow better design to improve their efficiency and decrease their work. The design team should also be able to share information back to these end users about limitations due to regulations, structure or cost so that they can adequately understand why all their dreams are not met (Thompson et al., 2012).

Patient safety

Patient safety has become the driving priority for patient care since the publication of the Institute of Medicine's monograph *To Err is Human: Building a Safer Health Care System* (Kohn et al., 1999). This report concluded that many errors in medicine are due to faults in systems or processes. Some of these errors have subsequently been titled "never events." These never events are defined by the National Quality Forum (NQF) as errors in medical care that are clearly identifiable, preventable, and serious in their consequences for patients, and that indicate a real problem in the safety and credibility of a healthcare facility (NQF, 2002). Some of these events include obvious problems such as operating on the wrong patient or sending a baby home with the wrong parents, but also include hospital-acquired infections.

Can design of the unit improve the risk of hospital-acquired infections? It can, both in obvious and subtle ways. Hand hygiene before entering a patient space, before touching the patient or their equipment, and after touching the patient or their equipment has been shown to decrease the spread of hospital-acquired organisms, many of which are resistant to standard antibiotic therapy. Convenient, unobstructed placement of sinks with the ability to turn the water on and off without using one's hands vastly improves compliance with appropriate hand-washing practices and maintains cleanliness. Close and convenient access to disinfectant hand gel is also imperative. Although there are fiscal arguments about providing sinks at every bedside, especially since disinfectant gels are as effective in controlling bacterial spread, sinks with "good old" soap and water are still the mainstay for hand hygiene, especially in pediatric intensive care units where exposure to body fluids is common. The goal is to make the right thing to do the easy thing to do. That is where good design is most helpful.

Another, less obvious example of where design can help is with the prevention of catheter-associated bloodstream infections. Catheters are commonly placed in critically ill pediatric patients for monitoring vascular pressures, blood sampling, and delivery of medications or nutrition that require stable intravenous access. These catheters can be a source of infection that, if one occurs, has been shown to increase hospital costs, length of stay in the ICU for the patient, and most importantly increase the risk of mortality. Bundles of procedures exist that when reliably performed can prevent these infections. These procedures include how to sterilely place or insert the line, change the dressing on the line, and change the tubing to the central line, among other processes. Again, with the goal of making the right thing to do the easy thing to do, good design can impact all these procedures. If the patient's room is too small and crowded with people and equipment, the risk of contamination of the line during insertion increases. If the very busy PICU nurse has to go to multiple different sites in the PICU to gather the proper equipment for a dressing or line change, her likelihood of performing the procedure completely goes down. Missing steps in the process can lead to increased risk of infection (NQF, 2002; Miller et al., 2011). A well-designed PICU would have a location for all the equipment needed for a dressing change or line change that is convenient to the bedside nurses and a clear area within the patient room to lay out equipment cleanly. The bedside nurses would need to provide input to the design team for what they think is "convenient" in the context of their daily workflow.

Patient and family-centered care

Pediatrics has always led the way when considering patient and family-centered care when compared to our adult colleagues. The presence of family definitely helps in the care of the child. But even so, the presence of family in our PICUs has increased over the past ten years as more and more units have been designed to accommodate one parent sleeping in the ICU room with their child. Many of these units have bathroom facilities, including showers for the family as well as areas with desks, sleeping sofas and even televisions for the parents. This has been a very positive move for family-centered care. However, these family areas can impact the patient care space if care is not taken. There are standards for the appropriate size of ICU rooms: the minimum for pediatric patients is currently 250 square feet. The family area should not encroach on this space. In fact with the increased utilization of mechanical support for many critically ill pediatric patients, 250 square feet is often inadequate. When ventilators, nitric oxide delivery systems, continuous renal replacement therapy, or even extra-corporeal membrane oxygenation systems are needed, functional space shrinks rapidly. Thus, although inclusion of family space in the ICU room is important it should not impact the functional space for the patient.

Family support areas outside the patient rooms that are easily accessible and have adequate space are important in the design of the PICU. Although families like having free access to the child's bedside, parents and other caregivers need to take breaks. These support areas can contain amenities such as private lockers for the family, shower space, kitchen areas with refrigerators and microwave ovens, play space for patient siblings, and wifi access.

Other thoughts

Medicines change rapidly and the types of care delivered change faster than ICUs can be designed and built. Therefore high flexibility needs to be planned in the ICU. That flexibility includes not only providing adequate patient care space, as I noted above, remembering that pediatric patients range from tiny infants to large adolescents but also plenty of computer and electrical support. Another major opportunity when designing a pediatric ICU rather than an adult unit is the ability to decorate using color to enliven the space. Although it may be easy to get carried away with too many or too vibrant colors for children, the opportunity exists to make a playful yet soothing space. Natural light is as important for children as adults and should be provided, taking care that power columns or equipment do not block it.

In summary, when designing a PICU, input from all levels of caregivers and end users is important. The issues of patient safety and patient and family-centered care directly impact design. Providing a light, lively, colorful space is an opportunity to design a functional and aesthetically pleasing space that improves the experience of the child, the family, and the ICU personnel.

References

Kohn, L.T., Corrigan, J.M., and Donaldson, M.S. (1999). *To Err is Human: Building a Safer Health System*. Committee on Health Care in America. Institute of Medicine.

Miller, M.R., Niedner, M.F., Huskins, W.C., Colantuoni, E., Yenokyan, G., Moss, M., and Brilli, R.J. (2011). Reducing PICU central line – associated bloodstream infections: 3-year results. *Pediatrics, 128*(5), e1077–e1083.

National Quality Forum. (2002). *Serious Reportable Events in Healthcare: A Consensus Report*. National Quality Forum, Washington, DC.

Thompson, D.R., Hamilton, D.K. et al. (2012). American College of Critical Care Medicine Guidelines for intensive care unit design. *Critical Care Medicine, 40*(5), 1586–1600.

2.5.4 Guidelines post-2004

Shortly after the 2004 Guidelines were published, an erratum followed with a minor change in Figure 2.5. In Table 1, under item II – Personnel, A – Medical director, 3b should read: "Has authority to provide consultation for any PICU patient on a daily basis" (N.A., 2005). The 2004 Guidelines were reaffirmed in May 2008 per AAP Publications Reaffirmed and Retired, February and May 2008 (N.A., 2008). The Guidelines were last affirmed in 2008; they expire after five years (2013) unless revised or reaffirmed. As of the submission date for this text an update has not been published.

2.6 PICU growth and characteristics

2.6.1 Number of PICUs

The number of PICUs increased dramatically in the 1980s, by 59 percent, and the number of beds also increased by 59 percent (Pollack, 1994). During that same period, almost 50 percent of the PICUs had fewer than six beds (Pollack et al., 1993). By 1993, 301 hospitals were identified as having PICUs (Pollack et al., 1993), followed by 306 in 1995, and 349 in 2001 (Randolph et al., 2004).

According to data from the American Hospital Association (2011) there are currently approximately 462 PICUs in the United States. Authors have noted (e.g. Randolph et al., 2004) that the growth in the number of PICU beds in recent years has exceeded the population growth. Although the various researchers who gathered this data have used different databases and analysis patterns, it is evident that the number of units is increasing (see Figure 2.7).

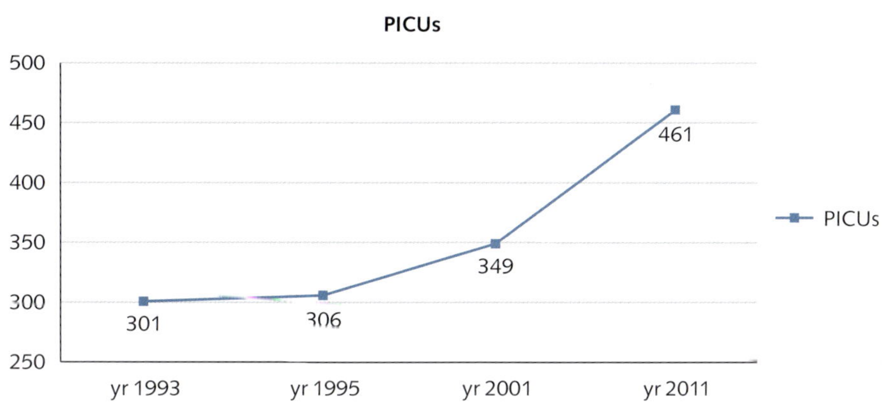

Figure 2.7: *Growth in number of PICU beds (Data sources: Pollack et al., 1993; Randolph et al., 2004; American Hospital Association, 2010)*

2.6.2 Number of beds per PICU

Surveys from 1993 and 2004 reveal a growth in the number of beds per PICU (see Figure 2.8). In a survey of 235 hospitals in 1993 (Pollack et al., 1993), researchers found that the average number of PICUs had four to six beds, while only 6 percent had more than 18 beds per unit. The most rapid growth between 1995 and 2001 was in PICUs with 15 beds or more (Randolph et al., 2004). A survey in 2003 to 2004 of medical directors in 257 out of 337 eligible hospitals reported a median of 12 beds (8–17 beds in the interquartile range, and a median of 59 admissions per bed) (Odetola et al., 2005a); in 2004 only 23 percent had units of six or fewer beds, and 20 percent of the PICUs had units of 19 beds or more. Six percent of these beds were co-located with adult units (Odetola et al., 2005a).

Odetola et al. (2005a) did not find any significant differences in admissions per bed between the small and the large units, although the therapeutic technology was more sophisticated in the larger units and the staff-to-patient ratio was higher in the smaller units.

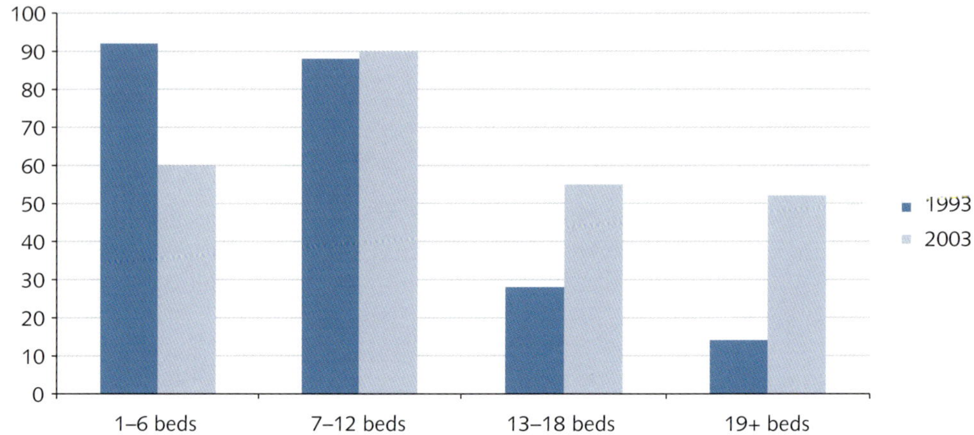

Figure 2.8: *Number of beds per unit, 1993 versus 2003 (Sources: Odetola et al., 2005a; Pollack et al., 1993)*

Odetola et al. (2005a) provide a snapshot of unit size and medical staffing in 2003 (see Figure 2.9). According to their data, the number of intensivists per bed decreases as the number of beds increase, although the PICU nurse-to-bed ratio appears to be quite stable, as is the nurse-to-patient ratio. As might be expected, the larger the PICU size, the more likely it is that the facility will have a pediatric cardiac unit.

Figure 2.9: *PICU data, 2003 (Source: Odetola et al., 2005a)*

	PICU size				
	All	*1 to 6*	*7 to 12*	*13 to 18*	*19+*
Admissions in 2003	662	300	500	900	1400
Admissions per bed	58.6	57.3	56.3	62.5	62.5
# of pediatric intensivists	4	2	3	4	6
Pediatric intensivist/bed	0.3	0.4	0.3	0.29	0.27
# 24 hour intensivist (%)	257	60	90	55	52
Nurse/patient ratio	1 to 2	1 to 2	1 to 2	1 to 2	1 to 2
PICU nurse/bed ratio	2.9	3.3	2.5	2.7	3.2
# w/cardiac ICU	25	1	2	10	12

2.6.3 Distribution and location of PICUs

The geographic distribution of PICUs varies across regions (see Figure 2.10), but ranges between 1/15,254 (West South Central) and 1/27,442 (New England) in 2001 (Randolph et al., 2004). Odetola et al. (2005b) observed that only 9 percent of counties in the United States have a PICU, and these units are typically located in cities.

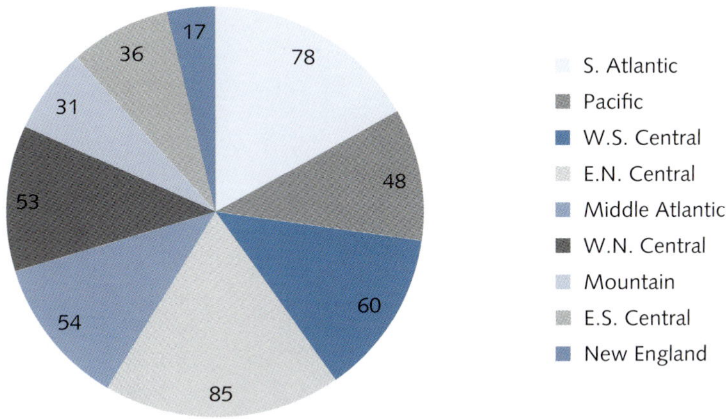

Figure 2.10: *Geographic distribution of PICUs (Source: Randolph et al., 2004)*

2.6.4 PICU demographics

Tilford and colleagues (2000) note that critically ill children admitted to PICUs are a very heterogeneous patient population. The demographic differences such as age and ethnicity/race vary broadly. The manner in which they are admitted (e.g. ER or surgery), their diagnoses, and insurance are other characteristics of interest impacting calculations of bed need. Regarding gender, there appears to be a preponderance of boys. Marcin and colleagues (2001) studied 32 PICUs with 11,165 admissions and reported that 57.4 percent of the population was male.

Regarding age, the mean varies by location and over time. In their 32 PICUs Marcin et al. (2001) found the mean age to be about 62 months in the study sample. Tilford et al. (2000) investigated the population in 16 PICUs and found the median age to be 36.9 months, ranging from 27 months to 60.5 months. Approximately 70 percent were emergency admissions (Marcin et al., 2001). PICU patients in the Tilford study were 35.4 percent surgical and 10.9 percent trauma.

Insurance coverage, gender, age, and diagnosis are important topics, as they appear to impact patient outcomes. Lopez and colleagues (2006) found that underinsured children had shorter lengths of stays, and greater physiological derangement when admitted, than did insured patients. Epstein et al. (2011) produced data which suggested that lack of insurance increased risk of mortality. According to this study, while gender, age, and diagnosis had an impact, illness-adjusted mortality and race/ethnicity did not play a role. Common categories of diagnosis are trauma, endocrine disease, oncologic disease, circulatory disease, congenital anomaly, infection, respiratory condition, and nervous system disease (Tilford et al., 2000).

Regarding racial distribution, Epstein et al. (2011) used the Virtual PICU Performance System to analyze the data of 80,739 children admitted to PICUs between 2005 and 2008. Fifty-five percent of the children in the survey were Caucasian/non-Hispanic, followed by 18 percent African-American, 17 percent Hispanic, and 3 percent Asian/Indian/Pacific Islander (see Figure 2.11). Turner and colleagues (2011) conducted a study in a Tennessee community of approximately 76.6 percent African-Americans and 41 percent non-Hispanic Caucasian children. The relative risk for African-American children compared to non-Hispanic Whites was 2.12 times greater.

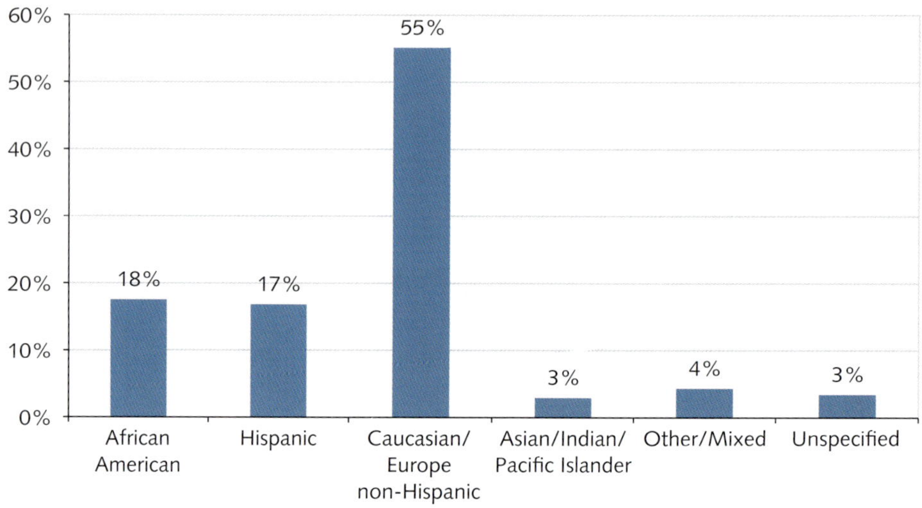

Figure 2.11: *PICU ethnic racial distribution (Source: Epstein et al., 2011)*

2.6.5 PICU length of stay

In the early 1990s, the average length of stay (LOS) in a PICU was a mean of 1.9 days, with the upper percentile of 12 days (Ruttimann and Pollack, 1996). This is somewhat less than the later work of Marcin et al. (2001), which found the mean LOS in a study of 32 PICUs to be 3.5 days, with a mean range of 1.8 to 6.0 days and a median of two days. Long-stay patients (LSPs) (>12 days) represented 4.5 percent of the population (see Figure 2.12). Tilford et al. (2000) recorded a median of 1.8 days.

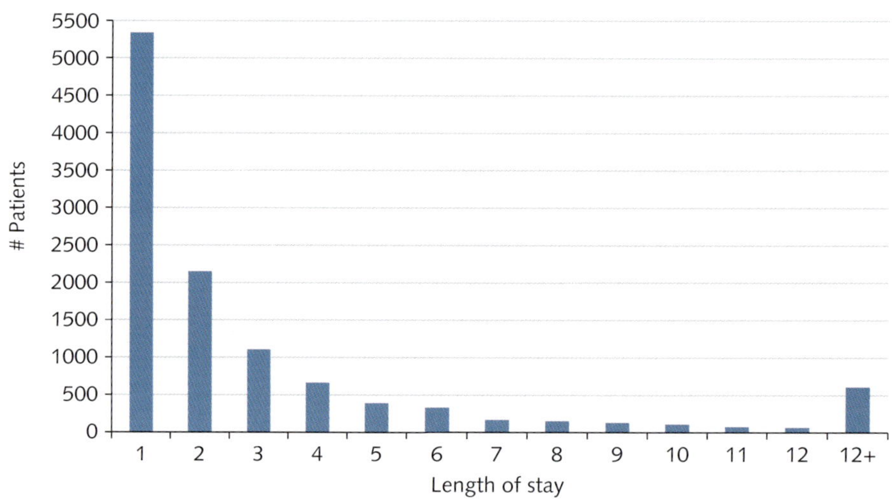

Figure 2.12: *PICU length of stay (Source: Marcin et al., 2001)*

The origins of pediatric critical care followed closely behind the creation of adult critical care units. A description of the staff and environmental needs of these units has evolved over the past 30 years.

References

American Hospital Association. (2010). *AHA Hospital Statistics 2011: The Comprehensive Reference Source for Analysis and Comparison of Hospital Trends*. Chicago, IL: Health Forum.

Bachman, L., Downes, J.J., Richards, C.C., Coyle, D., and May, E. (1967). Organization of an intensive care unit in a children's hospital. *Anesthesia Analgesia, 46*(5), 570–574.

Committee on Hospital Care and Pediatric Section (CHCPS) of the Society of Critical Care Medicine. (1983). Guidelines for pediatric intensive care units. *Pediatrics, 72*, 364–371, and *Critical Care Medicine, 11*, 753.

Committee on Hospital Care and Pediatric Section of the Society of Critical Care Medicine. (1993). Guidelines and levels of care for pediatric intensive care units. *Pediatrics, 92*(1), 166–175.

Costarino, A.T., and Downes, J.J. (2005). Pediatric anesthesia historical perspective. *Anesthesiology Clinics of North America, 23*, 573–595.

Downes, J.J. (1992). The historical evolution, current status, and prospective development of pediatric critical care. *Critical Care Clinics, 8*, 1–22.

Eldadah, M., Leo, S., Kovach, K ., Ricardo Argueta Morales, I., Pepe, J., Fakioglu, H., and DeCampli, W. (2011). Influence of a dedicated paediatric cardiac intensive care unit on patient outcomes. *Nursing in Critical Care, 16*(6), 281–286. doi:10:1111/j.1478-5153.2011.00455.x

Epstein, D., and Brill, J.E. (2005). A history of pediatric critical care medicine. *Pediatric Research, 58*(5), 987–996.

Epstein, D., Wong, C., Khemani, R., Moromisato, D.Y., Waters, K., Kipke, M.D., and Markovitz, B.P. (2011). Race/ethnicity is not associated with mortality in the PICU. *Pediatrics, 127*(3), e588–e597. doi:10,1542/peds.2010-0394

Lopez, A.M., Tilford, J.M., Anand, K.J., Dphil, J., Jo, C., Green, J., and Fiser, D. (2006). Variation in pediatric intensive care therapies and outcomes by race, gender, and insurance status. *Pediatric Critical Care Medicine, 7*(1), 2–6.

Marcin, J.P., Slonim, A.D., Pollack, M.M., and Ruttimann, U.E. (2001). Long-stay patients in the pediatric intensive care unit. *Critical Care Medicine, 29*(3), 652–657.

N.A. (2005). Erratum. *Pediatrics, 116*(2), 524. doi:10.1542/peds.2005-1512

N.A. (2008). AAP publications reaffirmed and retired. *Pediatrics, 122*, 450. doi:10.1542/peds.2008-1427

Odetola, F.O., Clark, S.J., Freed, G.L., Bratton, S.L., and Davis, M.M. (2005a). A national survey of pediatric critical care resources in the United States. *Pediatrics, 115*(4), 382–386.

Odetola, F.O., Miller, W.C., Davis, M.M., and Bratton, S.L. (2005b). The relationship between the location of pediatric intensive care unit facilities and child mortality from trauma: A county-level ecologic study. *Journal of Pediatrics, 147*(1), 74–77.

Pollack, M.M. (1994). Cost containment, the pediatric perspective. *New Horizons, 2*, 305–312.

Pollack, M.M., Cuerdon, T.C., and Getson, P.R. (1993). Pediatric intensive care units: Results of a national study. *Critical Care Medicine, 21*(4), 607–614.

Randolph, A.G., Gonzales, C.A., Cortellini, L., and Yeh, T.S. (2004). Growth of pediatric intensive care units in the United States from 1995 to 2001. *Journal of Pediatrics, 144*(6), 792–798.

Reisner-Sénélar, L. (2011). The birth of intensive care: Björn Ibsen's records. *Intensive Care Medicine, 37*(7), 1084–1086. doi:10.1007/s00134-011-2235

Rosenberg, D.I., Moss, M.M., and the American College of Critical Care Medicine of the Society of Critical Care Medicine. (2004). Guidelines and levels of care for pediatric intensive care units. *Pediatrics, 114*(4), 1114–1125. doi:10.1542/peds.2004-1599

Ruttimann, U.E., and Pollack, M.M. (1996). Variability in duration of stay in pediatric intensive care units: A multi-institutional study. *Journal of Pediatrics, 128*(1), 35–44.
Smith, T. (2012). A comparative study of occupancy and patient care quality in four different types of intensive care units in a children's hospital. *Work, 41*, 1961–1968.
Tarnowski, K.J., Rasnake, L.K., Linscheid, T.R., and Mulick, J.A. (1989). Ecobehavioral characteristics of a pediatric burn injury unit. *Journal of Applied Behavior Analysis, 22*(1), 101–109.
Tilford, J.M., Simpson, P.M., Green, J.W., Lensing, S., and Fiser, D. (2000). Volume-outcome relationships in pediatric intensive care units. *Pediatrics, 106*(2), 289–294.
Turner, D., Simpson, P., Li, S.H., Scanlon, M., and Quasney, M.W. (2011). Racial disparities in pediatric intensive care unit admissions. *Southern Medical Journal, 104*(9), 640–646.

Definition and history of neonatal intensive care environments 3

The birth of newborn intensive care does not begin at a single moment in time or a single hospital. Likewise, the architectural environment that supports these activities has evolved slowly and in parts. This chapter provides a definition of neonatal intensive care and discusses the complex evolution of the organizational and physical NICU environment.

3.1 Definition of neonatal intensive care

A neonatal intensive care unit (NICU) is an inpatient medical unit specializing in the care of ill or premature infants and their families. Intensive care is a level of care with equipment and staff dedicated to a higher level of treatment and supervision than in other inpatient units.

From a historical perspective, the precursor environments manifested as the space occupied by specialized equipment – such as respirators and incubators – that might have been present in a surgical suite, but were instead in use in an inpatient setting. Therefore, apart from higher levels of observation, laypersons might describe intensive care as a bridge between technology that supports surgery, and straightforward monitoring and patient care.

3.2 The history of the NICU: early incubators

The baby incubator is the seed and heart of the NICU. Sometimes referred to as an isolette, the purpose of both the early and contemporary incubators was to provide an environment that was more hospitable to the infant than the unfiltered environment outside of the womb. In the early years, incubators were located in a variety of settings. Eventually, small, dedicated units were provided, followed several years later by larger units with a wide variety of support spaces. This section discusses the invention of baby incubators and summarizes the subsequent prototypes.

The earliest incubators, which were inspired by poultry incubators, were in use in Russia and France in the 18th century (Antonucci et al., 2009). Their basic purpose was to keep the infant warm, but they were also known to improve outcomes (Baker, 1991). The poultry incubators after which they were fashioned may have been inspired by the inventions of ancient Egyptians (Marshall-Baker, 2011).

A more evolved baby incubator was built in 1880 and used at the Paris Maternity Hospital (Gartner and Gartner, 1992). Among the first incubators thought to have been in use in the United States in the late 19th century, it was on display at the 1898 Omaha Exhibition. For many years, baby incubators and the premature children receiving treatment within them were displayed as curiosities at fairs. This particular device, referred to as the Lion incubator, included a system for utilizing outside air for ventilation (Baker, 2000). The 1940s ushered in several advancements in incubator design, including more effective temperature, oxygen, humidity, and infection control. Plastic panels were introduced that were lighter and hermetically sealed, reducing the need for a metal frame (Marshall-Baker, 2011).

In 1938, the first modern incubator was developed by Charles Chapple at the Children's Hospital of Philadelphia (Downes, 1992). This isolette provided clean, humidified air, limited exposure to external contamination, and maintained a constant thermal environment (Downes, 1992). Additions over the past 75 years include improvements to air circulation, humidity controls, heating components, and sensors of the physical environment and the infants' physiological status (Ferris and Shepley, 2012).

The first incubator station was operational at the Chicago Lying-In Hospital in 1899 (Gartner and Gartner, 1992). The incubator station, which presumes the co-location of multiple incubators in a single location, was the precursor for the first NICU. Generally, early premature nurseries consisted of incubators in a narrow hall supported by servo-controlled infrared heat and a sink (Gluck, 1992).

A somewhat more elaborate environment, described as a "Premature Infant Station," was established at Sarah Morris Hospital in 1922 (Hess et al., 1934). The impact of this dedicated space was significant. Between 1922 and 1933, the survival rate of premature infants treated in this pre-NICU increased from 56 percent to 76 percent. The average length of stay for children who weighed less than 1,000 grams was 83 days, while children over 3,000 grams stayed an average of 15 days. The design of the Sarah Morris Hospital included four rooms; one for normal small newborns, one for infants who were about to be discharged (graduating infants), a third for infants with infections, and a fourth for breast pumping. The Sarah Morris Hospital, the location of the premature infant station described above, also included an oxygen station (Antonucci et al., 2009). The temperature in the graduating unit was lower than in the other rooms. A glass partition was located between the wet-nurse (mother) pumping station and the wards to allow for observation by the caregivers. Living quarters for these mothers were provided on the same floor.

Hess et al. (1934) observed that during this period, the only facilities using equipment for ventilating, heating, and humidifying the air of neonatal environments were the Boston Children's Hospital and the Yale Children's Hospital. The Sarah Morris facility featured double-hung windows with operable transoms, and radiators with thermostats to control room temperature. In addition, each infant was located in a water-jacketed heated bed in which the temperature could be modulated to meet each child's requirements. This arrangement promoted free air exchange similar to what would be appropriate for other nursing units. The average room temperature was 75 degrees Fahrenheit and, in order to achieve the appropriate humidity sheets were hung over ward screens. Figure 3.1 gives a list of equipment provided in this facility.

Over the next few decades, facilities transitioned in response to the need for improved infection control. In 1960, Wheeler listed the following as requirements for the nursery environment that focuses on this specific need:

- Heated beds
- Bassinets for graduates
- Oxygen therapy units
- Heated dressing table
- Sink and bathing table
- Shelves for toiletries
- Supply closet
- Scale
- Wet and dry bulb thermometer
- Hygrometer
- Time clock
- Electric heater
- Transportation ambulance
- Loaner heated beds for graduates

Figure 3.1: *Equipment in the Sarah Morris premature infant station (Source: Hess et al., 1934)*

- A limited number of infants sharing an air supply (four to six per unit).
  - Adequate distance between infants (30 square feet per four-infant unit).
  - Positive pressure ventilation (12 to 15 air exchanges).
  - Cohort and rotation system of admission and discharge.
  - Medical staff exposure (fewest persons in contact, same nurses caring for same infants, cultures of attendants, separation from contact with those exposed to staph or respiratory infection).

In the late 1950s, adult ICUs and rudimentary PICUs appeared (Gluck, 1992), paving the way for the development of NICUs. By the 1960s, the concept of a newborn intensive care unit began to take root (Yaffe, 1992). Pediatricians such as Clement Smith in Boston, William Silverman in New York, Paul Swyer in Toronto, and C. Evert Koop and Leonard Bachman in Philadelphia encouraged the co-locating of infants diagnosed with life-threatening conditions into special infant units. These units shifted the emphasis from environmental and nutritional support to system monitoring (Downes, 1992). Between 1960 and 1964, other units also appeared in Western Europe and South Africa (Downes, 1992). The first intensive care unit was opened in October 1960 at Yale-New Haven Hospital.

The first NICU, however, spawned a negative response from the medical community. Largely due to fear of the spread of staph infections, US laws prevented the integration of infants who were term with premature patients, well with sick, those born in the hospital with those born elsewhere, and medical with surgical care patients (Gluck, 1992). Data suggested that co-locating these populations did not increase the spread of infection. Allowing neonatal patients who would suffer from major lifelong disabilities to survive was also raised as a questionable practice (Gluck, 1992). Researchers, however, have contended that NICU care has resulted in improved outcomes for both preterm infants and those with critical medical or surgical conditions (Bode et al., 2001; Clement, 2005; MacDorman and Kirmeyer, 2009). Dr. Sumner Yaffe (Director of the Center for Research for Mothers and Children at the National Institutes of Health from 1980 to 2000) noted:

> Doctors now are able to save the lives of many premature or desperately ill newborns who in the past would have died soon after birth. The result is that the U.S. infant mortality rate has shown a steady decrease since the NICU first came into widespread use a quarter of a century ago and, concomitantly, survivors have fewer sequelae.
>
> (Yaffe, 1992, p. 3)

At the time that the Yale-New Haven Hospital was opened, however, there were few established neonatal intensive care techniques. Little equipment was available to support the scalar needs of babies. Newborns were ventilated with adult equipment and electrical equipment was not appropriately grounded (Gluck, 1992). Thus the Yale-New Haven NICU underwent a remodeling in 1964 due to a gift from Charles A. Dana, the grandfather of an NICU graduate. This first foray into the world of NICU design was not without its challenges, as noted by Gluck (1992).

> Almost immediately upon receipt of Dana's gift, a physically new perinatal center was planned, but did not open until early 1967. The delay occurred when the first three Yale architects resigned due to state and national (under Hill-Burton) hospital architectural regulations that prohibited large-room nurseries. The architect who eventually designed the center was not a hospital architect and was not familiar with the regulations. A compromise was made with the Hill-Burton regulations by dividing the 40 beds among four rooms, one of which accommodated 20 babies.
>
> (Gluck, 1973, p. 13)

Several innovations resulted from this new design, including the location of the medical gases and electrical systems in the ceiling, allowing for more flexibility around the isolette. The decentralization of supplies into sub-areas was another development. In addition, each baby station had its own monitors, infusion equipment, ventilation equipment, and supply storage.

Improvements in spatial provisions for newborns had not advanced dramatically for 60 years until the unit opened at the Yale-New Haven Hospital (Gluck, 1992). Since the 1960s, however, the number and design of newborn intensive care environments has grown dramatically; space requirements have accelerated, and the technology required to support very premature and ill newborns has improved significantly.

The primary focus of the physical environment of the early NICUs was to support life-saving treatments, and was not characterized by what would be described as a nurturing environment (White, 2011). Beginning approximately 30 years ago, a transition occurred, modifying the mission of the setting from the mere sustaining of life to the support of the development of preterm infants (Wielenga et al., 2007).

3.3 Advancements in NICU environmental design: emergence of single family rooms

The most radical development in the history of contemporary NICU design has been the increase in the number of single family-room (SFR) NICUs. Inspired by the provision of private rooms in intensive care units for adults and pediatrics, single family rooms have had a significant impact on the ability to provide developmental care for infants and privacy for families. For a summary of research on SFRs, see Chapter 5. Smith et al. (2004) note the following potential benefits of SFRs:

- Enhanced privacy and confidentiality.
- Improved control of noise, light, and temperature.
- Reductions in undesirable stimulation.
- Reductions in sedation medication.
- Decreased nosocomial infections.
- Improved staff and family satisfaction.
- Increased involvement of families.
- Reduced length of stay.
- Reduced cost per patient.
- Reduced movement of patient.

Among the first NICUs in the United States that dedicated a portion of the rooms to SFR care were the 30-bed facility at the Baptist Health Medical Center in Little Rock, Arkansas (1997), the Children's Regional Medical Center 19-bed NICU in Seattle, Washington (2000), and Blank Children's 35-bed NICU in Des Moines, Iowa (2001) (Smith et al., 2004).

From roommates to neighbors: a case study in the transition of open to private NICUs

Samuel Alan Black, AIA, ACHA, LEED AP

Diane R. K. Osan, FAIA, ACHA

Historically, neonatal intensive care units (NICUs) have been relatively small, dark, open-bay units. Noise was not a great issue because there was little equipment associated with the bassinet/warmer. Families were only allowed at the bedside for limited periods of time. As the importance of parent involvement in the care model was recognized, visitation hours were extended, causing crowding and introducing noise. As time progressed and technology advanced, more equipment made its way to the bedside, requiring larger spaces and bringing increased noise into the NICU. In recent years the significant danger to the infant caused by these elevated noise levels has been clearly documented. Along with the issue of noise, infection control in the NICU has demanded increased vigilance.

Physicians and staff in the units had grown accustomed to being able to see and hear everything that went on in the NICU. If an alarm went off or an infant was in distress, it was quickly recognized and help was close at hand. Caregivers became accustomed to having their colleagues nearby for backup. There was also a social element to staff being in an open environment. Nurses could chat as they went about their duties. Likewise there was a social aspect for patient families. Unit parents could bond and rely on each other for comfort, support, and encouragement during an extremely stressful time in their lives. Families and caregivers formed small communities working toward a common goal of healthy babies.

Moving to an all-private room environment addresses many issues, but also raises some concerns. It is a culture change for caregivers. There is fear of staff isolation – *"If I need help with a patient, will I be able to receive assistance? Will I lose the social connection with my colleagues?"* Another concern is the loss of control of the NICU – *"How will I know what is going on if I cannot see every baby?"* Because the space dedicated to each patient position has expanded, the travel distance to support space has also increased – *"Is this going to make it harder to care for my patients?"*

Cook Children's Medical Center case study

With the demands of ever-expanding population growth in the Dallas/Fort Worth area, Cook Children's Medical Center decided to replace their open bay NICU to accommodate not only increased bed capacity, but also to plan and build a unit that would incorporate best practices for increased patient safety and family-centered care. Cook Children's new NICU – one of the largest all-private units in the nation – opened in the fall of 2011 and comprises 106 private NICU beds on two full floors of a new 270,000-square-foot tower.

Private NICU rooms were a new concept for Cook Children's. Realizing that their environment transition is a great research case, the hospital made a point to capture and compare the data and document the results of both their open-bay and private care models. Cook Children's new NICU beds are in a combination of fully and partially enclosed (four walls and open doorway) patient rooms that include parent sleeping accommodation.

In regard to noise, decibel levels were measured in both the old and new units. Sound levels at the bedside were found to be 13 percent quieter in the new unit under normal conditions. Parent surveys showed that 78 percent more parents noted low noise levels in the new unit compared to the old unit. To address infection control concerns, a sink was located directly adjacent to the entry of each room to encourage hand washing by staff and families. Poured rubber terrazzo flooring was chosen for its ease of cleaning and lack of seams that could harbor bacteria. This flooring choice has the additional benefit of being durable and sound absorptive. Soiled linen and trash collection are completed through small doors along the corridor to avoid disturbing the patient and family, and to reduce traffic in and out of the room. Already low infection rates remain unchanged in the new unit.

A distinct family zone is separate from the patient and nursing zones of the room. The family is provided with a sleeper sofa, a television requiring use of headphones, a wardrobe and a chair. Privacy is provided by a curtain track and the family can control lighting in their area. This arrangement allows nursing staff to enter the room any time day or night without disturbing the family. Some rooms are connected by sliding doors to form "twin" rooms. Other rooms can be configured for triplets or quads so that parents can stay with all their babies in one room. Patient family satisfaction scores regarding privacy increased nearly 100 percent shortly after occupying the new unit.

Careful consideration was given to accommodation for families outside of the patient room as well. Each floor of Cook Children's NICU has laundry facilities for parent use. Shower facilities are provided adjacent to the family lounge. A large milk bank serving neonates is located on the main floor of the NICU to store and process mothers' breast milk. This program has been so successful that the hospital purchased two additional breast milk freezers within weeks of opening to accommodate the significant increase in milk production from breast-feeding mothers. A family care room is provided and serves as a palliative care space when needed. Child life has a special area equipped with an incubator to work with siblings. Offices are provided in units for chaplains, social workers, child life, and physical and occupational therapists. One floor below the NICU offers families a retreat with a new food court-style cafeteria, main dining-room, and other special amenities such as a Build-a-Bear Workshop, yogurt shop and a Starbuck's.

Moving to an all-private unit at Cook Children's caused some staff reservations about not being able to see all their patients and being isolated from other caregivers. To ensure visibility of each patient, bedside nursing stations with observation windows are placed between each room. The 18 to 24 beds in each unit are arranged in a "racetrack" configuration with a glass-enclosed main nursing station at the front. In addition to the main nursing station, an ancillary staff workstation is located at the back of each unit to ensure control of that area. This comprehensive coverage combination of workstations assures staff that their patients and their other team members are always within sight. Parent surveys revealed that families were 17 percent more satisfied with nurse attention, 22 percent more satisfied with how nurses answered their questions, and more than 25 percent more satisfied with the knowledge of their child's condition.

As a patient safety initiative, each patient room is designed for the patient to be admitted and discharged from the same room. In addition, patients are assigned to cohorts: cardiac, neurology, and metabolic. These two factors allow families to get to know caregivers in a particular unit. The nursing staff report that they are able to build a stronger rapport with families, helping to develop trust, and resulting in parents being more receptive to instruction, thus improving the quality of parent/family education which they provide. The survey of parents demonstrated that they were 17 percent more confident in the nurses that cared for their infant.

Another staff concern expressed was the increase in travel distances that the private NICU environment would produce. Measures taken to lessen travel distances and improve the caregiver experience include the decentralization and strategic placement of staff locker rooms among the units. Most supplies needed on a daily basis are kept in lockable carts inside the rooms. A bedside computer is provided in each room, in addition to the computer in the bedside nursing station in the corridor. A pedometer study performed before and after the unit move did chart increased walking distances. Charge nurse travel distances increased by 149 percent. Staff nurses walked 40 percent more in the new unit, while respiratory therapy staff walked 21 percent more. Travel distance for care partners increased by 77 percent (Greer, 2012). In an effort to allay fears of staff isolation caused by expanded travel distance, a unique staff amenity was added. A two-storey staff lounge connecting the two floors of NICU units is placed in the center of both floors, enabling staff from different units and floors to visit during breaks.

While there has been an adjustment period for the new private NICU care model, Cook Children's patient outcomes and family satisfaction have significantly benefited, as anticipated. As they continue to collect and evaluate their data, the hospital and its staff are motivated by the progress they have already made in propelling the care and quality of life for their most fragile patients. The future will bring more advancements as they examine, learn from, and share their research to create the optimum family-centered, evidence-based care environment.

Reference

Greer, B. (2012). *Cook Children's NICU: Design and Implementation by the NICU Leadership Team and Staff.* Presentation at the 2012 NICU Leadership Forum, Marco Island, FL.

3.4 Evolution of neonatal intensive care staffing and standards

NICU standards have developed in parallel with the evolution of the physical environment. The roots of neonatal intensive care lie in the mid-19th century through the practice of a small group of European and Russian physicians. The practice of newborn care appears to have become more formalized around the close of that century. According to Gartner and Gartner (1992), Dr. Martin A. Couney (born around 1865) was the father of neonatology, due to his specialization in the care for ill newborns. Couney studied under Pierre-Constant Budin, who in turn studied under Stephane Tarnier, described as the grandfather of neonatology (Gartner and Gartner, 1992). Subsequent to the Chicago Exhibition of 1914 which included displays of premature babies, a center for premature infants was created at the Michael Reese Hospital in Chicago (Downes, 1992).

These early activities garnered the attention of the medical establishment. In late 1937, the Executive Board of the American Association of Pediatrics met to establish the Committee on Neonatal Morbidity and Mortality to collaborate with a similarly named committee of the American Pediatric Society (CoFN, 2012). The two groups concurred that neonatal mortality and morbidity could be reduced and made recommendations on statistical methods, nomenclature for causes of death, protocols for autopsies, and enhanced collaboration with obstetricians. In 1938 the committee changed its name to the Committee on Problems of the Fetus and the Newborn Infant, and in 1941 it became the Committee on Fetus and Newborn. The Committee developed standards in 1949 and continues to function (CoFN, 2012). The initial efforts for the formalized care of premature babies began in the 1950s (Farah et al., 1996). Prior to this time, ill newborns were cared for on pediatric wards, typically by obstetric nurses (Gluck, 1992).

The subsequent history of neonatology reflects the contributions of a variety of individuals. One of them was Dr. Edith Jackson from Yale University who began promoting rooming-in and later supported skin-to-skin contact between mothers and babies after their birth. Although it was illegal, she began permitting parents to visit their children in the NICU as early as 1955 (Gluck, 1992).

3.4.1 *Early staffing protocols and training*

Following the success of the Yale-New Haven facility, other NICUs were instituted in the late 1960s, primarily in large teaching hospitals. At that time, NICUs were staffed by a single neonatologist, along with nursing staff, and a shortage of caregivers was apparent by the 1970s (Johnson, 2002). The limited residence hours of pediatricians, and of the consequent need for specialized nurses, gave rise to the establishment of the neonatal nurse practitioner (NNP) (Johnson, 2002). In 1973, a Blue Ribbon Commission was formed to discuss appropriate educational programs for these nurses, which resulted in the *Guidelines for Short-term Continuing Education Programs for the Nurse Clinician in Intensive Neonatal Care and the Nurse Clinician in Intensive Maternal-Fetal Care* (1975) (Johnson, 2002). The first certificate examination for NNPs was in 1983 (Samson, 2006).

The early NICUs were supervised by a small group of physicians, including Dr. Gluck, who had a special concern for frail infants, together with pediatric house staff (Honeyfield, 2009). The associated 24-month pediatric residency programs of the 1960s and 1970s typically included seven to nine months in a NICU (Honeyfield, 2009). Neonatology became an official subspecialty in 1975 (Johnson, 2002). While the expansion of education and certification of caregivers grew, in the 1980s protocols for pain management and developmental care were still not commonly practiced. Ventilation was accomplished through the use of traditional pressure ventilators, and little attention was applied to the adoption of universal precautions (Samson, 2006).

3.4.2 *Environmental standards*

On another front, with specific regard to the physical environment, in 1992 the first *Recommended Standards for Newborn ICU Design* were published, followed by iterations in 1996, 1999, 2002, 2006, and 2012. These recommendations, while not associated with levels of care, provided more detail about NICU environmental needs. Another important resource was the *AAP Guidelines for Perinatal Care*. The 6th edition was published in 2007 (AAP/ACOG, 2007).

Educational events and certifications are another indicator of the development and growth of a specialization. Regarding organizations and congresses associated with neonatal intensive care, the National Association of Neonatal Nurses was founded in 1984. The first of the Graven conferences, "The Physical and Developmental Environment of the High Risk Infant," took place in 1987, and this event was in its 26th year in 2013. In 1989 the first annual meeting of the European Society of Paediatric and Neonatal Care was held and the 24th meeting took place in 2013.

An examination of the timeline of the current history and development of NICUs shows a slow beginning in the 1960s and 1970s, followed by a flurry of education and certification activities in the 1980s, and the development and improvement of guidelines over the past 30 years (Figure 3.2).

3.5 Levels of NICU care

In the later 1960s, Paul Swyer expressed the need for regionalization of services and the transport of high-risk mothers to centers with perinatal and neonatal intensive care (Downes, 1992).

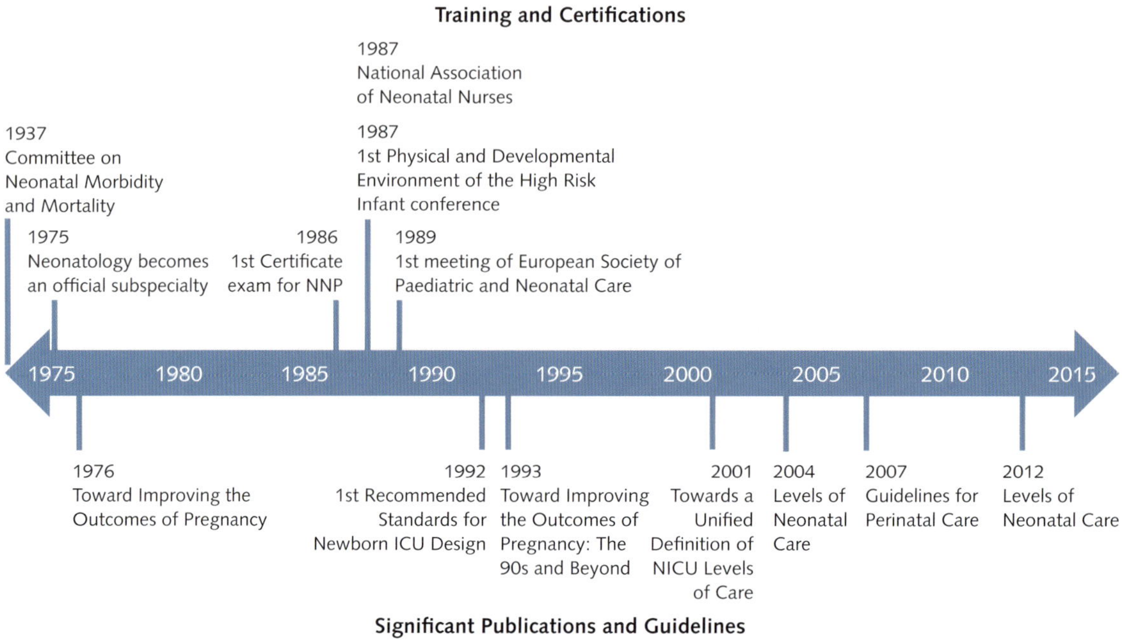

Figure 3.2: *Timeline of events in the history of neonatal intensive care*

According to the Committee on Fetus and Newborn of the American Academy of Pediatrics (AAP) (Stark, 2004), the notion of regionalization of services, as determined by levels of intensive care for newborns, was subsequently raised in 1976 in a publication by the March of Dimes, *Toward Improving the Outcomes of Pregnancy*. This document described three categories of care and made recommendations regarding referrals to higher care centers. The March of Dimes publication was updated in 1993 with *Toward Improving the Outcome of Pregnancy: The 90s and Beyond*, which created the designations of levels under the rubrics of basic, specialty, and subspecialty (CoFN, 2004). Subsequent to this, three important documents were generated that represented an expansion and evolution of the categories of care: the 2001 level definitions (Bhatt, 2001), the 2004 guidelines (CoFN, 2004), and the 2012 guidelines (CoFN, 2012). The definition of newborn intensive care is linked directly to the identification of theses levels of intensive care. These guidelines, provided by the Committee on Fetus and Newborn (CoFN) American Academy of Pediatrics (AAP), propose classifications based on intensity of care. The classification system is linked to complexity of care on the basis of functional and operational capabilities. The definition of levels of care also provides a structure for the regionalization of services.

The authors of the CoFN (2004, 2012) note four advantages of providing definitions:

1. Shared definitions allow for outcome comparisons and resource allocation.
2. Standardized nomenclature will help high-risk maternity patients understand levels of care options.

3. Consistent definitions, published by an authoritative organization, will reduce the cost to businesses which must develop standards of their own.
4. Standardized definitions will enhance standard consistency and service.

In 2001, a survey was conducted by the Section on Perinatal Pediatrics that resulted in recommendations for three levels, the highest of which was segmented into four categories. This was followed by a refinement in 2004 and, most recently, in 2012. The total number of levels and the number of sub-levels have varied over time. All three are described here, to provide a context for the facilities that were created in the associated timeframe. The next iteration or reaffirmation of the guidelines is likely to occur by 2020.

3.5.1 *Levels of care 2001*

An initial survey, published in 2001 (see Bhatt, 2001) resulted in the categories of basic neonatal care, specialty neonatal care, and subspecialty NICUs, the latter of which was divided into four levels. Level I was essentially well-baby care, and not technically an intensive care setting, although facilities and staff for resuscitation and the ability to stabilize frail infants were addressed. Level II might be compared to a step-down unit. An overview is provided in Figure 3.3.

Figure 3.3: *Definitions of levels of neonatal care, 2001 (Source: Bhatt, 2001)*

Level	*General category*	*Services*
I	Basic neonatal care	Well-newborn nursery
		Care of healthy newborns
		Resuscitation
		Stabilization prior to transfer to specialty
II	Specialty neonatal care	Special care nursery
		Care of infants ≥ 1,500 g
		Resuscitation
		Stabilization prior to transfer to ICU
IIIA	Subspecialty NICU	Mandated restriction and/or duration of mechanical ventilation
IIIB	Subspecialty NICU	No restrictions on mechanical ventilation
		No major surgery
IIIC	Subspecialty NICU	Major surgery on site
		No surgical repair of serious congenital heart anomalies that require bypass of ECMO
IIID	Subspecialty NICU	Major surgery including anomalies requiring bypass of ECMO

3.5.2 *Levels of care 2004*

In 2004 the CoFN conducted a detailed analysis of the literature, which was used to help redefine and detail the neonate care levels. The conclusions of researchers provided in the literature review were used to support their recommendations. This approach is an example of a process called evidence-based medicine, which uses research to inform the decision-making process. While normally applied to patient care decisions, the guidelines are also an appropriate application. Evidence-based design, which was derived from the concept of evidence-based medicine, also strives to use the best available data and experience to inform design decisions.

Based on the CoFN (2004) analysis, the three main categories previously proposed were maintained, but Level II was divided into two sub-levels, and Level III was reduced from four to three sub-levels.

In addition to the level classifications/modifications previously described, the CoFN makes several recommendations regarding protocols:

1. Perinatal care be provided in a regionalized system to ensure that neonatal care is appropriate for each child's needs and to facilitate optimal outcomes.
2. Uniform standards for related facilities and staffing, linked to the level classifications, are also needed. These components include personnel, equipment, ancillary services, and organization services such as transport and facilities.
3. Patient outcome data relating to mortality, morbidity, and outcomes should be gathered to support level-specific standards for patient volume by specialization.

The level descriptions are summarized in Figure 3.4.

Level I (basic). Level I is a nursery that has the appropriate staff and equipment to conduct resuscitation and care for healthy newborns. In addition, the staff must have the competency to care for stabilized infants between 35 and 37 weeks' gestational age and be able to stabilize infants of less than 35 weeks' gestational age until transportation to a higher level of care can be provided.

Level II (specialty). Level II is a special-care nursery with the capacity to treat infants of more than 32 weeks' gestational age and weighing at least 1,500 grams. Diagnoses addressed in the Level II nurseries were identified as being:

> physiologic immaturity such as apnea of prematurity, inability to maintain body temperature, or inability to take oral feedings; who are moderately ill with problems that are expected to resolve rapidly and are not anticipated to need subspecialty services on an urgent basis; or who are convalescing from intensive care.
>
> (CoFN, 2004, p. 1346)

Level II nurseries were divided into two categories. The primary function of Level IIA was to resuscitate and stabilize preterm and/or ill babies prior to transfer to a NICU. The higher level (Level IIB) was to have the capability of providing mechanical ventilation for up to 24 hours or continuous positive airway pressure.

Level III (subspecialty). A Level III neonatal intensive care unit is characterized by staff and equipment that provide continuous life support and comprehensive care to infants who are high-risk or critically ill. There are three categories within this level. Level IIIA supports infants of

Figure 3.4: *Definitions of levels of neonatal care, 2004 (Source: CoFN, 2004)*

Level	*General category*	*Services*
I	Well-newborn nursery	Resuscitation at every delivery
		Postnatal care for healthy newborns
		Stabilize care for stable infants 35–37 weeks
		Stabilize ill infants and those born <35 weeks until transfer
IIA	Special care nursery	Resuscitate and stabilize preterm and/or ill infants before transfer to a NICU
		Care for infants >32 weeks and ≥ 1,500 g who (1) have physiologic immaturity such as apnea, inability to maintain body temperature or inability to take oral feedings, or (2) who are moderately ill with problems expected to resolve rapidly and not anticipated to need subspecialty services urgently
		Patients who are convalescing after intensive care
IIB	Special care nursery	Same as level A plus ability to provide mechanical ventilation for <24 hours or continuous positive airway pressure
IIIA	Subspecialty NICU	Comprehensive care for infants >28 weeks and weighing >1000 g
		Sustained life support limited to conventional mechanical ventilation
		Minor surgical procedures such as placement of central venous catheter or hernia repair
IIIB	Subspecialty NICU	Comprehensive care for infants ≤ 28 weeks, ≤ 1,000 g
		Advance respirator support
		On-site access to range of pediatric medical subspecialists
		Advanced imaging with interpretation
		Pediatric surgical specialists and anesthesiologists on site or close to perform major surgery such as ligation of ductus arteriosus and repair of abdominal wall defects
IIIC	Subspecialty NICU	Same as IIIB but also has ECMO and surgical repair of complex congenital cardiac malformations

more than 28 gestational weeks and 1,000 grams in weight. Continuous life support is limited to traditional mechanical ventilation. Level IIIB nurseries care for infants less than 28 weeks' gestational age and weighing less than 1,000 grams. They must have pediatric surgical specialists and anesthesiologists on site or readily available. Care that is provided includes:

> advanced respiratory care such as high frequency ventilation and inhaled nitric oxide; prompt and on-site access to a full range of pediatric medical subspecialists; and advanced imaging with interpretation on an urgent basis, including computed tomography, magnetic resonance imaging, and echocardiography.
>
> (CoFN, 2004, p. 1346)

A Level IIIC NICU was defined as having the capabilities of Level IIIB plus extracorporeal membrane oxygenation (ECMO) and the staff and facilities to conduct surgical repair of cardiac malformations associated with cardiopulmonary bypass.

A full description of the 2004 guidelines may be found in the following document: Committee on Fetus and Newborn (CoFN), American Academy of Pediatrics. (2004). Levels of neonatal care. *Pediatrics, 114*(5), 1341–1347.

3.5.3 *Levels of care 2012*

In 2012, the AAP Committee on Fetus and Newborn reviewed the previously defined levels of care in the context of a meta-analysis of a literature review that covered the period between 1978 and 2010. In addition to information used to formulate the new guidelines, the results demonstrated improved outcomes for very low birth weight (VLBW) infants and those less than 32 weeks' gestational age who were born in Level III NICUs. Regardless of this apparent trend, the authors of the 2012 guidelines note an ongoing discussion regarding what the components of the various levels should be.

While the intention of the guideline levels is to support regionalization of services (i.e. placing lower intensity of care in less populated areas), the authors of the 2012 recommendations note the trend is in the opposite direction. Evidence that demonstrates a movement away from regionalization includes: (1) a growth in the number of neonatologists and NICUs that is not consistently linked to the number of high-risk infants by geographic region; (2) an increase in the number of small NICUs in the same districts as large NICUs; and (3) the failure of states to achieve the goal set by Healthy People 2010 that 90 percent of VLBW infants would be treated at Level III NICUs. The Healthy People initiative, which is now in its 2020 iteration, is sponsored by Health and Human Services and sets goals for health promotion and disease prevention (see healthypeople.gov). Related to the trend toward de-regionalization is an increase in early cesarean deliveries, pregnancy complications, and advanced maternal age (CoFN, 2012). Figure 3.5 shows the additions relative to the previous guidelines in bold, and the deletions are crossed out.

The primary differences between the 2004 and 2012 are as follows:

- *Level I.* Level I 2012 has not changed significantly from Level I 2004.
- *Level II.* The primary difference between 2004 and 2012 is the addition of a statement regarding the stabilization of infants ≤32 weeks' gestation and ≤1,500 grams until transfer to an NICU.
- *Level III.* Several modifications have been made to Level III, largely due to the transition from three levels with sub-components to levels III and IV. Level III nurseries must provide sustained life support and comprehensive care for infants younger than 32 weeks' gestation and less than 1,500 grams, and all critically ill infants. The unit must also provide advanced respiratory support, advanced imaging, and prompt access to a variety of specialists.
- *Level IV.* Level IV has the facilities and staff to address the surgical repair of complex cardiac

Figure 3.5: *Definitions of levels of neonatal care, 2012 (Source: CoFN, 2012) (items in* **bold** *are additions)*

Level	*General category*	*Services*
I	Well-newborn nursery	Resuscitation at every delivery
		Postnatal care for healthy newborns
		Stabilize care for stable infants 35–37 weeks
		Stabilize ill infants and those born <35 weeks until transfer
II	Special care nursery	Level I capabilities and:
		Resuscitate and stabilize preterm and/or ill infants before transfer to a NICU
		Care for infants >32 weeks and ≥1,500 g who (1) have physiologic immaturity such as apnea, inability to maintain body temperature or inability to take oral feedings or (2) who are moderately ill with problems expected to resolve rapidly and not anticipated to need subspecialty services urgently
		Patients who are convalescing after intensive care
		Same as level A plus ability to provide mechanical ventilation for <24 hours or continuous positive airway pressure
		Stabilize infants ≤32 week gestation and ≤1500 g until transfer to an NICU
III	Subspecialty NICU	Level II capabilities and:
		Provision of sustained life support
		Comprehensive care for infants of <32 wks gestation and <1,500 g, and all critically ill infants
		Advanced respiratory support such as high-frequency ventilation and nitric oxide
		Advanced imaging with interpretation including tomography, MRI, and ECG
		Provide prompt access to pediatric **medical** and surgical specialist and anesthesiologists and **ophthalmologists** on site or close to perform major surgery
IV	**Subspecialty NICU**	Level III capabilities and:
		Surgical repair of complex congenital cardiac malformations or acquired conditions
		Maintain a complete range of pediatric medical, surgical, and anesthesiologist specialists at the site
		Facilitate transport and outreach programs

conditions, and on-site pediatric medical, surgical, and anesthesiology specialists. Transport and outreach programs must be supported.

Access to the full set of guidelines is available at the Committee on Fetus and Newborn (CoFN), American Academy of Pediatrics (2012). Levels of neonatal care. *Pediatrics, 130*(3), 587–597. doi:10.1542/peds.2012-1999

3.6 Current NICU data

An overview of statistics provides a contextual picture of the status of NICUs in the early 21st century. The benefit of documenting current history is the insight it provides regarding future allocation of services. For the purposes of this book, a study was initiated to map the recent growth in the number of neonatal intensive care units and the number and geographical distribution of beds. In addition, a literature review has been conducted to address the demographic composition of NICU patients and their families, and their average length of stay.

3.6.1 Number of NICUs and neonatologists

There is little data prior to the 1980s regarding the growth in the number of NICUs, although Goodman and colleagues (2002) suggest that in the prior two decades, the number of neonatologists and number of NICUs grew rapidly. In 1982, Harper and colleagues reported the existence of 248 neonatal intensive care units. The SSCM estimated that there were 1,500 units in 2009.

In order to evaluate the recent growth of neonatologists and neonatology units, we statistically analyzed the data in the 1996, 1999, 2002, and 2011 editions of the *Directory of Neonatologists* (AAP, 1996, 1999, 2002, 2011). Some of these data are slightly different from data provided by the American Hospital Association (AHA), but the total numbers of units are within 3.4 percent of one another.

In 1996 there were 3,397 neonatologists, and in 2011 hospitals reported 4,665 neonatologists. During the same period, the number of NICUs grew from 832 to 1,007. This pattern, namely 4.08 neonatologists per NICU in 1996 versus 4.63 neonatologists per NICU in 2011, suggests increased levels of care, but is likely a reflection of an increase in the size of individual NICUs. In a review of current projects, several units exceeded 60 beds. Based on the total number of neonatologists (4,665) and the total number of beds (28,475) in 2011, there is one neonatologist per 6.1 beds. Figure 3.6 summarizes the recent trends.

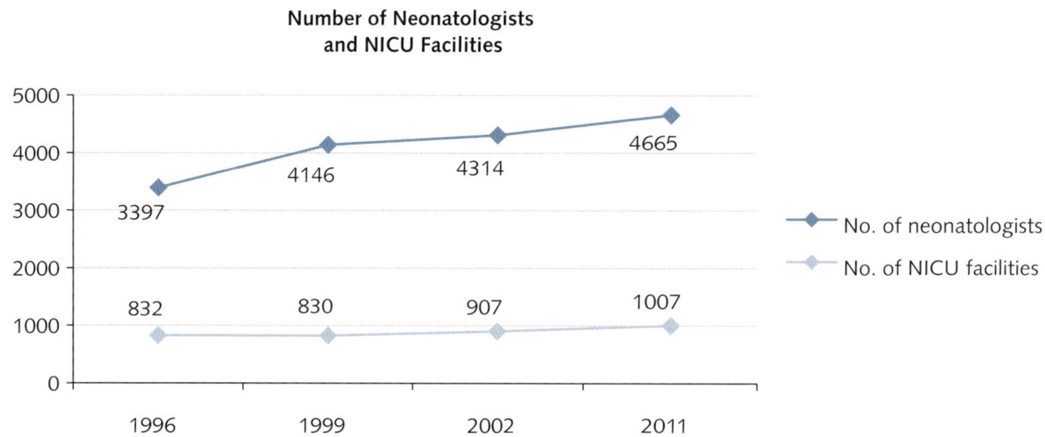

Figure 3.6: *Number of neonatologists and NICUs, 1996 to 2011 (adjustments made for some missing data in 1999) (Sources: AAP, 1996, 1999, 2002, 2011)*

Of the 1,006 NICUs in the United States and Puerto Rico in 2011, 16 percent of these were Level III nurseries. Wyoming reports no Level II and Level III beds, and several states only have Level II beds.

3.6.2 Number and location of NICU beds

There is a wide variation in the number of beds per capita in each state, ranging from 0.283 beds per 1,000 persons in Washington, DC to 0.056 beds in New Hampshire. When examining the regional data, they parallel the state data – the largest numbers of beds are in the South Atlantic region, and the fewest numbers of beds (with the exception of Puerto Rico) are in the New England States. A comparison of the relationship between the total number of NICU beds in the region and the NICUs per capita suggests larger NICUs in specific portions of the country. According to the data summarized in Figure 3.7, in 2011 the average number of beds per unit ranged from 22 to 32 (excluding Puerto Rico).

An analysis was done to try to estimate the ratio of newborns to number of beds. Using the AHA reported number of births in 2009 (the 2011 data were not available) and comparing it to the number of beds, the average per region ranged from 6.22 beds per 1,000 newborns in the Mountain states (Colorado, Arizona, Wyoming, Nevada, Utah, Idaho, Montana, New Mexico) to 8.31 beds per 1,000 newborns in the West South Central portion of the United States (Texas, Louisiana, Oklahoma, and Arkansas).

With respect to geographic distribution, more than 60 percent of the beds are located in four of the ten regions. Those regions are: the South Atlantic, the Pacific, the West South Central region, and the East North Central region (see Figure 3.8).

3.6.3 NICU demographics

Several factors influence the demographic characteristics of the NICU population and their mothers. Two important characteristics are maternal age and race/ethnicity. De Jongh et al. (2012) found that older mothers (35 to 49 years of age) were more likely than adolescent mothers to have babies that spent time in NICUs, and that the infants of Black/non-Hispanic mothers with private insurance were also more likely to be admitted. According to Figure 3.9, the percentage of adolescent mothers (14 to 18 years) whose babies were admitted to NICUs is relatively equivalent for all races, and the differences increase with the age of the mother. The De Jongh study concluded that private insurance did not mitigate the frequency of Black/non-Hispanic admissions.

The mortality rate is higher for some ethnic populations. In the United States, prematurity appears to be the leading cause of death for African-American babies (Ashton, 2006). In a study by MacDorman and Mathews (2011), researchers found that 78 percent of the elevated infant mortality rate of non-Hispanic Black women was due to preterm births. Claydon and colleagues (2007) in a Canadian study also provide data suggesting that minority populations are overly represented. Their study found a significantly high mortality rate among Aboriginal males and East Asian females.

Regarding the frequency of preterm births, the primary driver of the NICU census, data provided in the 2011 *National Vital Statistic Reports* (NVSR) makes evident the high level of premature

Figure 3.7: *Regional distribution of beds (Sources: AAP, 2011; American Hospital Association, 2010)*

	Data from Directory 2011						AHA data		
Region	*NICUs in region*	*NICU units*		*NICU beds in region*	*NICU beds*		*Births (1,000s) 2009*	*NICU beds per unit*	*NICU beds per 1,000 newborns*
		III	*II*		*III*	*II*			
West South Central	145	131	14	4671	4538	133	561.8	32.21	8.3143
East South Central	68	61	7	1911	1847	64	234	28.1	8.1667
West North Central	63	53	10	1922	1812	110	274.1	30.51	7.012
Pacific	169	137	32	4463	4159	304	645.1	26.41	6.9183
South Atlantic	181	151	30	5077	4817	260	736.1	28.05	6.8972
Middle Atlantic	134	111	23	3479	3285	194	481.9	25.96	7.2193
Mountain	63	53	10	1871	1782	89	300.6	29.7	6.2242
East North Central	128	111	17	3883	3738	145	569.7	30.34	6.8159
New England	48	33	15	1060	913	147	156.3	22.08	6.7818
Total	**999**	**841**	**158**	**28337**	**26891**	**1446**	**3959.6**	**28.37**	**7.1565**
Puerto Rico	7	6	1	138	126	12	Not available	19.71	
Grand total	**1006**	**847**	**159**	**28475**	**27017**	**1458**		**28.31**	
Percentage		**84.19**	**15.81**		**94.88**	**5.12**			

West South Central (TX, LA, OK, AR)
East South Central (TN, KY, AL, MS)
West North Central (MO, MN, IA, NE, KS, ND, SD)
Pacific (CA, WA, OR, HI, AK)
South Atlantic (FL, GA, NC, VA, MD, SC, DC, DE, WV)
Middle Atlantic (NY, PA, NJ)
Mountain (CO, AZ, NV, UT, ID, MT, NM, WY)
East North Central (IL, OH, MI, IN, WI)
New England (MA, CT, ME, NH, RI, VT)

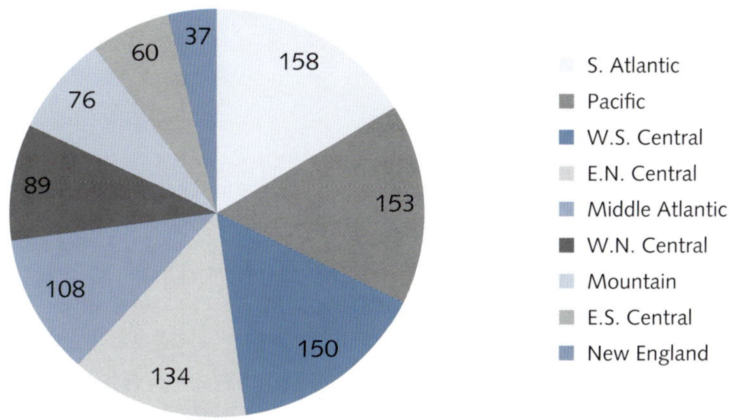

Figure 3.8: *Geographic distribution of Level II and III NICUs (Sources: AAP, 2001; American Hospital Association, 2010)*

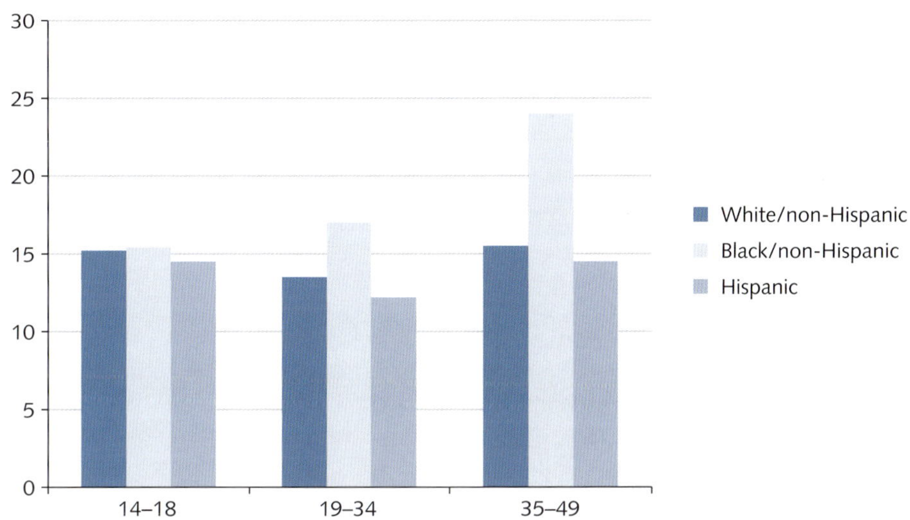

Figure 3.9: *Percentage of births by maternal age and race/ethnicity admitted to the NICU (Source: De Jongh et al., 2012)*

births among non-Hispanic Blacks. Figure 3.10 demonstrates this trend as well as the relative portion premature births represents relative to infant mortality among infants from this minority group.

While differences in the regional number of beds per infant have been described earlier in this chapter, there is no consistent relationship between neonatal mortality and the number of beds in a geographic region (Goodman et al., 2002).

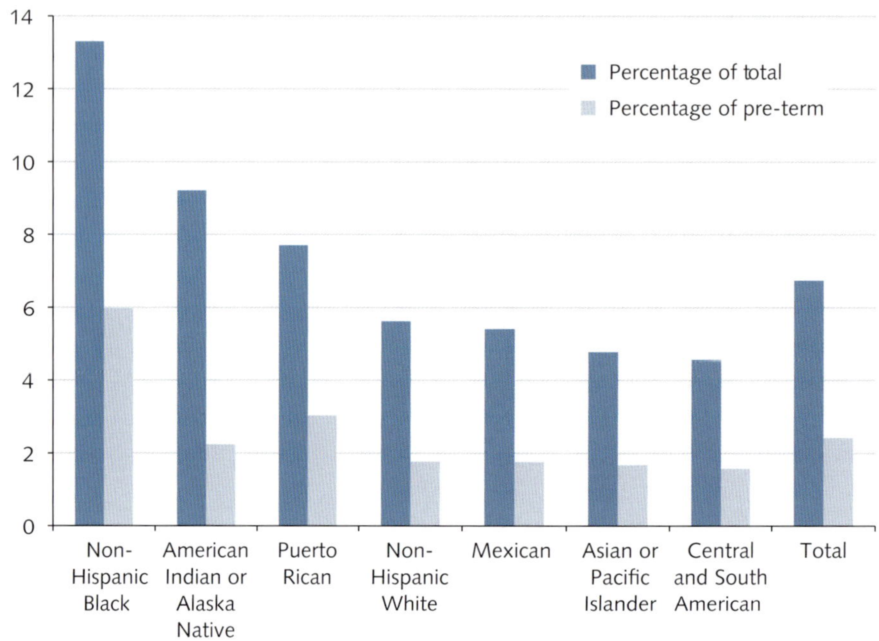

Figure 3.10: *Infant mortality and prematurity by ethnicity/race (Source: Mathews and MacDorman, 2011)*

3.6.4 NICU length of stay

No single source for average length of stay in a NICU was found in the literature, likely due to the wide variation created by the impact of LBW and premature babies. A premature baby is any child born before 37 weeks' gestational age and a very premature baby is born before 32 weeks (Browne, 2003). A low birth weight baby is less than 2,500 grams (5.5 pounds); a very low birth weight baby is under 1,500 grams (3.5 pounds), and an extremely low birth weight baby (ELBW) is under 1,000 grams (2.4 pounds) (Browne, 2003). In order to provide a general sense of what may be typical in a unit, the data reported in the research of six NICUs are summarized in Figure 3.11.

The average length of stay of VLBW children in a study by Melnyk et al. (2006) dropped from 60.12 to 51.81 days and preterm babies improved from 35.63 days to 20.16 days when protocols for parent engagement were in place. In a dissertation on the impact of private rooms, Smithgall (2010) found that children in private rooms remained in the NICU for 22.40 days as opposed to children in open bays, who were there for 18.23 days. These few studies make it clear that VLBW infants stay considerably longer than other infants.

Chapters 2 and 3 have provided a summary of developments in the definition and design of PICUs and NICUs. These environments have evolved in sophistication and focus, particularly within the past decade. The purpose of these summaries was to create a context for the next two chapters, which describe design issues and research regarding pediatric and neonatal critical care.

Figure 3.11: *Average length of stay reported by researchers*

Citation	*Subject*	*#*	*ALOS (days)*	
			Interven	*Control*
Bender, G.J., Koestler, D., Ombao, H., McCourt, M., Alskinis, B., Rubin, L.P., & Padbury, J.F. (2013). Neonatal intensive care unit: Predictive models for length of stay. *Journal of Perinatology*, *33*(2), 147–153.	Newborn	615	28	
Berns, S.D., Boyle, M.D., Popper, B., & Gooding, J. S. (2007). Results of the premature birth national need-gap study. *Journal of Perinatology*, 27, S38–S44.	Preterm	502	20.16	
Melnyk, B.M., Feinstein, N.F., Alpert-Gillis, L., Fairbanks, E., Crean, H.F., Sinkin, R.A., & Gross, S.J. (2006). Reducing premature infants' length of stay and improving parents' mental health outcomes with the Creating Opportunities for Parent Empowerment (COPE) neonatal intensive care unit program: A randomized, controlled trial. Pediatrics, *118*(5), e1414–e1427.	Preterm VLBW	241 90	31.86 51.81	35.63 60.12
National Perinatal Information Center. (2012). V.12.1 Special report: Very low birth weight neonates. Retrieved from http://www.npic.org/Services/V121_Special_Report_SAMPLE.pdf	VLBW special care*	81	57.8	
Smithgall, L.M. (2010). *Perceptions of maternal stress and neonatal patient outcomes in a single private room versus open room Neonatal Intensive Care Unit environment.* Retrieved from ProQuest Dissertations & Theses (PQDT). (ProQuest document ID 848129604)	Newborn	52 each	22.40 private	18.23 open
Stone, P. W., Gupta, A., Loughrey, M., Della-Latta, P., Cimiotti, J., Larson, E., & Saiman, L. (2003). Attributable costs and length of stay of an extended-spectrum beta-lactamase-producing Klebsiella pneumoniae outbreak in a neonatal intensive care unit. *Infection Control and Hospital Epidemiology*, *24*(8), 601–606.	Newborn	486	18.8	

* Include both NICU and NINT (neonatal intermediate care)

References

American Academy of Pediatrics (AAP). (1996, 1999, 2002, 2011). *Newborn Intensive Care Units (NICUs) and Neonatologists of the USA & Canada*. Elk Grove Village, IL: American Academy of Pediatrics.

American Hospital Association. (2010). *AHA Hospital Statistics 2011: The Comprehensive Reference Source for Analysis and Comparison of Hospital Trends*. Chicago, IL: Health Forum.

Antonucci, R., Porcella, A., and Fanos, V. (2009). The infant incubator in the neonatal intensive care unit: Unresolved issues and future developments. *Journal of Perinatal Medicine, 37*(6), 587–598.

Ashton, D. (2006). Prematurity – infant mortality: The scourge remains. *Ethnicity and Disease, 16*(2 Suppl. 3), 58–62.

Baker, J.P. (1991). The incubator controversy: Pediatricians and the origins of premature infant technology in the United States, 1890–1910. *Pediatrics, 87,* 654–662.

Baker, J.P. (2000). The incubator and the medical discovery of the premature infant. *Journal of Perinatology, 20*(5), 321–328.

Bender, G.J., Koestler, D., Ombao, H., McCourt, M., Alskinis, B., Rubin, L.P., and Padbury, J.F. (2013). Neonatal intensive care unit: Predictive models for length of stay. *Journal of Perinatology*, *33*(2), 147–153.

Berns, S.D., Boyle, M.D., Popper, B., and Gooding, J.S. (2007). Results of the premature birth national need-gap study. *Journal of Perinatology*, *27,* S38–S44.

Bhatt, D. (2001). Towards a unified definition of NICU levels of care. *Perinatal Section News, 7,* 12.

Bode, M.M., O'Shea, T.M, Metzguer, K.R., and Stiles, A.D. (2001). Perinatal regionalization and neonatal mortality in North Carolina, 1968–1994. *American Journal of Obstetrics & Gynecology, 184*(6), 1302–1307.

Browne, J. (2003). New perspectives on premature babies and their families. *Zero to Three, 24*(2), 4–12.

Claydon, J.E., Mitton, C., Sankaran, K., Lee, S.K., and the Canadian Neonatal Network. (2007). Ethnic differences in risk factors for neonatal mortality and morbidity in the neonatal intensive care unit. *Journal of Perinatology, 27,* 448–452. doi:10.1038/sj.jp.7211766

Clement, M.S. (2005). Perinatal care in Arizona 1950–2002: A study of the positive impact of technology, regionalization and the Arizona perinatal trust. *Journal of Perinatology, 25*(8), 503–508.

Committee on Fetus and Newborn (CoFN), American Academy of Pediatrics. (2004). Levels of neonatal care. *Pediatrics, 114*(5), 1341–1347. doi: 10.1542/peds.2004-1697

Committee on Fetus and Newborn (CoFN), American Academy of Pediatrics. (2012). Levels of neonatal care. *Pediatrics, 130*(3), 587–597. doi: 10.1542/peds.2012-1999

Committee on Perinatal Health. (1976). *Toward Improving the Outcome of Pregnancy: Recommendations for the Regional Development of Maternal and Perinatal Health Services*. White Plains, NY: March of Dimes National Foundation.

Committee on Perinatal Health. (1993). *Toward Improving the Outcome of Pregnancy: The 90s and Beyond*. White Plains, NY: March of Dimes Birth Defects Foundation.

De Jongh, B.E., Locke, R., Paul, D.A., and Hoffman, M. (2012). The differential effects of maternal age, race/ethnicity and insurance on neonatal intensive care unit admissions rates. *BMC Pregnancy and Childbirth, 12*(1), 97.

Downes, J.J. (1992). The historical evolution, current status, and prospective development of pediatric critical care. *Critical Care Clinics, 8*, 1–22.

Farah, A., Bioda, A., and Shiao, S. (1996). The history of the neonatal nurse practitioner in the United States. *Neonatal Network, 15*(5), 11–21.

Ferris, T., and Shepley, M. (2012). A multidisciplinary human-centered approach to the design of incubation systems. In A. R. Andre (Chair), *Proceedings of the 2012 Symposium on Human Factors and Ergonomics in Health Care* (pp. 187–192). Santa Monica, CA: Human Factors and Ergonomics Society.

Gartner, L.M., and Gartner, C.B. (1992). The care of premature infants: Historical perspective. In *Neonatal Intensive Care: A History of Excellence* (NIH Publication No. 92-2786). Bethesda, MD: National Institutes of Health.

Gluck, L. (1973). The perinatal center: Special care nursery for the newborn infant at risk. In H. Abramson (ed.) *Resuscitation of the Newborn Infant* (3rd edn) (pp. 198–207). Maryland Heights, MO: C.V. Mosby.

Gluck, L. (1977). Why P/N? *Perinatology and Neonatology*, July/August, pp. 8, 52.

Gluck, L. (1992). Conceptualization and initiation of a neonatal intensive care nursery in 1960. In *Neonatal Intensive Care: A History of Excellence* (NIH Publication No. 92-2786). Bethesda, MD: National Institutes of Health.

Goodman, D.G., Fisher, E.S., Little, G.A., Stukel, T.A., Chang, C.H., and Schoendorf, K.S. (2002). The relation between the availability of neonatal intensive care and neonatal mortality. *New England Journal of Medicine, 346*, 1538–1544.

Harper, R.G., Little, G.A., and Sia, C.G. (1982). The scope of nursing practice in Level III neonatal intensive care units. *Pediatrics, 70*(6), 875–878.

Hess, J.H., Mohr, G.J., and Bartelme, P.F. (1934). History of the organization and development of the premature infant station. In *The Physical and Mental Growth of Prematurely Born Children* (pp. 3–11). Chicago, IL: The University of Chicago Press.

Honeyfield, M.E. (2009). Neonatal nurse practitioners: Past, present, and future. *Advances in Neonatal Care, 9*(3), 125–128.

Johnson, P. (2002). The history of the neonatal nurse practitioner: Reflections from "under the looking glass." *Neonatal Network, 21*(5), 51–60.

MacDorman, M.F., and Kirmeyer, S. (2009). Fetal and perinatal mortality, United States, 2005. *National Vital Statistics Report*, *57*(8), 1–19.

MacDorman, M.F., and Mathews, T.J. (2011). Understanding racial and ethnic disparities in U.S. infant mortality rates. *NCHS Data Brief, 74*, 1–6.

Marshall-Baker, A. (2011). Healthful environments for hospitalized infants. *HERD*, *4*(2), 127.

Mathews, T.J., and MacDorman, M.F. (2011). Infant mortality statistics from the 2007 period linked birth/infant death data set. *National Vital Statistics Reports,* 59(6). Hyattsville, MD: National Center for Health Statistics.

Melnyk, B.M., Feinstein, N.F., Alpert-Gillis, L., Fairbanks, E., Crean, H.F., Sinkin, R.A., and Gross, S.J. (2006). Reducing premature infants' length of stay and improving parents' mental health outcomes with the Creating Opportunities for Parent Empowerment (COPE) neonatal intensive care unit program: A randomized, controlled trial. *Pediatrics, 118*(5), e1414–e1427.

National Perinatal Information Center. (2012). V.12.1 Special report: Very low birth weight neonates. Retrieved from http://www.npic.org/Services/V121_Special_Report_SAMPLE.pdf

Owens, A.M. (October 14, 2004). Stahlman named distinguished alumna. *Reporter: Vanderbilt University Medical Center's Weekly Newspaper*. Retrieved from http://www.mc.vanderbilt.edu/reporter/index.html?ID=3553

Samson, L. (2006). Perspectives on neonatal nursing: 1985–2005. *Journal of Perinatal and Neonatal Nursing, 20*(1), 19–26.

Smith, J., Bajo, K., and Hager, J. (2004). Planning a developmentally appropriate neonatal intensive care unit. *Clinics in Perinatology*, *31*(2), 313–322.

Smithgall, L.M. (2010). *Perceptions of maternal stress and neonatal patient outcomes in a single private room versus open room Neonatal Intensive Care Unit environment*. Retrieved from ProQuest Dissertations & Theses (PQDT) (ProQuest document ID 848429604)

Stark, A.R. (2004). Levels of neonatal care. *Pediatrics*, *114*(5), 1341–1347.

Stone, P.W., Gupta, A., Loughrey, M., Della-Latta, P., Cimiotti, J., Larson, E., and Saiman, L. (2003). Attributable costs and length of stay of an extended-spectrum beta-lactamase-producing Klebsiella pneumoniae outbreak in a neonatal intensive care unit. *Infection Control and Hospital Epidemiology*, *24*(8), 601–606.

Wheeler, W.E. (1960). Infections and nursery problems. *Archives of Pediatrics and Adolescent Medicine, 99*(6), 772.

White, R.D. (2011). The newborn intensive care unit environment of care: How we got here, where we're headed, and why. *Seminars in Perinatology, 35*, 2–7.

Wielenga, J.M., Smit, B.J., Merkus, M.P., and Kok, J.H. (2007). Individualized developmental care in a Dutch NICU: Short-term clinical outcome. *Acta Paediatrica, 96,* 1409–1415.

Yaffe, S. (1992). Foreword. In *Neonatal Intensive Care: A History of Excellence* (NIH Publication No. 92-2786). Bethesda, MD: National Institutes of Health.

Part Two: The physical setting

PICU and NICU design

4

The design of PICUs and NICUs is a complex task in the context of a complex healthcare setting. Apart from the technological and medical requirements that must be integrated into the design of intensive care units, the needs of some of the most frail patients in the healthcare system and the most challenged families must be supported. All resources must be brought to bear to achieve the most appropriate environments – resources that include both experience and research. Since the advent of evidence-based design (EBD), however, there has been a heated discussion about the relationship between practice experience and scientific data.

Clearly, the pioneers of EBD did not intend to exclude experience as a reliable tool for designers – after all, research only touches on a limited number of topics. To adequately serve patients as designers and members of design teams, though, we must be familiar with the current state of practice, as well as with evidence-based design research. This chapter attempts to blend the two and generate recommended guidelines specific to these settings. Chapter 5 will focus on design research more directly.

4.1 Theoretical approaches

Healthcare design strategies originate from a variety of disciplines, ranging from environmental and social psychology to finance. Planetree design, issues associated with environmental congruence, and positive distraction are three of the most prominent from the fields of environmental and social psychology. Concepts of return on investment and target value design are derived from the fields of organizational management and finance.

4.1.1 The role of Planetree in pediatric and neonatal ICUs

Planetree is the organization dedicated to patient-centered care that was founded by Angelica Thieriot in the late 1970s (Frampton et al., 2008). Planetree partners with healthcare organizations to achieve an organizational culture and physical environment intended to enhance the patient experience through patient-centered care. Frampton and Charmel (2008) outline the essential components of Planetree patient-centered care as access to information; involvement of patients, families, and volunteers; nutrition; diversity; complementary practices; and healthy communities. Two additional components of Planetree and other approaches to healing environments involve the introduction of art and healing environments. The first Planetree model unit was opened in 1985 and incorporated some of the design features that have become trademarks of Planetree facilities: removal of partitions between staff and patients, soothing colors, individualized room décor, patient lounge with resource center, and a family- and patient-accessible kitchenette (Frampton and Charmel, 2008).

In the *Patient-centered Care Improvement Guide* (Frampton et al., 2008), a collaborative effort between the Picker Institute and Planetree, the authors list a number of environmental requirements in their tool for assessing patient-centered care. As part of the evaluation process, these items are each awarded a point value depending on whether the item has been fully incorporated throughout the facility or is partially incorporated. These requirements are as follows:

- The lobby, emergency entrance, parking areas, information desk and nurses' stations "create a first impression of welcome, comfort, and healing."
- Patients are provided privacy while registering, changing, and being treated.
- If a hospital has shared rooms, accommodation is provided for private conversations.
- Patients are personally able to adjust the lighting and temperature in the room.
- Patient rooms offer views to the outdoors.
- Lounge areas are provided for patients and visitors.
- Diversions for patients and families are provided, in addition to television.
- Overhead paging is limited to emergencies.
- Cleaning materials are non-toxic and have a pleasant odor.
- Signage addresses the language needs of the primary groups served.
- Wayfinding from parking areas to one's destination is clear.

In reviewing the Planetree site, I did not find any children's hospitals that had achieved Planetree designation; however, there are a few general hospitals on the Planetree list that appear to have intensive or intermediate care services for children and neonates, including the Fauquier Hospital in Warrenton, Virginia, which has an intermediate care nursery; the NICU and PICU in the Hospital Israelita Albert Einstein in Sao Paulo, Brazil; the NICU at Kadlec Regional Medical Center in Richland, Washington; the NICU at the Longmont United Hospital in Longmont, Colorado; the NICU at Northern Westchester Hospital in Mount Kisco, New York; and the Stamford Hospital NICU in Stamford, Connecticut.

4.1.2 Environmental congruence

In keeping with the Planetree model of patient-centered care, environments should be congruent with the needs of patients, staff, and families. One of the early pioneers of this idea, Powell Lawton, addressed the need to modulate dimensions of the sensory environment to meet the psychological and emotional resources of the individual experiencing the environment. This theory holds particular resonance for healthcare environments. Patients, staff, and families in a hospital setting may well experience a lower level of competence due to the inherent stress of the situation (see Figure 4.1). Thus, using Lawton's Environmental Press-Competence Model (Lawton and Nahemow, 1973), the environment should be clearer and less challenging than the typical environment.

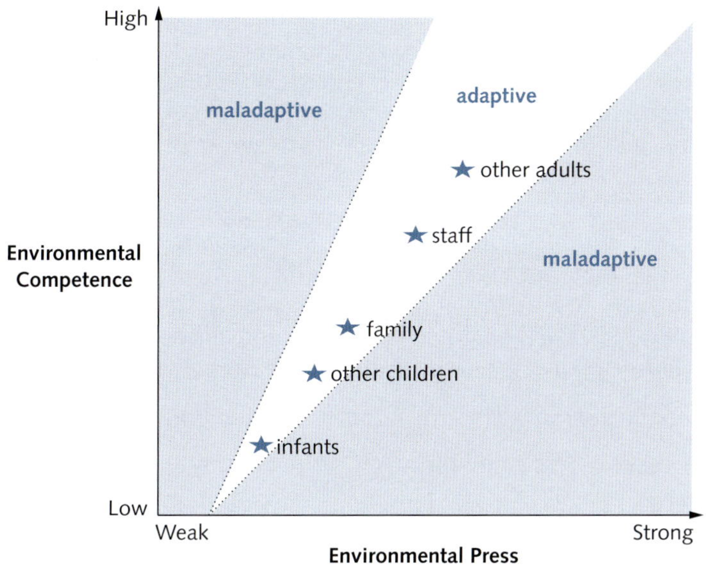

Figure 4.1: *Environmental competence press theory applied to PICU and NICU settings (Source: Lawton and Nahemow, 1973)*

Environmental dimensions of particular concern in creating these compatible settings are sound and light levels. A variety of recommendations, which are discussed later in this chapter, deal with the negative impacts of inappropriate noise levels, poorly designed electrical lighting, and inadequate provision of daylight – both insufficient light and too much direct light or glare.

4.1.3 Positive distraction

The notion of positive distraction was first incorporated in the Recommended Standards for Neonatal ICU Design in 2006. Other official guidelines have addressed this topic to varying degrees in general hospital settings, which in turn have impacted the PICUs and NICUs that are located within them.

The following section focuses on general recommendations regarding positive distraction. A description of the research in support of positive distraction is provided in Chapter 5. Essentially, the purpose of positive distraction is to alleviate stress by helping patients or family members shift their focus from experiences that challenge their ability to make choices and their sense of control to experiences that have a positive effect. Positive distractions include art, access to nature, music and other supportive sounds, entertainment/activities of daily living (ADL) support, and social interaction.

4.1.3.1 Art

Many researchers and design practitioners embrace the use of art for the purposes of positive distraction in healthcare settings. Based on the current research literature, a conservative approach to art installations in pediatric and neonatal settings would be to provide soothing realistic or abstract art. As there is some disagreement regarding the effectiveness of abstract art, preapproval by staff, families and patients would be helpful. Apart from the style of the art (e.g. abstract, realism, primitivism), and the medium (e.g. sculpture, painting, photography, digital prints, serigraphy, lithography), the subject matter should be broadly discussed with design team members. Using nature themes for content appears to be a reliable approach, regardless of genre.

In the case of PICUs, the art must address a broad range of viewers – families, staff, and children ranging from infants to older teenagers. The audience for NICUs is limited primarily to adult visitors and staff, although, if a sibling playroom is provided, the art selection should reflect the children and adolescents in that location. Blumberg and Devlin (2006) noted that childhood symbols, such as teddy bears and balloons in hospital hallways and lobbies, were not appealing to children aged 12 to 14, although strong color was positively evaluated. Due to the wide range in tastes, an art cart may be the best solution; this cart holds a variety of works of art from which family members can choose. This is an approach advocated by Planetree.

The art and graphics found in a home nursery are not appropriate for a NICU. Much of the design in a home nursery is intended to stimulate the visual development of an infant, and most NICU infants lack the visual acuity or visual access (due to the incubator) to benefit from this approach. In actuality, adults in NICUs are the primary audience for artwork and benefit from stress-reducing art; stress reduction is more likely achieved with nature scenes than teddy bears. Recent NICU facilities identified by Smith et al. (2010) as incorporating more effective themes included elements such as pianos and harps, a faux fireplace, fiber optic stars and clouds, and fiber optics on nurse stations and art programs.

Regarding PICUs, Eisen et al. (2008) studied art preferences in hospitalized children and found that nature art was highly preferred by 60 percent of children aged 8 to 17, and 50 percent of 5- to 7-year-olds. A frequent approach in PICUs is to commit to a theme, for example, sports, or the seashore. Establishing specific thematic parameters expedites the design process and, if flexible enough, will support multiple ages of children.

4.1.3.2 Access to nature

Access to nature is important in healthcare settings. While direct access to the outdoors, atria, or gardens may not be available adjacent to the PICU or NICU environment, having options somewhere within the hospital and in the path of travel from the entrance of the building to the intensive care setting is recommended. To study the role of gardens in children's hospitals, Pasha (in press) used site evaluations, interviews, surveys, and observation techniques to evaluate satisfaction and garden visitation duration and frequency in children's hospitals. She concluded that satisfaction was related to the presence of garden amenities, and that the frequency and duration of visitation was related to the presence of amenities such as shading, seating options, landscaping, amenities focused on children, and playfulness. Although there are no studies specifically relating access to nature in PICUs and NICUs, several researchers have studied the use of gardens by families and staff who might use hospital-wide garden amenities. These studies are summarized in Chapter 5.

Two excellent references with regard to healing garden design are Cooper Marcus and Barnes

(1999) and Cooper Marcus and Sachs (2013). With regard to the latter, the authors provide the following programming and site guidelines:

1. Evaluate the whole site as a healing environment.
2. Incorporate the landscape architect at the inception of the project.
3. Involve a landscape architect who is trained in therapeutic design.
4. Consider all types of patients.
5. Design for health outcomes and support programs that address those outcomes.
6. Educate staff about the garden.
7. Consult with specialists (e.g. therapists) for specific programs.
8. Provide at least one space dedicated to staff.
9. Incorporate nature indoors.
10. Make the primary garden visible and accessible from interior public spaces.

With specific regard to gardens in children's hospitals, Pasha (2011) recommends the following:

- Provide comfortable, movable, and a variety of seating options.
- Incorporate a range of sculptures, colors, and signage.
- Include a hierarchy of paths.
- Provide shade and plantings that support a cooling microclimate.
- Incorporate play amenities for children.
- Provide proximity to patient rooms.
- Provide proximity to staff areas.
- Provide information to enhance familiarity with the garden.
- Include exclusive outdoor space for staff.
- Integrate gardens with the daily routines of staff and patients.
- Locate gardens so that they are readily encountered by visitors.

PICU children, and NICU and PICU staff and families should have views to the outdoors either on or adjacent to the unit. PICU patients are required to have windows in their rooms, but the content of the views from these windows should include aspects of nature. Staff and family lounges would also greatly benefit from the natural light and nature views offered by windows. When the location of the unit prevents this, skylights and nature art may enhance the experience (Shepley, 2006).

Gen X architecture: tales of an expanding pediatric intensive care unit

Peter Syrett, AIA, LEED AP BD+C

Breeze Glazer, LEED AP BD+C

"Generation X" typically describes people born from the 1960s through the early 1980s (Jackson, 2010), following the post-World War II baby boomer generation (Dobransky-Fasiska, 1994). They also have another distinction; they are the first generation of people that may have spent time in a Pediatric Intensive Care Unit (PICU), as the first one in North America opened in the Children's Hospital of Philadelphia (CHOP) in 1967 (Children's Hospital of Philadelphia, 2012). In the 45 years since, they have become ubiquitous to the hospital program – providing a care environment to a wide range of pediatric patients, from toddlers through young adults. Pop culture has also dubbed Generation X as the "MTV Generation"; describing a group that is intentionally disconnected from the natural world – preferring to plug into a digital alternative. The unhealthy consequences of this behavior are ever-expanding waistlines and increasing energy intensities. These generational traits and their consequences may also be used to describe the design evolution of the pediatric intensive care unit whose inherent space and program requirements have led to a trend of supersizing, and over-reliance on mechanical systems.

In recent years, a distinct "Return to the Past" trend has occurred within our own wellness vocabulary; a desire to connect to the outdoors and seek healthier, more natural lifestyles. At the same time, healthcare development experts predict that the recent shifts in the U.S. healthcare system will inform areas within hospitals to become more "mission critical," leading to a growing trend in renovation and adaptive reuse of inpatient projects. The same critical analysis that we place on improving human health may be applied to PICUs and inform a more sustainable typology that reduces its environmental and economic impacts while simultaneously supporting improved health outcomes.

To start the endeavor, one must first critically examine the PICUs across the existing hospital building stock in the United States. A primary classification division is by construction type – new, ground-up construction versus renovations, retrofits, and adaptive reuse projects. Through this initial filtering, stark differences begin to emerge. In particular it is clear that PICUs retrofitted in pre-World War II buildings are quite different than those built recently in a new hospital. Many of the retrofitted PICUs exist in dense urban environments such as New York City, where architects typically must work within existing, historic buildings because the opportunities to design for new, ground-up construction are limited.

The floor plates of the pre-World War II hospital buildings are significantly narrower than those we are used to today, as they relied primarily on natural, and not mechanical, systems to bring light and fresh air into the building. They tend to be just wide enough for a central, double-loaded corridor flanked by patient rooms on either side that typically have operable windows. This configuration allowed for cross-ventilation and for natural light to reach the most interior parts of the building. This approach differs radically from the floor plates of PICUs in newer buildings that often locate the nursing and support cores deep into the middle of a wide floor plate, without visual access to the exterior environment. Some interesting beneficial design solutions emerge from looking at older nursing unit designs, for instance, by locating satellite nursing stations within alcoves adjacent to the central corridor, increased levels of observation and care are possible. While this layout can potentially pose some operational challenges, it does enable all occupants – staff, patients, and visitors – to have access to daylight and views to nature when provided by site conditions. In the foreseeable future it is likely that operable windows remain closed during typical hospital operations but can provide an added level of resiliency to allow for passive survivability during catastrophe when there is a loss of power and failure of mechanical ventilation systems. Because available square footage is typically more limited in an existing building, efficiency dictates the planning of family support and sleep areas that are located within the patient room. A centralized approach may also be used, providing additional family sleep, lounge, and meeting areas that are co-located and shared at each patient floor. As such, the narrow floor plates and historic envelopes often inherent to adaptive reuse healthcare projects can be recalibrated from a deficit to instead become an asset that provides added value and opportunity.

A recent study by researchers from the University of Chicago revealed that the healthcare sector is responsible for approximately 8 percent of the United States' total carbon footprint, with hospitals directly contributing as much as 3.2 percent of that total; emitting 80 million tons of carbon dioxide annually (Chung and Meltzer, 2009). According to the DOE, 10 to 15 percent of the average hospital's annual energy consumption is spent on electric lighting (Taddonio, 2011). By allowing daylight in and incorporating sensor controls and reduced lighting power densities, the reliance on electric lighting can be greatly reduced and inform energy and carbon reductions and related operational cost savings. Most importantly, enhanced access to daylight and views of nature for patients in intensive care units can support and improve health outcomes. A wide range of research studies have demonstrated that patient benefits can include reduced requests for pain analgesics, reductions in patient stress and delirium, and resulting increase in recovery times, and reduced length of stay. The benefits aren't limited to just patients, as a 2005 study of a 141 nurses in Akdeniz University Hospital in Antalya, Turkey found that exposure to daylight for at least three hours a day resulted in less stress and higher satisfaction at work (Alimoglu, 2005). As many healthcare administrators have noted, the health, wellness, and satisfaction of staff is critical in achieving the same for patients under their care.

The United States' healthcare system is undergoing the most radical changes in its history. Under these conditions it may be more cost-effective for health systems to renovate than build new, which should inform a rise in adaptive reuse projects. Rather than be seen as a limitation, these projects can benefit from the design and operational opportunities provided by existing buildings; in particular pre-World War II structures. As such, there is no better time to critically examine the design of pediatric intensive care units to understand how they can be improved to reduce their environmental impacts while supporting improved health outcomes.

References

Alimoglu, D. (2005). Daylight exposure and the other predictors of burnout among nurses in a university hospital. *International Journal of Nursing Studies, 42*(5), 549–555.

Children's Hospital of Philadelphia. (2012). *Anesthesiology and Critical Care Medicine History*. Retrieved from www.chop.edu/service/anesthesiology-and-critical-care-medicine/historical-highlights.html, October 12, 2012.

Chung, J.W., and Meltzer, D.O. (2009). Estimate of the carbon footprint of the US healthcare sector. *Journal of American Medical Association, 302*, 1970–1972.

Dobransky-Fasiska, D. (1994). *A discriminant analysis of entrepreneurial personality characteristics for each of three generational cohorts: The silent generation, the baby boomers, and generation X*. Doctoral dissertation, University of Pittsburgh.

Jackson, R.L. (2010). *Encyclopedia of Identity*. Thousand Oaks, CA: Sage, p. 307.

Taddonio, K. (2011). *Energy Efficient Lighting Strategies Pay Off Quickly*. Washington, DC: US Department of Energy.

4.1.3.3 Music, mothers' sounds and nature sounds

The three main topics when discussing positive audial distraction are music, nature sounds, and, in the context of the NICU, sounds associated with a baby's mother. The research regarding this topic is provided in Chapter 5. In general, there are a few reliable conclusions designers can lean on when considering the incorporation of these elements:

- Music can be used as a distraction for older children and adults, particularly if the listener has control over the source, the content, and the volume. Some scientific data and common belief support the notion that, under these circumstances, music has the potential to positively impact patient and staff outcomes. Live music may also be beneficial in reducing stress reactions (Arnon et al., 2006; Gilad and Arnon, 2010). The impact of music on neonates is unclear and likely influenced by the condition of the child.
- Taped nature sounds have typically been provided in association with views or images of nature. Most agree that this tool can be used for positive distraction, if the individual can control access. Both of these distractions should be used judiciously so as not to disturb other patients, and in the case of staff, the sounds should not impede alarms or communication.
- Some evidence exists that piping the sounds of the mother (heartbeat, etc.) may have a positive effect on a neonate. The usefulness of this technique may vary depending on the age of the child. According to Hartline (2013), full-term birth babies prefer the mother's voice, followed by another female voice, followed by music. Suggested guidelines for preterm infants are: limit ambient noise, speak or sing during gentle handling, and play music at ambient levels (no directly applied speakers) (Hartline, 2013).

4.1.3.4 Family entertainment/activities of daily living/sibling play

In treating the family unit, multiple amenities come into play: movies, music, access to the internet, and so on. Areas in which siblings can play may also be relevant. One approach is to provide features that help to simulate the activities of daily living (ADL) home life. Access to the internet and computers may enable parents to maintain their connections to their jobs and their families. Access to healthy food will promote a healthy diet for family members. Entertainment such as music, movies, and computer games may help deflect stressful thoughts.

4.1.3.5 Social interaction

Social interaction is a form of distraction, while not in and of itself an environmental component. Nonetheless, by creating spaces that support social interaction, we facilitate its occurrence. There is a strong body of literature to indicate that providing social support is beneficial to both the giver and the receiver (e.g. Christensen et al., 1999; Brown et al., 2003). Spaces that support social interaction include lounges, education seminar rooms, family kitchens/shared eating areas, and laundry spaces.

The work of Hilal Ozcan (2006) provides important insights into the design of PICUs relative to social interaction. Ozcan used behavioral maps, participant observation, in-depth interviews, and floor plan analysis to obtain data on the relationship of the physical environment to positive social interaction in a cross-cultural analysis of PICUs in Turkey and the United States. In terms of defining needs to support social interaction, she found they clustered in the categories of programmatic, functional, symbolic, environmental, social, and psychological (see Figure 4.2). Ozcan's research is phenomenological. This approach emphasizes a broad understanding of the nature of behavior and environments in support of a conceptual framework for examining an issue. This framework may either be used to generate future quantitative and qualitative studies or serve as a format for addressing a design problem.

4.2 Lean process, lean design, and return on investment

An important conversation when discussing contemporary approaches is the economic impact of these design decisions. At the same time that the healthcare industry is experiencing rising expectations for the development of high-quality, economically effective, environmentally sustainable facilities, Lean design – an approach to project delivery that focuses on cycles of continuous improvement to reduce waste and add value – has gained traction in the construction community. Using this technique, healthcare facility design projects are reporting success in terms of reduced project cost, streamlined duration, and minimal litigation (Kulkarni et al., 2012; Rybkowski et al., 2012). Healthcare facility owners now require architects to demonstrate proficiency in their understanding of lean processes.

There are multiple books that address lean process in healthcare, such as *Sustaining Lean in Healthcare: Developing and Engaging Physician Leadership* (Nelson, 2011) and *Leading the Lean Healthcare Journey: Driving Culture Change to Increase Value* (Wellman et al., 2010), and some journal articles that specifically address lean process in PICUs, including Vats et al. (2012), who explored lean rounding processes, and Dick (2011), who used simulation to examine lean approaches to PICU bed availability.

Likewise, there are publications that address the aspects of physical lean hospital design more generally, such as Grunden and Hagood's *Lean-led Hospital Design: Creating the Efficient Hospital of the Future* (2012). With particular regard to children's hospitals, *Lean and Green Healthcare Facilities: Improving the Delivery Process in Children's Hospitals* (Enache-Pommer, 2008) and Bilec and colleagues' "Analysis of the design process of green children's hospitals: Focus on process modeling and lessons learned" (2009) discuss this topic. However, the literature on the use of lean principles to drive the physical design of pediatric and neonatal intensive care

Figure 4.2: *PICU categories for designing socially supportive healing environments (Source: Ozcan, 2006)*

Categories	*Sub-categories*	*Definition*	*Low*	*High*
Programmatic	Provisional	Presence and location of spaces that support interaction	Activity not present, inhibiting social interaction	Present, influential, allows for privacy and interaction
	Scale	Size, scale, proportion	Intimate	Monumental
	Location	Relational interactions and spatial ordering	Compact, moderate walking	Extended spatial arrangements
Functional	Functionality	Efficient provision of functions	Locally generated function and aesthetic	Complicated; universal aesthetic
	Flexibility and accessibility	Multifunctional spatial order	Activities singular and monotonous	Diverse layout, good wayfinding
	Technology	Access to and dependency upon technology	Low tech; imported from foreign countries	High tech, locally generated and accessible
	Rest and relaxation	Opportunities for rejuvenation	Functions absent; low nature	Central to design; access to nature
Symbolic	Materiality	Symbolic quality of materials	Local materials, but institutional looking	High tech materials but friendly and homelike
	Transparency	Degree of visibility	Concealed activities	Visible
	Form language	Geometry, image, symbolic value	Assertive, unforgiving	Friendly, respectful
Ambience	Comfortable and familiar	Dwelling and healing	Institutional	Homelike
	Image and character	Form character and innovation	Monotonous layout	Sophisticated, high tech, diverse
	Nature responsiveness	Access to nature and stress reduction	Lack of window and nature views	Views, natural systems
	Other positive distractions	Water, play, music, pets	Does not address healing arts	Pluralist use of healing approaches
Social	Social and organizational support	Social systems, requirements and services	Informal support; inappropriate communication	Scheduled meetings and group activities, FCC
	Social interaction	Social and professional interactions	Formal and professional	Natural, intimate, trustworthy
	Staff collaboration	Professional and work relationships	Limited communication	Intense knowledge sharing
Psychological	Privacy	Privacy and enclosure	Lack of privacy and respect	Privacy and respect for personhood
	Personalization	Individuality	Impersonal	Self-expression, need satisfaction
	Healing art	Self-expression	Little self-expression	Art to reveal oneself
	Spiritual	Self-transformation, ego transcendence	No spiritual space functions	Spiritual functions and expressions of belief

units is minimal. Exceptions are the research by Rybkowski et al. (2012) on NICUs and target value design, and the work described by Anderson and Weber (2012) on the NICU design process. Rybkowski comments on overcoming the capital cost challenges of evidence-based design in her guest author essay.

Overcoming the capital cost hurdle of evidence-based design: lean construction and target value design

Zofia K. Rybkowski, PhD, LEED AP

Healthcare facility owners may readily agree that implementing evidence-based design (EBD) interventions in healthcare facilities makes logical sense. After all, even without seeing data, most of us have experienced the therapeutic, health-giving benefits of exposure to live foliage and sunlight or the quiet presence of supportive family members who remain beside us during times of need. For some owners, the challenge of EBD has less to do with agreeing that it works than with the very real possibility that every time an additional window with a sunlit view or special seating area for supportive family members is introduced, there is a potential cost premium associated with that decision.

To this owner, I say: Your frustration is understandable. However, are you aware that the cost premium associated with higher quality design does not have to be so? In fact, there is a community of healthcare facility owners, designers, engineers, and constructors who are collectively lowering the capital cost of quality healthcare facility design and construction by up to 20 percent. They are doing this by practicing target value design, a design-to-budget-based methodology introduced by the lean construction community. Derived from and similar to lean manufacturing (also known as Toyota Production Systems), lean construction practitioners identify waste and value present in an existing system, and then proceed to eliminate that waste while simultaneously proposing opportunities that augment value.

Target value design (TVD), a brainchild of lean construction researchers, formally emerged in 2007 from collaboration between not-for-profit Northern California-based Sutter Health and lean construction researchers at the University of California, Berkeley. Sutter Health needed to design and then construct a new hospital in San Francisco – the 850,000-square-foot Cathedral Hill California Pacific Medical Center (CPMC) – to a budget which the owner could afford. The owner had fired the first architect, engineering, and constructor team for creating a design that was over budget and, trying again with a brand-new team of architects, engineers, and constructors, decided to experiment with a new design and delivery method which they called target value design. Team interactions would be guided by an innovative legal contract – the integrated form of agreement (IFOA) – that would allow risk to be more equally shared than is customary with traditional contracts. The owner, architect, engineering, and constructor (OAEC) team collectively established a non-negotiable allowable cost which team members would be incentivized to reach, and engaged a full-time estimator who continuously recalculated the building's capital cost during each new iteration of the design process.

The transformation of OAEC stakeholders into an integrated team requires mastery of both soft and hard skills. Soft skills include developing and nurturing a culture of cooperation, collaboration, transparency, and trust. Hard skills involve translation of the Toyota Production System's lean manufacturing tools to reduce waste and add value during the design and construction process, including *kaizen* (continuous improvement), cell design, pull versus push or just-in-time, small batch sizes, *heijunka* (workload leveling), and mistake-proofing, etc. Unlike traditional design-bid-build delivery which places the architect as the prime professional, lean construction engages a form of integrated project delivery where a third-party facilitator solicits design ideas from all members of the core OAEC team. Roles typical to most traditional delivery processes are expanded, and because the team meets on a regular basis – or even co-locates – waste due to misunderstandings that are common during traditional forms of delivery is eliminated. The more complex the project, the greater the benefits from the implementation of TVD. In fact, because healthcare facility projects are so complex, they are arguably the project type that benefit the most from application of TVD.

The Cathedral Hill CPMC project experimentation – and the over $100,000,000 in calculated savings – paved the way for Sutter Health to repeat the process with other projects.

Since then, experimentation with TVD has expanded, not only with Sutter Health projects, but with those of other healthcare providers as well. Although project names are still confidential at the time of writing, preliminary results from some of this experimentation are listed in Figure 1. Note the savings garnered by each project team.

Figure 1: *Examples of cost results following target value design exercises on reduction of capital cost (Source: Glenn Ballard, personal communication, 2012)*

Name of project (SF)	*Market cost ($ millions)*	*Final cost ($ millions)*	*Reduction of cost (%)*
Project A (368,882 SF)	98,000,000	89,200,000	9
Project B (114,000 SF)	13,533,179	11,717,000	13.4
Project C (75,362 SF)	13,600,000	11,200,000	17.6
Project D (230,000 SF)	22,000,000	17,900,000	18.6

The IFOA contract, developed by Will Lichtig, legal advisor during the Cathedral Hill CPMC project, went on to serve as a guide for the development of two new forms of contract – the AIA Integrated Project Delivery contract and the AGC Consensus Docs – legal contracts that are increasingly being implemented in the United States for the very reason that owners want to build higher quality facilities at reduced cost. Twenty years of results from lean construction experimentation conducted by collaborative teams of academics and practitioners is freely available on the website of the International Group for Lean Construction (www.iglc.net).

The ultimate point is that healthcare facility owners need not be discouraged by the potential capital cost premium-associated implementation of EBD. Early results from experimentation with TVD by the Lean Construction community suggest that EBD is not only good in theory; it can also be realizable in practice for even financially constrained healthcare facility owners. This should be greeted as good news for owners in China as well as those from other regions of the world who are looking to realize a vision of better quality healthcare facilities.

References

Ballard, G. (2011). Target value design: Current benchmark (1.0). *Lean Construction Journal*, 79–84.

Forbes, L.H. and Ahmed, S.M. (2011). *Modern Construction: Lean Project Delivery and Integrated Practices*. Boca Raton, FL: CRC Press/Taylor & Francis Group.

Macomber, H., Howell, G., and Barberio, J. (2008). Target value design: Nine foundational practices for delivering surprising client value. Retrieved from http://www.aia.org/nwsltr_pm.cfm?pagename=pm_a_112007_targetvaluedesign website, July 30, 2008.

Rybkowski, Z. (2009). *The application of root cause analysis and target value design to evidence-based design and the capital planning of healthcare facilities*. Doctoral dissertation, University of California, Berkeley.

Tjell, J. (2010). *Building information modeling (BIM) in design detailing with focus on interior wall systems*. Masters thesis, Technical University of Denmark.

With regard to the notion of return on investment, a concept applied to the potential savings of implementing strategies of evidence-based design (Berry et al., 2004), analysts have conducted a few studies that allow for calibration of the financial implications. Stone et al. (2003) found that the fiscal cost of an infection outbreak in a NICU was more than $340,000 due primarily to additional healthcare worker time in direct patient care (2,489 hours). In addition to the fiscal impact, these children had a 48.5 longer mean LOS than a national sample. Were the facility to consist of SFRs, a projection could be made in terms of the reduction in infection, which could be linked to reduced worker time and a financial return on investment.

In *Evidence for Innovation*, Sadler et al. (2008) discuss the business case for better pediatric hospitals. Although this does not focus specifically on PICUs and NICUs, the discussion is generalizable to these sub-settings. The concept of pay-for-performance (P4P) is serving as a motivator to improve the effectiveness of healthcare delivery. Likewise, the notion of not charging for errors, and the requirement through Hospital Consumer Assessment of Healthcare Providers and Systems (HCAHPS) for patients to report their experiences, are forcing hospitals to manage their systems more closely (Sadler et al., 2008). Several strategies that have cost-reduction implications have been studied in health facilities, such as the introduction of ceiling lifts, the location of washing dispensers in every patient's room, and design features that reduce falls. These features also apply to pediatric environments and a business case for PICUs and NICUs in those settings as well.

The economics of hospital NICU design

Blair L. Sadler, JD

One of the biggest barriers to building NICUs that provide optimal benefits to patients and staff is the myth that better design costs more. The reply to evidence-based design innovations is still too often: "we would like to but we cannot afford it." Zofia Rybkowski, Mardelle Shepley, and Glen Ballard have done an excellent job in partially puncturing this balloon with their analysis of target value design. They show that initial design and construction costs ("first costs") can be significantly reduced using their recommended methodology.

Equally important, I believe, is the impact of good, evidence-based design on ongoing operating costs. The relationship of capital costs to operating costs is essential to making prudent design and construction decisions. As a leader of Rady Children's Hospital in San Diego for 26 years, I grew to understand this relationship all too well. As important as it is to reduce one-time construction costs, I believe the real financial win is in reducing multi-year operating costs, which dwarf one-time construction costs when one takes a long-term, life cycle perspective. For example, in my last year at Rady Children's (2006), our annual capital budget was $40 million and our annual operating budget was $400 million. It's like comparing a golf ball to a basketball. If a modest, one-time increase in design/construction costs (the golf ball) yields a decrease in operating costs year after year (the basketball), the conclusion is obvious. But, until recently, no one had made a systematic attempt to examine this relationship and to quantify the impact.

This is what the Fable Hospital is all about. In 2004, a multidisciplinary team created a mythical 300-bed hospital (a Fable) that incorporated the leading, accepted evidence-based design principles based on actual experience in the published literature. We then analyzed the one-time incremental costs of incorporating these designs, and the reduction in operating costs. The results were profound – the incremental construction costs were offset by operating cost savings in just two years, creating a powerful return on investment (Berry et al., 2004). In 2011, we updated our analysis and published Fable 2.0. Despite being even more conservative in our assumptions of operating cost benefits, the business case was even stronger. The costs of preventable infections, patient falls, medication errors, unnecessary patient transfers, longer lengths of stay compounded by dark, depressing patient rooms, sleep deprivation due to noise, nurse and other staff fatigue and burn-out all increased (Sadler et al., 2011).

While the Fable analysis was applied to a general acute care hospital, the basic framework applies equally well to the NICU setting. Not all design innovations are relevant but many are. Specific research is needed on NICUs and the good news is that there is a lot out there (NACHRI and the Center for Health Care Design, 2008). The importance of environmental design in the NICU is enormous. Robert White has phrased it well: "a case can be made that no other part of the hospital is providing an optimal physical environment more important than in the NICU, because nowhere else will the adverse effects of noxious physical elements have more profound effects than there" (White, 2012).

An excellent example of recent research is the comprehensive comparison of open-bay and single family-room (SFR) NICUs at Sanford Children's Hospital by Stevens et al. (2011) It showed that the SFR design increased sleep time for babies, lowered direct costs of care by 15.5 percent, and caused no increased risks to neonates. The SFR design also provided enhanced ability to control sound and light, improved parent satisfaction with care, improved staff perception of care, and improved neonatal nutritional outcomes (Stevens et al., 2011).

But research alone is not enough. We are all creatures of habit. Making significant changes in hospital design that change how work is performed requires a change in the culture of an organization. Data alone won't do it. Visits to places that have made changes and seeing them at first hand are essential. Having "bilingual" conversations between clinicians and financial managers is essential to overcome preconceived notions.

A straightforward four-step framework can often help. First, identify the harm to be reduced or avoided and agree on the number by when. Second, identify the improvement target (aim) and dollars that could be saved. Third, identify the needed specific clinical and administrative strategies, as well as evidence-based design strategies, and estimate associated costs. Fourth, calculate the return on investment (ROI) by subtracting improvement costs from savings achieved (Sadler et al., 2009). This is the kind of analysis that CEOs and CFOs understand and that boards of trustees will support.

Healthcare leaders today are confronted by unprecedented challenges. Healthcare systems are moving from the single aim of improved patient care (and the patient experience) to the triple aim of improved population health, and lower costs per capita. Patients and families have better access to information to make choices about where they receive their care.

Improved environmental design that enhances care and the care experience, reduces costs, increases market share, and provides a less stressful, more joyful place to work has become a key survival strategy. Healthcare leaders, architects, and clinicians ignore this reality at their peril. Besides, whether a patient is in our care for an hour, a day, a week, or a year, they deserve an optimal healing environment. This goes double for our tiny neonates.

References

Berry, L.L., Parker, D., Coile, R.C., Hamilton, D.K., O'Neill, D.D., and Sadler, B.L. (2004). The business case for building better buildings. *Frontiers in Health Services Management*, *21*(1), 3–21.

NACHRI and the Center for Health Care Design. (2008). Evidence for innovation: Transforming children's healthcare through the physical environment. Downloaded from www.children'shospitals.net and www.healthdesign.org.

Sadler, B.L., Berry, L.L., Guenther, R., Hamilton, D.K., Hessler, F.A., Merritt, C., and Parker, D. (2011). Fable Hospital 2.0: The business case for building better health care facilities. *Hastings Center Report*, *41*(1), 13–23.

Sadler, B.L., Joseph, A., Keller, A., and Rostenberg, B. (2009). Using evidence-based environmental design to enhance safety and quality. Institute for Healthcare Improvement. Downloaded from www.ihi.org/IHI/Results/WhitePapers/UsingEvidence-BasedEnvironmentalDesignWhite Papaer.htm

Stevens, D.C., Helseth, C.C., Thompson, P.A., Pottola, J.V., Khan, M.A., and Munson, D.P. (2011). A comprehensive comparison of open-bay and single-family-room neonatal intensive care units at Sanford Children's Hospital. *Health Environments Research and Design*, *5*(4), 23–39.

White, R. (2012). Small comforts: Evidence-based design comes to the NICU. *Health Environments Research and Design*, *5*(4), 3–4.

4.3 Sustainability

The introduction of sustainable features may be framed as part of the business case for good design. Some of these features may not cost more, such as the appropriate selection of materials (Sadler et al., 2008), and those that do are likely to involve operational savings.

One of the most focused discussions on sustainability in children's hospitals is provided by Gottlieb and Dickeman in *NICQ 2007: Improvement in Action* (2007). Gottlieb and Dickeman identify the primary issues of contamination in hospitals to be waste, climate change, food systems, cleaning and disinfecting, building materials, and exposure to di-2-ethylhexyl phthalate (DEHP). The authors describe the case of enhancing the sustainability of the Seattle Children's Hospital in a program called the Clean, Green Initiative; one of the primary settings for this initiative was the NICU. The NICU took the lead in phasing out the use of materials with DEHP.

Steps to accomplish sustainable objectives included the following:

- Evaluating medical devices containing PVC and DEHP, and subsequently phasing out IV and feeding tubes containing these chemicals.
- Recycling and waste reduction.
- Conserving energy.
- Emphasizing sustainable foods.
- Specifying green cleaning products.
- Exploring the potential use of organic linens.
- Addressing staff transportation and climate change.
- Using non-contaminating building materials.
- Being aware of contaminants in electronics.
- Regulating pharmaceutical waste (Gottlieb and Dickeman, 2007).

There are several Leadership in Energy and Environmental Design (LEED) certified NICUs and PICUs that either achieved their certification as independent construction projects or as part of the broader facility certification. Examples of such facilities are Aspirus Wausau Hospital, Asante Hospital, Dell Children's Hospital, Rady Children's Hospital, Portneuf Medical Center, Women and Infants Hospital of Rhode Island, Children's Hospital of Pittsburgh, Hershey Children's Hospital, and Tampa General Hospital.

Regarding sustainability in PICUs, there is limited literature. Pate (2012) notes that the environment of the PICU is potentially detrimental to staff as well as to patients; and materials in a PICU may be contributing to the high level of asthma in nurses. Pate (2012) makes a series of suggestions for the greening of the PICU.

Unit operations:

- Verify that medical supplies and toys do not contain polyvinyl chloride which includes DEHP. The compound, when in tubing, leaches into the fluids as they enter patients.
- Work with vendors who work with PICU staff to reduce packaging and unneeded supplies in kits.
- Confirm that the hazardous waste bags are not being used for other kinds of refuse.
- Support radiation safety for staff, patients, and families.
- Monitor the use of mercury thermometers.
- Initiate a recycling program.

Design features:

- Specify recycling bins in family areas with multilingual signage.
- Specify a dishwasher in the staff lounge to limit the use of paper, Styrofoam and plastic cutlery, plates, and cups.
- Provide natural light to reduce electrical use and support orientation.
- Use non-toxic paints, glues, sealants, and carpeting.
- Provide single family rooms to control infection and support privacy.

Guest authors Annie Coull and Greg Mare has provided a clear discussion on the greening of PICUs.

Toward a healthier PICU

Annie Coull and Greg Mare

Evidence-based approaches to creating optimal environments for critical care have resulted in design directions that address reduction of stress, promotion of safety, and support of healing. However, the conversation about human and ecological health in the hospital is still in its infancy. For example, in California, hospital entries are required by state law to post this sign: "WARNING: This area contains chemicals known to the State of California to cause cancer and birth defects or other reproductive harm." It is an irony that the very buildings and units dedicated to upholding the Hippocratic Oath which states "First, do no harm," and to providing healthcare to our most vulnerable patients – critically ill infants and children – are known to contribute to some of our greatest health problems. As designers, what can we do to avoid this paradox?

While the building industry has made a start on considering environmental criteria in choosing building materials, such as recycled content, recyclability, low levels of volatile organic compound (VOC) emission, no added formaldehyde, and wood certified by the Forest Stewardship Council (FSC), we have not yet really tackled the long-term impacts of materials on human health.

Material selection criteria

Design teams and owners usually filter building materials for healthcare based on seven criteria:

1. Code compliance.
2. Cost.
3. Performance and durability.
4. Comfort.
5. Maintainability.
6. Ease of replacement.
7. Aesthetics.

In PICUs, comfort for parents who "move in" with their child is an especially important evaluation factor, and the interior material selection process for the patient room is likely to benefit from family input.

Adding human and ecological health filtering criteria to this list makes materials selection more challenging because it adds another layer of data collection and filtering on top of an already information-overloaded process. However, applying human health criteria to materials planned for use in the PICU environment where care is being delivered to young, developing children is appropriate and should not be considered discretionary.

Human health and ecological health criteria

On an ecological level, materials filtering criteria focus on eliminating or reducing toxicity to the air, water, and soil of local and global environments. In planning and design of the PICU environment, especially the patient room, human health criteria take center stage in materials selection for reducing toxicity to patients, families, and staff. Priority human health criteria to be considered for measurement include demonstrated carcinogenicity, endocrine disruption, mutagenicity (toxins that cause DNA malformations in fetus development), teratogenicity (toxins that cause birth defects which are not necessarily gene mutations), and reproductive toxicity. Unfortunately at this time there is no proven system of researching and testing materials that are potentially harmful to the health of building inhabitants. Often full disclosure of material content is not available from manufacturers due to closely held trade secrets, and research findings are in disagreement from report to report. Chemists such as McDonough Braungart Design Chemistry (MBDC) are working with design teams to develop filtering criteria and to test building materials against these criteria, as was done on the UCSF Medical Center at Mission Bay currently under construction in San Francisco. In addition, resources for identifying known toxic and potentially harmful substances are being developed to make this process easier in the future. For example, the Healthy Building Network's Pharos Project (pharosproject.net) is a Web-based tool that provides "critical health and environmental data about the manufacture, use, and end-of-life of building materials specified and used every day."

The PICU patient room: interior finishes and materials

The pediatric patient in the PICU is critically ill and already in a compromised state by virtue of medical condition. PICU patients are likely to spend nearly 100 percent of their

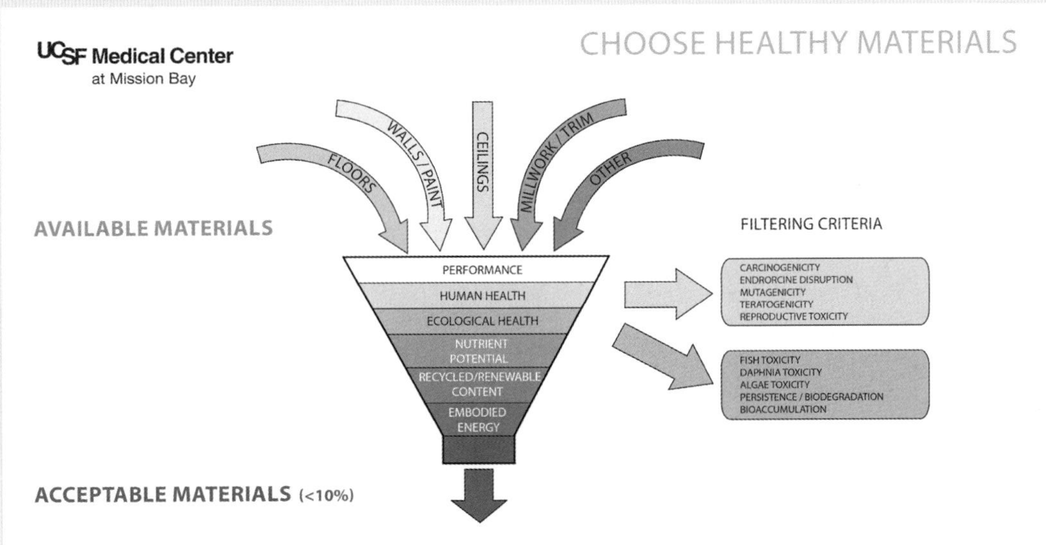

Figure 1: *Materials filtering criteria of UCSF Medical Center at Mission Bay (Source: © and courtesy William McDonough + Partners and MBDC with Stantec)*

critical care stays in their rooms, and their families and caregivers also spend a significant amount of time at the bedside or in the patient room. Young children, even those that are critically ill, may be more likely to touch, smell, lick, or even chew on a material in the environment and possibly absorb toxins through their mucous membranes. It follows that every attempt should be made to reduce toxicity in this environment, and that room finishes must be selected with extraordinary care to promote both human and ecological health.

Lessons learned so far

The results of materials testing for the selection of interior finishes in the new UCSF Benioff Children's Hospital at Mission Bay, including 44 pediatric critical care patient rooms, were interesting and gave the design team significant insight into sources of toxicity. The team was surprised to discover that the worst offenders usually appeared as additives and optional extras to finish materials. For example, fabrics were satisfactory on their own, but the applied flame retardants were a source of toxicity. Similarly, carpets ranked adequately, but the stain-resistant finishes did not, and flooring materials tested fine, but the sealers did not score well in terms of toxicity. This led to an effort to make better choices in order to reduce the need for these coatings, such as specifying rubber floors or linoleum that does not need sealing. While a 100 percent toxin-free environment for the PICU is unachievable today, we must continue to strive for this goal by using the best finish material options today, and asking the right questions to put pressure on manufacturers to change for tomorrow.

The goal is to have a different sign at the entry to the PICU: "GREAT NEWS! This PICU contains only products considered to be extremely beneficial to your health."

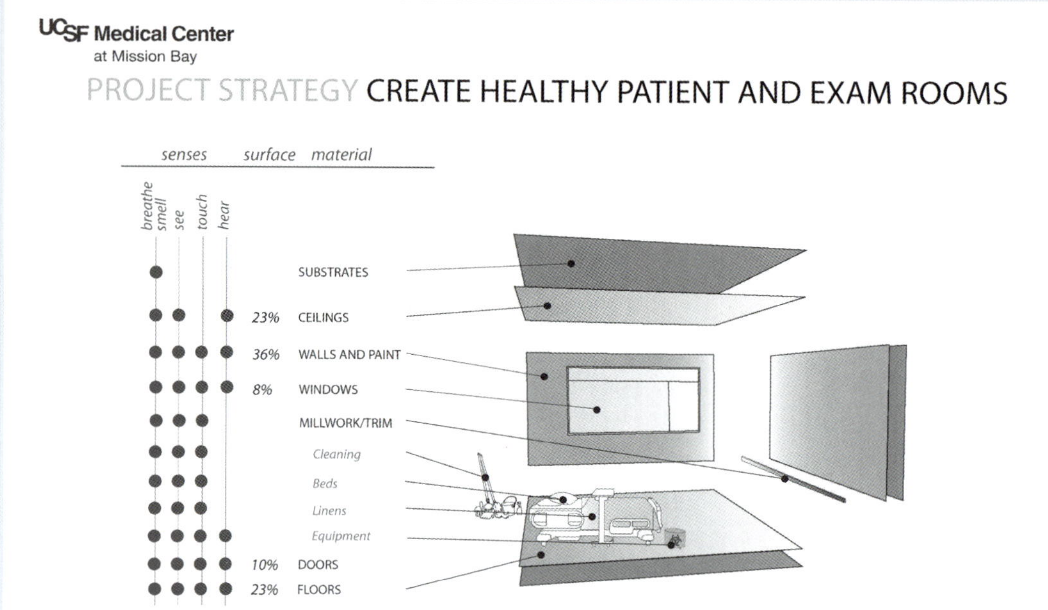

Figure 2: *Relationships between interior materials and senses of UCSF Medical Center at Mission Bay (Source: © and courtesy William McDonough + Partners and MBDC with Stantec)*

Because of the acute sensitivity of neonates, protecting newborn infants from toxins from the built environment in NICUs is paramount – both toxins that are encountered during care and those that are sources of infection (White, 2011a). Potentially toxic substances include volatile organic compounds, electromagnetic radiation, airborne substances (cleaning agents' vapors, dust, alcohol wipes), contact (iodine, chlorhexidine), or materials placed within the body (feeding and intravenous tubes) (White, 2011a). These toxins may negatively impact the development of the newborn directly, or cellular growth and brain development (White, 2011a). The current Recommended Standards for Newborn ICU Design include recommendations for the designation of recycling areas and avoiding materials "known to be teratogenic, mutagenic, carcinogenic, or otherwise harmful to human health" (White, 2006). Along these lines, Kaiser Permanente has eliminated the purchase of products containing mercury (Marshall-Baker, 2006). Marshall-Baker (2011) recommends the use of alternative materials in the NICU setting, particularly with regard to those made from PVC. In addition, not all reusable materials are good. Nylon and polyethylene, as she points out, may be reused, but are made from petroleum, so may not be appropriate.

4.4 Safety

Developmental differences, pediatric-specific disease patterns, and variable drug metabolism characteristics may make children particularly vulnerable to error and harm (Scanlon and Bauer,

2011, quoted in Bauer et al., 2011). In addition, appropriate human factors engineering dedicated to enhancing the safety of children in healthcare settings is limited (Scanlon et al., 2007). Montgomery (2006, 2007) notes that the complexity of the environment and potential staff fatigue can adversely impact the effectiveness of medical staff in the PICU. PICU care takes place in an unpredictable, high-tech environment relying on skilled staff, who require constant communication – factors that set the stage for potential errors (Montgomery, 2007).

Bauer et al. (2011) conducted a survey of physicians who treated pediatric intensive care patients and found that their primary safety concerns aside from medication errors appertain to ineffective communication, poor hand washing, and inadequate training. The researchers define an adverse event (AE) as an unintended injury or complication contributing to death, and a critical incident (CI) as an event that could or did lead to harm but did not cause death. In this study no AEs occurred in PICUs. However, pre-PICU AEs resulted in death in the PICU. CI events occurred throughout the medical process.

Coull and Mare (2011) recommend the following to reduce medical errors in PICUs:

- Use standards of care.
- Examine processes before events take place.
- Implement better communication.
- Create workstation and bedside environments that support a zone of silence and use task lighting.
- Place supplies and equipment near patient.
- Increase technologies that reduce need for human review.

According to Miller and Zhan (2004), pediatric patients, particularly those who are youngest and poorest, are most likely to experience medical errors. Thus the need to enhance safety in NICUs is essential. Errors are most common in premature babies, particularly those weighing less than 1,500 grams and those who have achieved less than 30 weeks' gestation (Samra et al., 2011). The risk of this population is enhanced because of their severe illnesses and need for more medical care, including medications, monitoring, and nutrition.

Critical errors of focus in NICUs are patient identification, communication, medication administration (McGrath, 2005), and hand washing. The latter three are particularly susceptible to attributes of the physical environment. Communication is enhanced by reduced noise levels and spaces dedicated to the sharing of information. Staff who administer medication are significantly impacted by noise and light levels. Hand washing is impacted by the number of devices/sinks and their locations.

4.5 Lighting and acoustics

Lighting and acoustics impact sleep. The psychological and physiological changes associated with interrupted sleep decrease the ability of a critically ill infant or child to adapt to hospitalization, thereby hampering recovery (Corser, 1996). Stimuli of light, noise, and staff activity are negatively correlated with sleep state (Corser, 1996). No literature was found regarding problems with lighting on PICUs, although issues that adults face, such as lack of ability to control lighting or glare, may be similar.

Researchers indicate that noise impacts both patients and staff in PICUs. In studies on noise levels in PICUs, researchers have found mean night-time sound at the bedside to be frequently greater than 50 dB with spikes up to 120 dB (Al-Samsam and Cullen, 2005; Bailey and Timmons, 2005; Carvalho et al., 2005; Cureton-Lane and Fontaine, 1997). Researchers on PICU patients found that when the noise level exceeds 75 dB for more than three minutes, awakenings occurred in 57 percent of these events (Al-Samsam and Cullen, 2005). Pediatric patients are not the only individuals negatively impacted by PICU noise levels. Regarding staff, they were found to have an increase in stress in association with increments in sound. In a study by Morrison et al. (2003), for every 10 dB increase the nurse's average heart rate increases by six beats per minute.

Recommendations regarding light and acoustics in PICUs include the following:

- Emphasize the day/night lighting patterns of home life on the unit (Evans and Madsen, 2005).
- Standardize light schedules (Schieveld et al., 2007).
- Provide light controls (both daylight and electrical light) readily available to patients and families.
- Encourage parental interaction in combination with musical intervention (del Olmo et al., 2010).
- Install a dosimeter to monitor noise levels (Jousselme et al., 2011; Shaffner, 2011).
- Use materials with low sound reflectivity (Shaffner, 2011).
- Reduce alarm noise (Shaffner, 2011).
- Reduce bedside discussion through safety glasses with head-up display that show alarms, paging and communications (Shaffner, 2011).

These recommendations would be equally beneficial for NICUs, and medical professionals have made clear the need to address light and sound in NICUs (e.g. White and Newbold, 1995). According to Stevens and colleagues (2007), one of the most effective ways to modulate light and sound is to provide single family rooms. These rooms allow staff to provide the amount of stimulation that is appropriate for the individual child. To support developmental care, the lighting should be located so that the baby is not positioned looking directly at a daylight or electric light source. The use of circadian rhythms may be appropriate, although the appropriate duration of daytime light is unclear for premature babies (White, 2011a). According to White (2011a), newborns need daylight levels of a minimum of 300 lux for a minimum of eight hours and a reduction at night to a minimum for 200 lux lower than daytime levels.

Vandenberg (2007) makes the following recommendations regarding light in NICUs:

- Avoid direct light except in procedure areas.
- Avoid overstimulation.

- Provide multiple options for lighting at each infant location to allow for customization.
- Provide equipment that supports circadian lighting.
- Provide adjustable lighting.

Sound levels should be less than 50 dB to support sleep and interaction with human voices (Philbin, 2004), and acoustical materials and room volume should be considered to minimize reverberation. In addition, attention must be directed at separating rooms from traffic and noisy work areas; for example, receptacles and storage can be located in a panel in the hallway rather than against the wall to reduce traffic in the patient room (White, 2011a). Care practices and equipment are sources of sound (Thomas and Uran, 2007); protocols encouraging quiet conversations and the specification of equipment that includes sound-absorbing or acoustically isolating components are recommended.

4.6 PICU design issues

Designers of pediatric and neonatal intensive care units encounter a variety of options with respect to the locations and presence of specific spaces on the unit. Many of these spatial relationships are controversial. For example, storage may be predominantly centralized or decentralized. Likewise, nursing stations may be predominantly centralized or decentralized. The purpose of this section is to discuss the recurring design options in the development of PICUs. For a thorough summary of PICU design issues, please see the guest author essay by Laura Poltronieri.

Key considerations in design of the PICU environment

Laura Poltronieri, AIA

You are a father and you have just received a call that your daughter has been in an accident … You are the mother of a child with a serious chronic disease, and this is your son's 20th admission to the ICU … You are a parent whose seemingly healthy 4-year-old has quickly developed serious complications from what you thought was a simple case of the flu, and the ED doc tells you they are admitting your child into the PICU.

You are a brother and your mom has just told you she is on her way to the hospital because your sister has been admitted to the ICU (… you are not sure what that is). She cannot stop to explain now, but a babysitter is on the way until your aunt gets there, and she will explain everything to you later. Try not to worry, everything will be all right.

You are a child drifting in and out of consciousness in a strange place with bright lights, unfamiliar beeping sounds (… is this a real-life video game?), bad smells, and many people in strange outfits coming and going. Some are there to talk to you, but you don't really know what they are saying, it all seems in slow motion. Others just pass you by, you don't understand where you are, you feel heavy, you are … asleep … again …

You are a nurse who has dedicated your life to caring for critically ill children. You want to minimize their pain, and with your experience and skill nurse them back to health.

You are all in a pediatric intensive care unit.

You are a designer. You idealistically believe that design can help support all of these people. What do you need to know?

For many decades the designs of pediatric intensive care units were physician- and technology-driven models patterned after adult ICUs. But recent research has shown that the presence of the family can improve safety, increase patient comfort, aid in reducing lengths of stay, and improve patient outcomes (Buechler et al., 2010). These **findings were strong enough to convince the Joint Commission on Accreditation of Healthcare Organizations (JCAHO)** to add family-centered care practices as a requirement for accreditation (The Joint Commission, 2010).

Designing to support the family

When a child is in an intensive care environment maternal instincts take over. These overwhelming parental impulses often mean that parents initially feel a need to be present 24/7 at their child's bedside. Most leading children's hospitals have evolved patient room designs that support the family's 24/7 presence at the PICU bedside. In fact, some children's hospitals even allow parents to be present in the room during code events. This potentially constant presence of family at the bedside obviously requires supportive space and furnishings.

For some parents, leaving the room, at all, under any circumstances, seems out of the question and overwhelming; but in most cases once some time has passed there is a need for parental respite spaces away from, but not too far away from, the grueling bedside vigil. These spaces are most useful when they are perceived by parents as being within the confines of the PICU, within a stone's throw of their child's bedside. These spaces do not need to be large or elaborate and should contain support amenities (e.g. kitchenette, laundry facilities) to encourage chance social support encounters with other PICU families.

In addition to being present at the bedside, some parents find comfort in "nesting behavior," by surrounding their children with favorite and familiar objects and photos from home. Designers can support this nesting impulse by providing appropriate places and surfaces within the patient ICU room to display such items.

Additional key issues required to support families in the PICU include the following:

- Appropriate and comfortable furnishings, such as a chair at the bedside that can be easily positioned next to the bed or crib, that allows parents to touch or hold hands with their child.
- Design of an accommodating in-room family zone that can serve to either connect or separate parents from children depending upon the need and time of day or night. While parents want maximum connection to their children during the day, they also need a comfortable sleeping place within the child's room at night. Thus the "family zone" needs to be separated by a cubicle curtain or other privacy device. At night this zone divider needs to shield parents from the ongoing activity, noise and lighting of ICU equipment to the greatest extent possible. The current popular design approach which locates the sleeping area next to the exterior wall window is often problematic due to the coldness and condensation of the window.

- Storage for clothing and other parent items, either within the room or in a separate family locker room.
- Many children's hospitals also provide separate hotel-like room accommodation for those parents choosing to leave the bedside for the night in order to catch up on needed sleep. Mothers and fathers, or other family members, will often trade off nights with one parent sleeping in the room while the other person catches up on deeper sleep. These accommodations need to be located as close to the unit as possible. There are often more families requesting these "hospital hotel" accommodations than there are rooms available, so these programs often pose management challenges for the hospital's administration.
- Patients in ICUs are usually being cared for by dozens of different nurses and other clinical team members. Insuring correct continuity of information is a key issue in giving parents a feeling of confidence about the quality of care their children are receiving. It is imperative to plan and design for inroom information and communication systems that keep the family well informed and updated on current staff assignments, patient status, and upcoming treatment schedule. Parents can also leave notes with questions or concerns for future clinical team clarification. Information is also needed regarding available community support amenities, from local restaurants to hospital-sponsored educational programs and services.
- Toilets and showers need to be provided for the use of the family. Some hospitals allow parents to use the facilities provided in their children's rooms, while others limit bathroom use to only patients due to infection prevention concerns. In those cases centralized family bathrooms and showers are provided. Again, these support amenities ideally need to be located within the confines of the unit.
- The family also needs to be supported by services outside the confines of the ICU, including sibling play and child life education areas, cafeteria, admissions, social work, chapel, etc. Thoughtful placement and access to these supplementary functions in relation to the PICU need to be carefully considered.

Designing to support the patient

While many patients in the ICU are sedated, there are still times when they are very much aware of their surroundings. Patients may be physically immobilized but drifting in and out of consciousness, and disoriented in their new and unfamiliar yet busy surroundings. Designers need to imagine themselves as a child in an ICU bed. Waking up in an ICU environment is often disorienting and stressful for adults, and is frequently even more distressful for children. Every attempt should be made to provide views from the patient bed that are calming. These views should be toward the child's favorite items from home, from calming scenes through the windows, to familiar faces in the family zone, and reassurance from their assigned nurses. Designers should try to eliminate or limit views to other patients, medical equipment, and general unit activities and bustle.

In family workshops parents frequently comment on the prominence and importance of the PICU room ceiling design for their children's well-being. They understand that this is the one place their children routinely view, yet the ceiling and cornice are frequently underutilized as design opportunities by healthcare designers. Ceiling lighting, cubicle curtain design, and cornice zone are also important potential design elements. Visual privacy from onlookers needs to be provided through the strategic location of cubicle curtains during disturbing procedures. Once children are ready to be transferred to less intensive units they may have to wait for hours to be officially discharged from the PICU. Providing elements on the unit for them to visit, perhaps just a small but accessible window seat, are welcome additional amenities to celebrate that they are feeling better.

Designing to support the staff

Without a doubt, nurses have the most direct and continuous interaction with patients and families in the PICU environment. There is also no doubt that being a PICU nurse is an extremely high-stress job. Nurses must deal with critically ill children and their families on a daily basis. One effect of this ongoing and sometimes irresolvable stress is "compassion fatigue."

How can we as designers best support nurses and minimize their stress and burnout? How can we support nurses in providing the highest and most compassionate level of clinical care to their patients while reducing medical errors and adverse events?

Throughout the unit

- In a recent research study nurses ranked abundant natural light above all other environmental factors as the most import positive contributor to helping them provide quality care (Poltronieri and Schleien, 2010). Thus, providing abundant daylight, wonderful views, and adequate differentiation between day- and night-time light cycling are all key factors in supporting nurses as well as patients and families.
- Provide easy access to on-unit staff support suites that include a dedicated staff lounge with kitchen, staff lockers, bathrooms with showers, as well as adjacent teaching space. Like parents, PICU nursing staff members do not like to be too far from their patients' rooms.
- Enhance visibility throughout the unit by providing service cores with transparency (e.g. glazed partitions) and support zones with low-height partitions that allow increased visibility to other nurses throughout the unit.
- Provide resilient flooring to help reduce leg and back strain; also, attention needs to be paid to infection control and acoustic properties of flooring materials.

At the bedside

- Maximize decentralization of supplies and equipment to the patient's room and bedside in order to minimize the time, distance, and number of steps involved in the most frequent and repetitive nursing tasks, such as diaper weighing and changing.
- Implement consistent adherence to a repetitive "universal" design approach to patient care rooms, head walls, storage, and supply locations to support and reinforce consistent repetitive operational protocols, no matter which room they are assigned to.
- Provide superior quality procedure lighting at bedside.
- Select comfortable work seating with full back support; nurses often prefer stool-height seating and workstations in order to maximize visibility to patients.

- Address issues of information management coordination during the planning phase of PICU projects to ensure seamless integration of operational models with unit design and communication technologies and alarms.

Excellence in PICU design is achieved when the essential needs of all four key constituencies – patients, families, nursing caregivers, and required technologies – are appropriately addressed and balanced. While nursing and family concerns in the PICU are sometimes seen as competing with one another, a more useful model sees them as complementary and supportive of one another, both full team members in support of care of the child. In this way children receive the best of everything, and outcomes improve.

References

Buechler, B., Garris, B., Vaught, D., and White, R. (January 2010). A journey to decentralized care in a private room NICU; New Hanover Medical Regional Medical Center, Betty H. Cameron Women's & Children's Hospital. Graven's Conference on the Physical and Developmental Environment of the High Risk Infant. Clearwater, FL.

Joint Commission, The. (2010). *Advancing Effective Communication, Cultural Competence, and Patient- and Family-centered Care: A Roadmap for Hospitals*. Oakbrook Terrace, IL; The Joint Commission.

Poltronieri, L. and Schleien, C. (March 2010). PICU design and influence on patient outcomes, staff and family satisfaction. National Association of Children's Hospitals and Related Institutions, Creating Connections Conference. San Diego, CA.

The design of PICUs has been lock-stepped with adult ICUs for many years. In 1996 a research team compared the physical environments of pediatric and adult inpatient units and found little or no differences between the two (Curry et al., 1996). However, there are multiple important distinctions. Coull and Mare (2011) have identified the following characteristics that distinguish this specialty:

- Family-centered design. While families are sometimes engaged in adult care, they are more frequently involved in pediatric care; accommodations should include bedside seating; a family storage area, sleeping area, and bathroom; separate lighting; and additional sleep areas and lounges. Family amenities might include a family great room and strolling garden, and areas for family members to eat together (Coull and Mare, 2011). Also important are a family resource center, spiritual and emotional support area, amenities for siblings, and access to outside meditation spaces (Coull and Mare, 2011). While historically there has been resistance to family participation in the PICU setting, research suggests that family presence during procedures, even critical ones, may be of benefit both to the parent and the child (Powers and Rubenstein, 1999).
- Age-appropriate design. Patients are typically up to 18 years of age but could be older due to diseases of childhood etiology (Coull and Mare, 2011). This variation in age means that designers need to be sensitive to differing visual preferences.
- Security. As in the NICU, the potential exists for abduction in a PICU. Security/safety starts at the entrance lobby where a badge may be required before allowing access to the elevator (Coull and Mare, 2011).

- Storage. Beds and cribs must both be accommodated (Coull and Mare, 2011), as well as a variety of equipment that serves a population ranging from infants to young adults.

4.6.1 PICU configurations

An analysis by the author of 10 PICUs built between 1990 and 2012 produced four configurations: racetrack (loop with a core), L- and V-shaped two-corridor, U-shaped three-corridor, and/or neighborhood/cluster/pod (see Figures 4.3, 4.4, 4.5, and 4.6). The majority of the new SFR units employ the racetrack design. A few smaller units use a single-loaded corridor scheme with rooms on one side and services on the other. The predominant configuration was the racetrack – the most common layout for an adult ICU as well. In the early 1980s, when PICUs were less common, there appeared to be more experimentation with different styles. In the past several years, however, design teams appear to support the racetrack configuration, followed by L-shaped configurations. My observation is that the design of these units in general hospitals is driven by the configuration of the adult ICU and acute care units. Likewise, those PICUs that are located in children's hospitals are highly influenced by sharing stacked floor plans with pediatric acute care units.

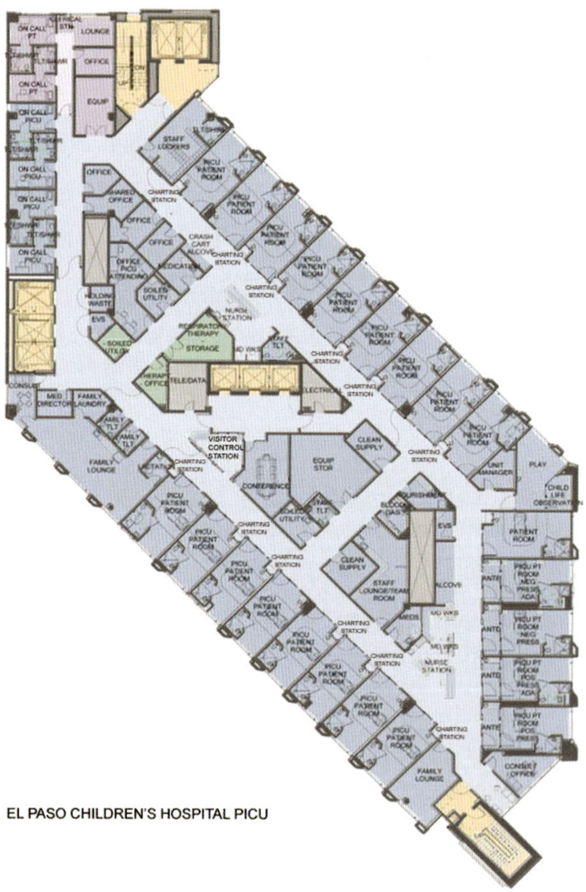

Figure 4.3: *PICU loop with a core design (Source: El Paso Children's Hospital PICU, El Paso, TX. Plan courtesy of KMD Architects)*

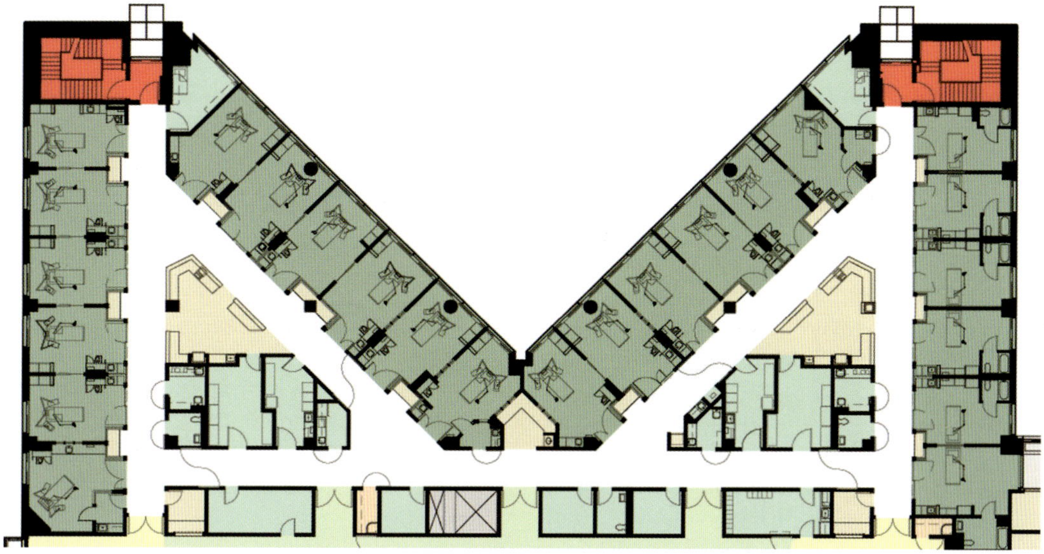

Figure 4.4: *PICU V-shaped corridor design (Source: Mattel Children's Hospital UCLA PICU, Los Angeles, CA. Plan courtesy of Perkins+Will (executive architect) and Pei Partnership Architects (design architect))*

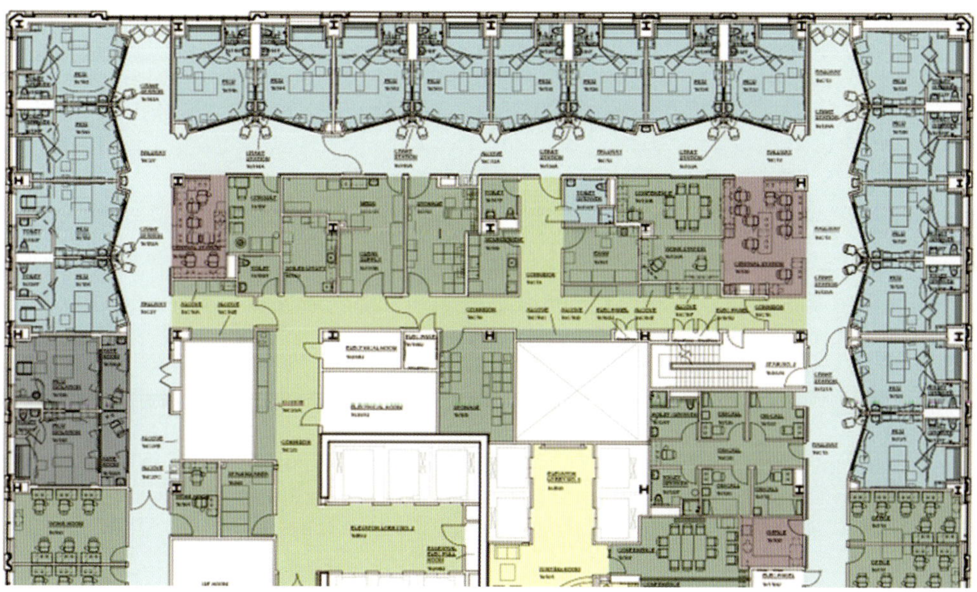

Figure 4.5: *PICU U-shaped three-corridor design (Source: Ann & Robert H. Lurie Children's Hospital of Chicago PICU, Chicago, IL. Plan courtesy of ZGF Architects LLP, Solomon Cordwell Buenz, Anderson Mikos Architects, Ltd.)*

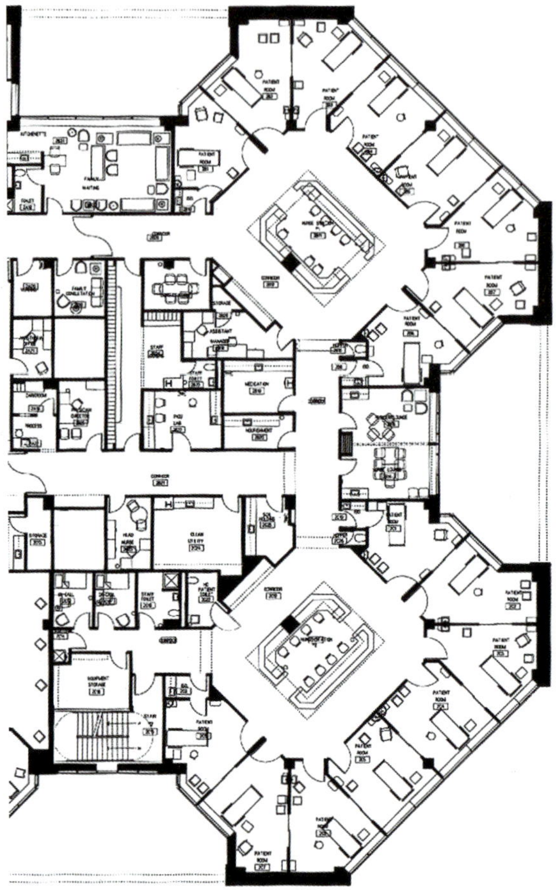

Figure 4.6: *PICU neighborhood/ pod/cluster design (Source: Hasbro Children's Hospital PICU, Providence, RI. Plan courtesy of Shepley Bulfinch)*

In Jim Diaz's history of ICU design (Diaz, 2000), he notes that the drivers for configuration have been (1) the transition from cubicles enclosed with curtains to enclosed rooms; (2) the number of rooms per unit; (3) the provision of bathrooms in patient rooms; and (4) the increased size of rooms.

The range in number of beds in a unit does not seem to have changed dramatically over the past 20 years. Wrench and Vyas (1995) recommend between eight and ten beds. Units smaller than six are not economical (Driscoll et al., 1993), as they have too few patients with whom medical staff can work and in so doing generate and maintain special critical care skills. Units with more than 16 beds are difficult to manage unless broken into clusters (Driscoll et al., 1993).

4.6.2 PICU spaces and their relationships

4.6.2.1 Patient spaces

Multiple articles have been written about topics associated with family-centered care (FCC) patient rooms, including the provision of zones for staff, patient, and families, and the need for family storage, relaxation, and work areas. The issues surrounding the debate about same-handed versus mirrored rooms in PICUs are identical to those of ICUs. Results as to the effectiveness of same-handed rooms are conflicting. Pati et al. (2010) did not find evidence of ergonomic benefits to same-handed rooms, while Watkins et al. (2011) discovered from staff and patient surveys that same-handed rooms had lower noise levels, the ergonomic benefits of more frequent approaches to the beds from the right, better patient sleep, and higher satisfaction with the workspace design. It would seem logical that rooms that are same-handed/identical would support the ergonomic actions required in an emergency, but they might present a problem regarding supervision from a single nurse substation.

Regarding adjacencies to other spaces, families need to be able to move from the patient room to the nourishment kitchen and lounge without disrupting unit activities. Likewise, medical staff require proximity from patient rooms to other functions such as charting areas (if not at the bedside) and storage and utility areas, so that as much time as possible can be spent with the child and family. In addition to a visual or physical link from the patient room to the nurse station(s), Ozcan (2006) recommends a direct link connecting as many patient rooms as possible to allow staff to arrive quickly when necessary. Direct links between adjacent rooms may facilitate care by a nurse who is working with two patients simultaneously, as long as privacy can be maintained. Patients may occasionally have to leave the unit to go to imaging, so the rooms should be located in a way that does not intersect with the public or highly active areas.

The need for surveillance and the desire for family privacy can be in conflict at times. This topic is addressed in Lauren Johnson's guest author essay.

The challenge of visibility and privacy

Lauren Johnson, MS, RN, CNS-BC

Balancing the need for continual visibility of the critically ill child with the privacy needs of the child and the family in the pediatric intensive care unit (PICU) is sometimes a challenge. It is essential that healthcare staff members are able to clearly view ill children but it is also essential that we ensure patient privacy. As children's hospitals build or renovate PICU spaces, architects, designers, and users frequently encounter a conflict when trying to plan for both during the design phase. As we planned and built a new 24-bed PICU, we created a room and unit design that demonstrated our ability to meet both privacy and visibility needs.

First, before program planning began, the project steering group developed overall guiding principles for the design and construction of a replacement children's hospital. The overarching principle was to create the best environment to receive and provide children's healthcare; a major design goal was to optimize the patient and family experience and to foster patient and family-centered care. Throughout the design and construction phases of the project we referred back to these principles when making decisions.

Second, we considered the staff requirement for visibility. The medical staff, nursing, and other staff members emphasized that children in the PICU require constant monitoring, observation, and visualization by one or more members of the healthcare team. With current staffing practices and varying acuity of patients' illnesses, nurses are sometimes assigned to care for patients in adjacent rooms. In our PICU, the nurse–patient ratio is 1:1 about two-thirds of the time. The rest of the time children's conditions are slightly less acute and one nurse is able to care for two patients. In these cases the nurse can leave the room for short periods of time, but the ability to still visually monitor the child, his or her immediate surroundings, and equipment from outside the patient's room remains imperative.

Third, we explored the concept of patient and family privacy. In new hospital construction today, inpatient rooms are single-occupancy, allowing for greater privacy. The Patient Bill of Rights (Minnesota Hospital and Healthcare Partnership, 2007) prescribes that patients have a right to privacy and that it is respected during treatment and personal hygiene activities. The principles of patient- and family-centered care state that people are treated with dignity and respect, including a respect for patients' and families' privacy (Institute for Patient and Family Centered Care, 2012). Rosenberg and Moss (2004) identify provisions for patient privacy as an essential element in the physical PICU design.

Over 16 months from program planning through the end of the design phase, PICU clinicians from multiple disciplines discussed how to address privacy and visibility satisfactorily in the unit. Members of the Parent Advisory Board, which included parents whose children had been hospitalized on the PICU, met monthly with key project leaders, architects, and designers to review the plans and provide input into the hospital and unit design. Discussions among clinicians and parents showed that both groups had a clear understanding of the need for the PICU room design to provide options for both full visibility and privacy. In addition, we needed to consider that four of the 24 PICU rooms would be designed for care of critically ill, immuno-compromised children undergoing blood and marrow transplant (BMT rooms).

Clinicians and parents met multiple times in the PICU mock-up room to get a real view and feel of the patient rooms they were designing. Many suggestions and changes occurred during these visits to the mock-up. For example, the decision to install large windows with integral blinds between all patient rooms was made after testing locations and sizes in the mock-up. We tested wide- and narrow-slat integral blinds in the mock-up. The clinicians determined that the slats measuring 1.5 inches wide rather than 1 inch or less provided a better view of the patient. We also used time in the mock-up room to identify where to locate privacy curtain tracks and where to store the privacy curtains when they were not in use. There was discussion about whether or not to place a privacy curtain for the small family zone in the PICU patient room. Both clinicians and parents agreed that family privacy was important and we installed privacy curtains to separate the family zone if desired. In the final design of the PICU rooms there were two privacy curtains in the patient room: one between the bed and the door to the corridor and one near the family zone. The four BMT rooms do not have privacy curtains; all windows and glass doors have integral blinds.

With windows, curtains, and integral blinds we successfully addressed the needs for patient/family privacy and visibility of the ill child in the PICU. By involving frontline staff and members of the Parent Advisory Board in designing the patient/family space in the PICU we ensured that both needs were fully understood and incorporated into the patient room design. Today, in the ongoing operation of the unit, staff members involve patients/parents in their care and explain the need for visibility, and why curtains or blinds need to be left open in certain situations. To date there has been no conflict between families and staff regarding the use of curtains. Our example supports that design with continued input from PICU patients/families and healthcare staff better balances the sometimes conflicting needs for privacy and visibility.

References

Institute for Patient- and Family-Centered Care. (2012). *Core Concepts of Patient- and Family-Centered Care*. Retrieved from http://www.ipfcc.org/faq.html, June 30, 2012.

Minnesota Hospital and Healthcare Partnership. (2007). *Patient Hospital Bill of Rights. Health. state.mn.us*. Retrieved from http://www.health.state.mn.us/divs/fpc/consumerinfo/mn_pts_rights_eng_reg.pdf, June 30, 2012.

Rosenberg, D.I., and Moss, M.M.. (2004). Guidelines and levels of care for pediatric intensive care units. *Pediatrics*, *114*(4), 1114–1125.

4.6.2.2 Family spaces

Coull and Mare (2011) and guest authors Michele Moss and Laura Poltronieri make several recommendations about family spaces. Apart from the identification of spaces that support FCC, the discussion here and in the literature focuses on the location of these elements, which can be complex. If, for example, the family resource center is too far from a child's room, parents are unlikely to use it (Ozcan, 2006). Conversely, in the case of the family waiting room, family members require a separate quiet room that provides acoustical isolation while being nearby. Similarly, play spaces for siblings should be provided near the unit but with sufficient acoustical isolation. Locating this space near the waiting room, with visual access from the seating areas, would promote family supervision.

4.6.2.3 Staff spaces

The relationship of staff spaces to the unit also presents some conflicts, as a variety of spaces need to be in direct proximity to one another. An adjacency diagram would likely show the nurse station or substations surrounded by multiple patient rooms, supply spaces, utility rooms, and charting areas – a physical impossibility!

The debate regarding centralization versus decentralization in acute care nurse stations is ongoing. In general, the trend is toward decentralized nursing stations with a centralized communication center. When studying medical-surgical units, Gurascio-Howard and Malloch (2007) found that registered nurses (RNs) were able to spend more time with patients, while Zborowsky et al. (2010), did not find any benefits with decentralized nurse stations regarding the frequency of observation of patients or decrease in noise. At the same time, they found less interaction among staff in the decentralized model. The literature suggests both benefits and disadvantages to decentralization for standard acute care units, but the need for more focused supervision in intensive care settings makes a strong argument for decentralized nursing.

Rothman and Ramanathan address the transition from nurse station to caregiver work station in their guest author essay.

From nurse station to caregiver workstation

Martha Rothman, FAIA, LEED AP

Uma Ramanathan, AIA

The evolution of the "nurse station" from central command center to collaborative "caregiver workstation" reflects the evolving roles of healthcare providers, the changing dynamics of the care provider team, and the impact of technology.

There was a time when the nurse station was a central station where patient charts were kept in notebooks. The doctor took the notebook to a private work area, reviewed the patient chart, and handwrote or dictated notes that were later transcribed into the record. For teaching hospitals, the central command station served not only as the repository of patient charts, but also expanded to accommodate other healthcare professionals who were encouraged to discuss the care plan from multidisciplinary points of view. The care team encompassed representatives from other disciplines such as pharmacy, nutrition, and social services, as well as physicians and nurses. The Planetree model turned the nursing station inside-out conceptually – that is, families were invited to participate with the professionals in the care planning and delivery.

At a point in the early 2000s, the computer changed how charts and notes were recorded and how the care team communicated. The central workstation, although not abandoned, has given way to a decentralized concept of nursing care. Decentralized workstations enable nurses to be closer to the patient bed while having access to patient information electronically. As the patient room changed from a two-bed room to a private room and travel distances consequently increased, the concept of having the workstation adjoin the patient room was viewed as a benefit both to patients and to nurses who are spared walking long distances. More direct care benefits the patient. Although staff initially expressed concern about isolation from other caregivers resulting from the decentralized workstation, additional team work areas alleviated this concern. Hybrid solutions have been developed, either combining central work areas with decentralized stations at the patient room, or locating workstations to serve a pod of rooms. One hospital reported a 51 percent reduction in steps walked daily by nurses when a workstation was located within each pod of 12 beds.

With the Affordable Care Act ("Healthcare Reform") signed into law in 2010, several initiatives significantly shifted the care team dynamic; consequently, the use and design of the nurse station further evolved into the caregiver workstation. Two initiatives to cite are, first, the focus on patient safety and reducing preventable medical error; and second, "meaningful use" of the electronic health record (EHR). Access to patient information, while controlled by privacy regulations, is open to healthcare providers beyond only the physician. Doctors, nurses, and other members of the care team have access to information which becomes a core component in reducing medical error. No longer is information entered and then transcribed by others; information is now immediate, with notes entered "on the spot" in real time. Alerts are embedded in the information; alarms sound when pharmacy doses, for example, are entered incorrectly. Although access to digital information no longer requires that all members of the care team are concentrated in a central workstation, open communication and collaboration engendered by physical proximity are factors in reducing medical error, particularly during hand-offs or transitions in care.

In the design of the patient floors at the new John R. Oishei Children's Hospital in Buffalo, the architects, Shepley Bulfinch, initiated a workshop with hospital leadership to analyze the functions of the workstation and determine whether the centralized or the decentralized model was the appropriate one for the new hospital. After the workshop, observations and recommendations were documented that informed the design:

- The workstations are not just "nurses'" stations. They are "caregiver workstations," designed for all caregivers: nurses, respiratory therapists, physicians (attending, consultants, residents), support staff (social work, patient management, nutrition, pharmacy), and students (medical and nursing). The name was changed to "caregiver workstations."
- Caregiver workstations serve multiple purposes: multidisciplinary collaboration – informal one-on-one encounters and formal huddles or debriefs; review of patient information and documentation; hand-offs/change of shift; points of contact with families and visitors.

Caregiver workstations should meet the following needs:

- Provide close proximity to patients.
- Provide access to patient information.
- Maximize sight lines between work areas and patient rooms.
- Decrease unnecessary steps; increase time for direct patient care.
- Maintain patient privacy.
- Allow for documentation at bedside: CPOE, medication administration, real-time documentation of vitals and assessments.
- Provide for interdisciplinary and multidisciplinary collaboration, in small and large groups.
- Reduce distractions and interruptions.
- Control noise levels.

The recommendation emerging from the workshop was to adopt a "hybrid" caregiver workstation model: central workstations and satellite workstations. The satellite workstations are either alcoves in the patient rooms or smaller workstations decentralized on the patient floor. A central caregiver workstation provides a highly visible place that patients, families, and visitors can readily identify and approach; and it must provide private areas for huddles and step-in areas for CPOE where interruption is minimized. The hybrid model also offers choice, depending on the specific activity the caregiver is engaged in; and it acknowledges different work styles among professionals.

The caregiver workstations at John R. Oishei Children's Hospital were designed to address the varied functions identified. The final design of the patient floor includes multiple workstations: a station visible from the entry to the unit that serves primarily as the information center, providing a check-in center for families, attending physicians and consultants, and other healthcare professionals on the floor; another, an inner core quiet

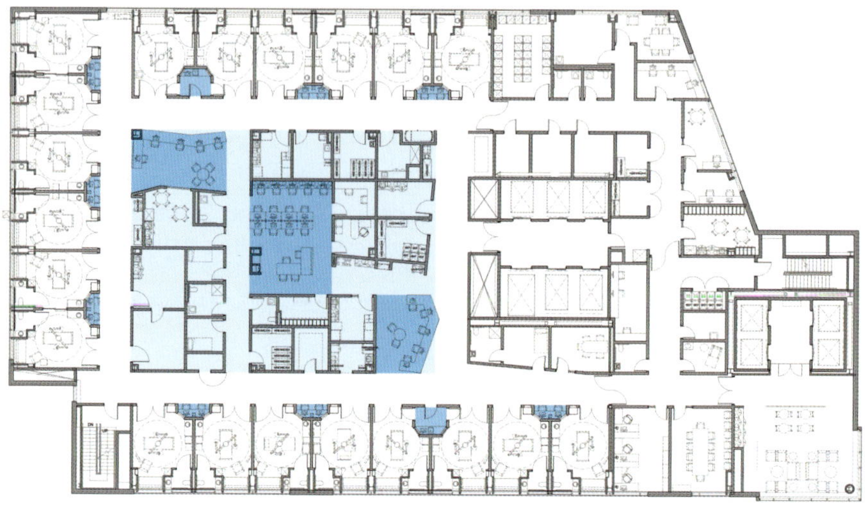

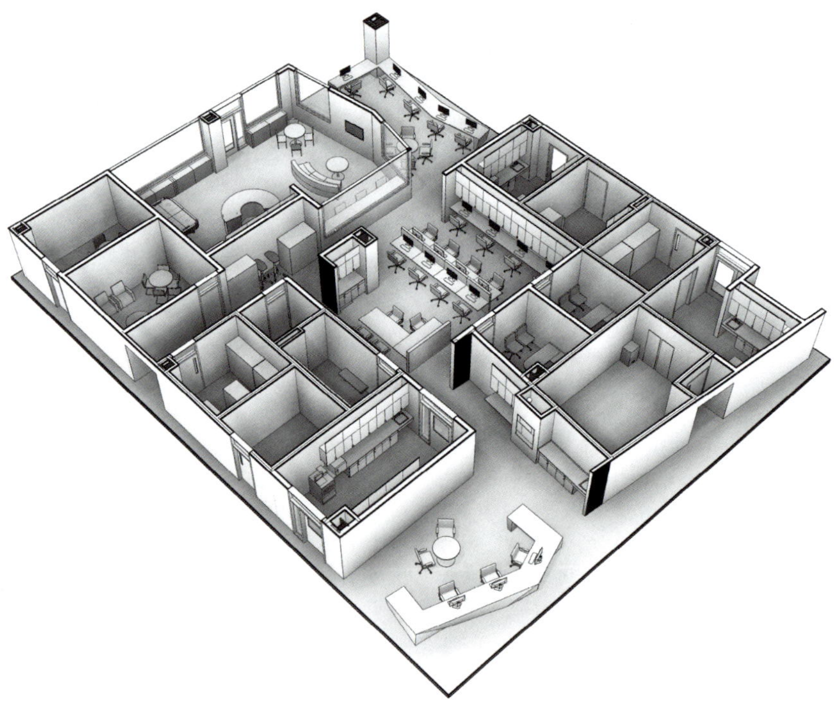

Figures 1 and 2: *The plan and perspective rendering of the patient floor at John R. Oishei Children's Hospital at Buffalo, NY (Source: Courtesy of Shepley Bulfinch)*

zone, where professionals work individually or together, open yet removed from the general circulation on the floor; and decentralized stations at each pair of beds, bringing the nurses close to the patient in the acute and intensive care environments. The inner core quiet zone has been designated as a "no patient care zone" where a hydration station is located for staff who are not permitted to eat or drink in patient care areas but need water during the day without having to retreat to a staff lounge. The outer caregiver stations allow for care team collaboration as well as interaction with families.

Recognizing the pace of change within healthcare, caregiver workstations must also allow for future flexibility and change. While much has been written in the past few years about the aging workforce in nursing, little has been suggested about what a new emerging workforce might bring to the profession, how a generation that has grown up with digital information and social media may communicate in the future. The change from a central computer mainframe to desktops to laptops to tablets to whatever is coming next and how these are used in the healthcare delivery process will require new thinking in what the caregiver workstation will become and how it will be designed.

Space changes must be accompanied by cultural change, a lesson learned in the change from an individual office environment to an open office environment. Design of the caregiver workstation in the future will grow out of observation and analysis of how staff can work more effectively. The design of future caregiver workstations will require observation and analysis of new patterns and cultural change to continually improve work patterns.

With regard to the adjacency of social spaces, Ozcan (2006) identified a conflict regarding the staff lounge. On the one hand, placing it on the unit means that staff don't have to travel far to use the space. On the other hand, administrators are sometimes concerned that the proximity may tempt staff away from patients. There is little research on this topic, and in light of the extensive distances that staff must travel during the day, location on the unit may be the better option.

4.6.2.4 Support spaces

For the most part, recommendations from the various codes adequately describe the adjacency requirements for support spaces. Satellite diagnostic systems is one of the most frequently recurring topics in the literature. For instance, researchers have made a strong argument in favor of having a satellite pharmacy on the PICU in order to reduce medication errors (Tisdale, 1986). When possible, a satellite laboratory space is also recommended (Rosenberg and Moss, 2004).

Regarding equipment and supply rooms, more space is needed for PICUs than for adult ICUs. This is due to the broad range in the sizes of the equipment needed to support children of varying ages (Wrench and Vyas, 1995). Multiple authors have recommended ceiling-mounted or pendant systems to allow access to patients. The equipment needed is shown in Figure 4.7.

4.6.2.5 External relationships

External relationships should also be considered. Among the recommended adjacencies are proximity to elevators, operating rooms, the emergency room, the recovery room, the physician on-call room, the nurse manager's office, the medical director's office, and the waiting room

Figure 4.7: *PICU equipment (Rosenberg and Moss, 2004)*

Emergency cart	Beds
Procedure lamp	Infant warmers and incubators
Ultrasonography device	Heating and cooling blankets
Infusion pumps	Bilirubin lights
Defibrillator and cardioverter	Transport monitor
Electrocardiography machine	EEG machine
Suction machine	Isolation cart
Thermometers	Blood warmer
Blood pressure apparatus	Pacer
Otoscope and ophthalmoscope	Other small equipment
Bed scale and patient scales	Respiratory support equipment
Cribs	

(Rosenberg and Moss, 2004; Wrench and Vyas, 1995). In some hospitals, adjacency to adult intensive care units may provide the opportunity to share staff and services.

Entries to units are particularly troublesome. I frequently see the arrival zone, usually at the elevator, some distance from a nurse or clerk station, which causes visitors to become lost and potentially interfere with the privacy of other patients.

Access to gardens is recommended. While this component is not likely to be directly accessible from the unit, garden access should be easily located and not a significant distance from the PICU.

4.7 NICU design issues

Several factors have been found to influence the historical development of the physical environment of NICUs. Some of these factors include the following:

- Awareness of infant sensitivity to environmental stimuli. During the early development of NICUs, the pervasive view was that newborns were not sensitive to external stimuli (White, 2011b). Because of this, most medical practitioners assumed that newborns were not significantly impacted by the physical environment, including sensitivity to pain (Browne, 2003). A vast body of research, however, demonstrates that noise and light levels have a profound impact on physical outcomes. While some of the sensory systems of infants are relatively well developed (e.g. smell and taste), radical ordering changes are occurring, particularly in the visual and auditory systems. In the context of the uterus, the visual system develops toward the end of gestation (Browne, 2003). Overwhelming stimulation in a young fetus may impact behavioral and physiological organization so as to influence the responsiveness during subsequent interaction with their families (Browne, 2003).
- Awareness of the critical impact of maternal separation at birth (White, 2011). This awareness is related to acceptance of the impact of the external environment, be it human or

architectural. Separation from the womb, particularly premature separation from the womb, suggests that the extra-uterus environment simulate the previous experience or allow for a gradual transition.

- Access to daylight. The importance of providing daylight for staff and families has been clarified by research. Diurnal variation in lighting may be beneficial to many infants, although clear requirements have not been established for very premature babies. While many NICUs in the twentieth century had no access to daylight at all, current designers try to introduce natural light into staff and family spaces in their design proposals.
- Access to nature. The positive impact of nature on stress reduction has also been demonstrated by research. Contemporary NICUs address the impact of views of the outdoors on unit design. Many new hospitals incorporate healing gardens that are accessible to families and staff within the medical facility.
- Advances in technology. The amount of equipment available for the treatment of high-risk infants grows annually. As a result, additional storage is required in common areas on the unit, in decentralized locations, and off the unit.
- Decentralized nursing. Decentralized nursing stations have been in evidence in adult units for many years. With the transition to private rooms and the resulting enlargement of NICUs, decentralized stations are common.
- Developmental care. Developmental care requires environmental (sound, light, temperature) control. Environmental control appears to be best accomplished in a private room (Smith et al., 2004). The physical environment should support opportunities for skin-to-skin care, avoid toxins, have the appropriate lighting, avoid inappropriate noise, and facilitate family presence (White, 2011a). The Neonatal Individualized Developmental Care and Assessment Program (NIDCAP) is intended to support developmental care for newborns and their families with the intention of improving neuro-developmental outcomes (Antonucci et al., 2009).
- Family-centered versus family-integrated care. The presence of families in NICUs has driven the need for additional spaces such as sleep rooms, family consultation rooms, family training rooms, family areas near the infant, and breast-feeding rooms. FCC is an approach to the planning, delivery, and evaluation of healthcare that is based upon a partnership between healthcare professionals and families of patients (Griffin, 2006). FCC involves four principles: information sharing, dignity and respect, family involvement in care, and family collaboration (Ahmann et al., 2003). The disruption of the relationship between the infant and the family is significant (Talmi and Harmon, 2003), and FCC tries to mitigate this. Family integrated care (FIC) takes this one step further by creating a setting and protocols where parents provide the majority of the care for their infants, while being taught by nurses (O'Brien et al., 2013). A preliminary study by O'Brien and colleagues (2013) found an increase in infant weight gain and incidence of breast discharge. In addition, parental stress decreased significantly from enrollment in the program to leaving the hospital, and parents reported satisfaction with the program. Barriers to extended parental participation are lack of privacy, inadequate space and layout, sibling and family issues, and lack of opportunity to engage in caretaking.
- Evolution of the incubator. Major modifications took place until the mid-twentieth century, but changes have been moderate since that date. Current proposals suggest modifications in terms of communication systems, sustainability, and ergonometric appropriateness. While

space requirements may not increase, appropriate infrastructure must be provided to support the equipment. A description of the history of incubators is provided in Chapter 3.

- Increase in population. The growth in the NICU baby population is the result of increased survival rates, and an increase in drug-dependent babies, among other factors. Units are becoming larger or more prevalent. As units increase in size, multiple challenges crop up in terms of supervision and level of ambience of the spaces.
- Infection control, privacy, and single family rooms (SFRs). Infection control and the need for privacy have driven the increase in adult private patient rooms. The same factors apply to NICUs, and SFRs are being identified as best practice.

The uniqueness of NICUs relative to other intensive care settings is self-evident. Specialized aspects include the following:

- The link to the mother's health post-partum. It is not uncommon for a baby who is placed in a NICU to have a mother who is coping with her own health challenges.
- The frequent presence of parents in the unit. While this is almost as common as the presence of families in the PICU, the importance of the family's presence is linked to creating a bond between parent and child at a critical stage.
- The frailty of the patients and the urgency of care provision.

4.7.1 NICU configurations

Approximately 90 examples of neonatal intensive care unit plans were collected from architecture firms throughout the United States, the Netherlands, Europe, and Canada. Plans were analyzed regarding room configuration, total area, area per baby, and space program components.

A study of these plans demonstrated the following. Historically, many of the original NICUs were divided into multiple multi-bed rooms based on the diagnosis of the child. This was likely a result of the initial opposition to co-locating children who were in-born and out-born, diagnosed with infections and not diagnosed with infections, and surgical versus non-surgical. Some of these original facilities (e.g. the old San Francisco General Hospital NICU) started with a few babies in each of several rooms, but wound up with a denser population as the need for beds increased. Some of the earliest units – such as the Sarah Morris premature infant station – had a similar arrangement, with children who were about to be sent home clustered in a single room.

The next phase of NICU design included open-bay units, which facilitated supervision. Most of the open-bay units had or have one or more private rooms serving to support isolation or extra-corporeal membrane oxygenation. Open-bay configurations are expressed in several themes, depending on the number of beds, the depth of the floor plate, and the area per infant. These configurations include a central open bay with support services clustered at the perimeter, a perimeter open bay with support services at a central location, and baby station clusters in the form of pinwheels and other geometric configurations. There are multiple hybrids of these configurations.

The NICU solutions are highly varied, and parallel the precedents found in adult ICUs. Configurations include the loop with a core arrangement (Figure 4.8), L- or Y-shaped corridor designs (Figure 4.9), open-bay layouts (Figure 4.10), and neighborhood/cluster/pod designs (Figure 4.11). The design of the SFR units faces the same challenges as adult ICUs, principally responding to the increased size of the unit and its impact on supervision and staff walking behavior.

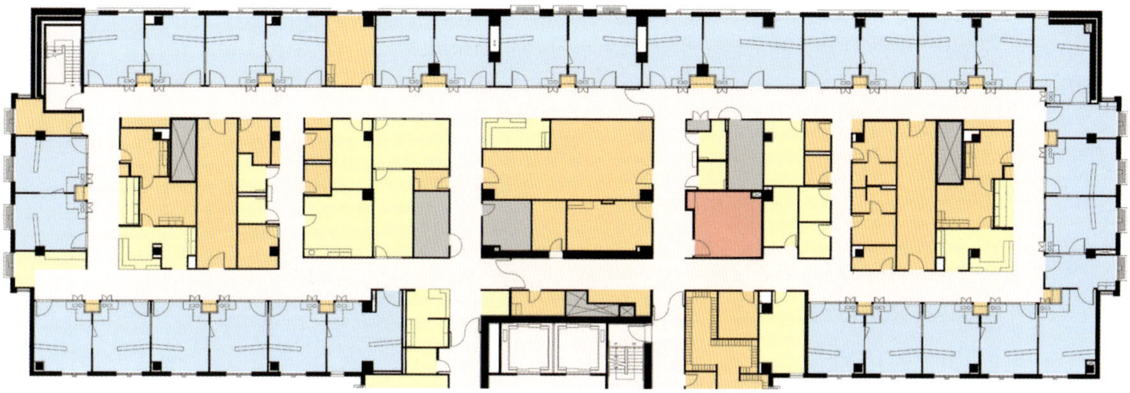

Figure 4.8: *NICU loop with a core design (Source: Le Bonheur Children's Hospital NICU, Memphis, TN. Plan courtesy of FKP Architects)*

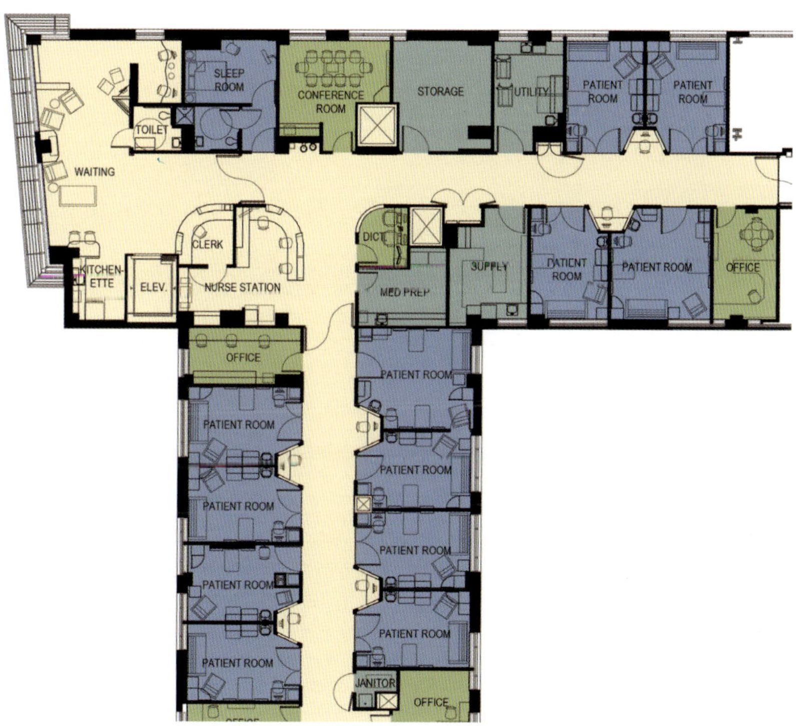

Figure 4.9: *NICU L-shaped corridor design (Source: Aspirus Wausau Hospital NICU, Wausau, WI. Plan courtesy of Plunkett Raysich Architects)*

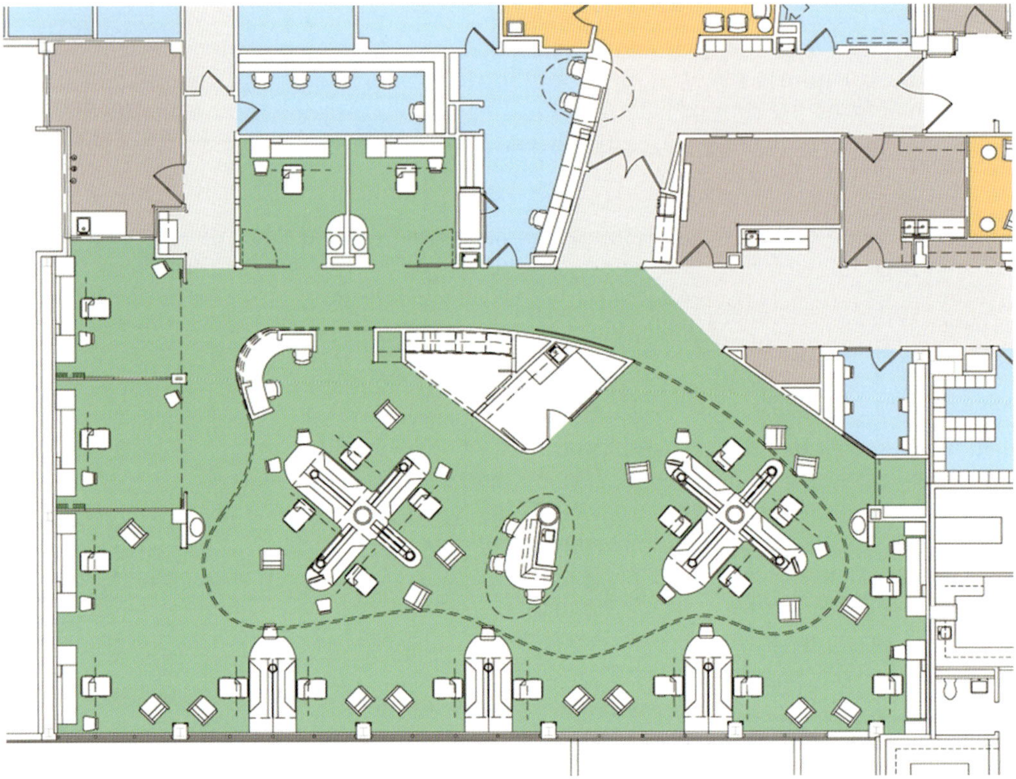

Figure 4.10: *NICU open-bay design (with perimeter and pinwheel components) (Source: Shands Hospital for Children at UF NICU Renovation, Gainesville, FL, 2004. Plan courtesy of Flad Architects)*

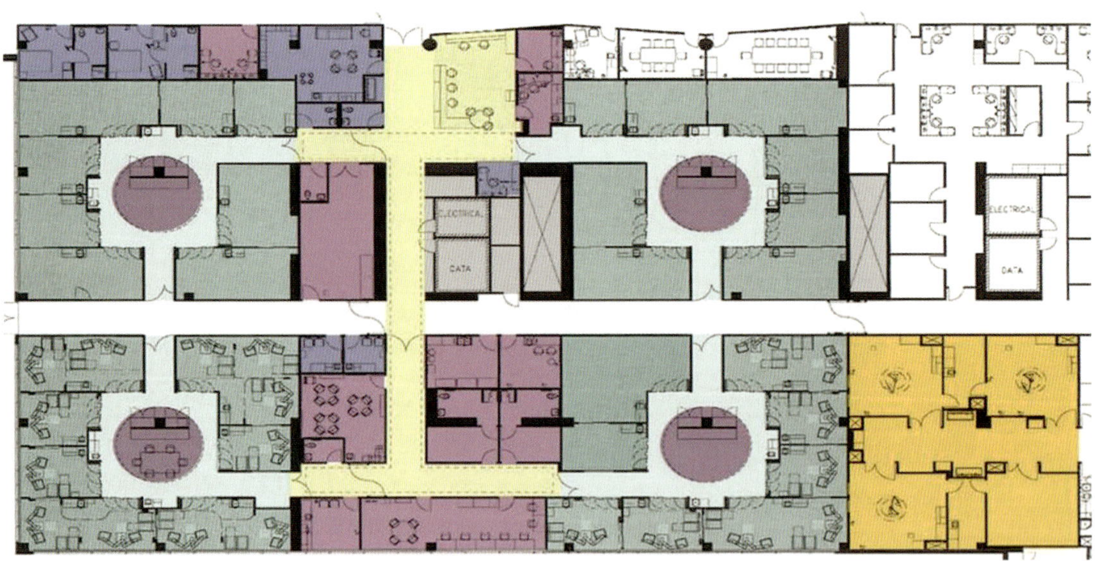

Figure 4.11: *NICU neighborhood/pod/cluster design (Source: Intermountain Healthcare NICU, Salt Lake City, UT. Plan courtesy of Stantec)*

4.7.2 NICU spaces and their relationships

4.7.2.1 Patient spaces

Patient units usually include larger or adjoining rooms for twins and triplets, as approximately 20 to 25 percent of the NICU population are multiple births (White, 2011b). Units of eight or fewer beds, whether private rooms or open bays, may negatively impact staffing collaboration, while larger clusters will require frequent patient transfers to maintain ratios (White, 2011b). Clusters larger than 12 rooms may be geometrically challenging. While Chapter 5 discusses research studies involving single family room care, a variety of authors have provided case studies and informal descriptions of this experience (e.g. Bruns and Klein, 2005; Carlson et al., 2006; Cone et al., 2010; Henry Bowie et al., 2003; McGrath, 2005; Milford et al., 2008).

4.7.2.2 Family spaces

NICU families and visitors experience high levels of stress and are very vulnerable to the critical care environment (Leibrock and Harris, 2011). Families often spend extended time in NICUs due to the long length of stay of some infants. As such, the needs of these families are significant. White (2004) proposes the following environmental features in support of family spaces:

- Access to the baby that doesn't conflict with equipment.
- Care area with privacy.
- Space to participate in rounds and a place to sit while engaged in conversations with the physician.
- Location to leave written or verbal messages for staff.
- An area where a family member can make phone calls, take a nap, get a midnight snack.
- Family sleep space.
- Places to meet with extended family that include refreshments, educational library, and play area for siblings.
- Ceiling-mounted equipment or equipment on articulating arms to provide ready access of families to babies (White, 2004).

4.7.2.3 Staff spaces

The issues discussed previously regarding centralized versus decentralized nurse stations in PICUs apply equally to NICUs. Historically, the nurses' station was directly integrated with the incubators in an open bay. Decentralized nursing stations are now more commonly distributed throughout an open bay or distributed near SFRs. One of the biggest challenges to SFRs has been assuring nurses that through decentralization and remote observation infants can be adequately cared for.

Working in a NICU is a highly stressful job. Provision of respite spaces in this context is likely more important than any other inpatient setting. Lounge spaces and access to nature away from the public may be an effective way of enabling staff to recuperate from intense experiences on the unit.

4.7.2.4 Support spaces

As with PICUs, satellite pharmacies have been recommended for NICUs to reduce errors (Kaushal et al., 2001; Lobas et al., 1991; Raju et al., 1989). In terms of supplies, a variety of models exist regarding centralized versus decentralized location, although some decentralization is present in all contemporary units. Neither central nor satellite laboratories may be the right solution for NICUs. Evidence suggests the effectiveness of an in-line point-of-care testing device (Alves-Dunkerson et al., 2002), as a means of reducing over-drawing that results in anemia.

4.7.2.5 Equipment

As equipment has become more advanced, parents have become more marginalized (Marshall-Baker, 2011). The protocol of skin-to-skin care, or kangaroo care, has been institutionalized in many settings, partially in response to this distancing between family and child resulting from the incubator. In addition to enhancing the emotional interaction between mother and child, researchers have reported improvements in the baby's perceptual-cognitive and motor development and improved parenting skills (Feldman et al., 2002; Whitelaw, 1990).

The primary piece of equipment in the NICU is the baby incubator. Recommended alterations to this equipment include the introduction of color and pattern to support individualization, arm rests, areas underneath for seating, less institutional material, and the ability to raise and lower the device to enable pulling a chair up to the isolette (Marshall-Baker, 2011). Antonucci et al. (2009) suggest that contemporary incubators have not resolved issues regarding temperature, noise, light, and electromagnetic fields. Ferris and Shepley (2012) describe incubator proposals generated by students who gathered ergonomic and social factor data at a NICU (see Figure 4.12). The design of the equipment in a NICU must be part of a systems approach, as described in Ferris' guest author essay.

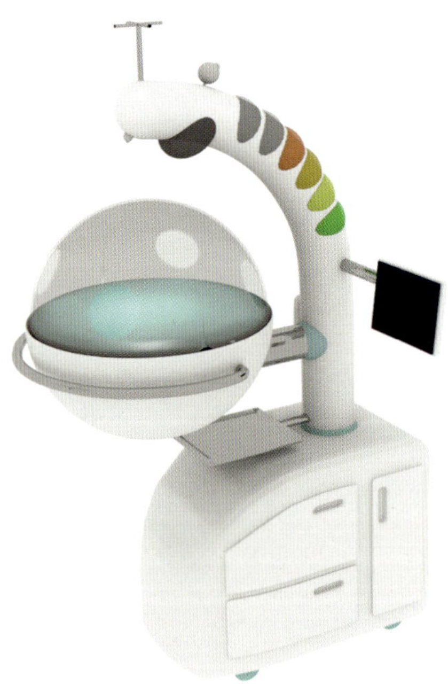

Figure 4.12: *Example of incubator designed by engineering and architecture students (Source: Author. Design by Cameron Christian, Tanya Singh, and Kara Wetzel)*

Systems-oriented design considerations for the NICU

Thomas K. Ferris, PhD

A mother's womb is a complex system. The primary goals of this system – the healthy growth and development of the fetus – are achieved when several biological subsystems "work together" in concert to provide the necessary environmental conditions and perform necessary care functions effectively. Similarly, a NICU may be thought of as a prosthetic womb in which the environmental conditions and care functions are provided by a system of humans and technologies within a controlled care setting. The growth and development of preterm or ill infants being cared for in a NICU depends in large part upon how effectively the synthetic system (human caregivers and technologies in the care setting) replicates the environment and functions of the biological system (the womb).

With the growing emphasis on evidence-based design approaches in healthcare (e.g. Ulrich et al., 2008), it is important to note that the qualities of interest in this branch of design – such as patient outcomes, worker productivity, patient and worker satisfaction, and safety – are not solely attributable to individual "components" of a healthcare system; instead, these qualities need to be considered as emergent properties of the entire system, viewed holistically. To understand how components of the NICU system – such as clinical care providers, patients, family members, technologies, care tasks, organizational culture, and the physical NICU environment – contribute to systems-level properties, the components should not be studied in isolation, but rather in a context that also analyzes the relationships and interactions among them. At the system level, the role of each component is defined as much by these relationships and interactions as by its individual characteristics.

For example, to understand how replacing an existing technology with a "new and improved" version would impact a system-level property such as quality of care, one must first understand how each technology is currently being or would be used by different user groups (e.g. nurses, physicians, perhaps family members or patients themselves) within the care setting of interest. These patterns of use represent one type of interaction among at least three system components (human users, technologies, and the environment). The outcome of this interaction is a degree of positive or negative support for the performance of cognitive and physical tasks that ultimately contribute to the overall quality of care. Often a technology may indeed be "new and improved" when a side-by-side isolated comparison is made with an existing technology, but from a systems perspective the new technology may not improve the overall quality of care (or, worse: it may diminish the quality).

This perspective reflects a problem-solving approach known as *systems thinking*, a dogma central to the emerging fields of systems engineering and systems-oriented design, and also familiar to a family of design fields that include human factors: engineering, human–computer interaction, and user-centered design (e.g. Wickens et al., 2004). To guide systems-oriented analysis and design in a NICU, PICU, or similar system, one may find it useful to consult systems models that have been tailored for analysis in the healthcare domain. One example, the Systems Engineering Initiative for Patient Safety

(SEIPS) model (Carayon et al., 2006), provides a framework to facilitate understanding of how patient safety is an emergent property of many components of the healthcare work system as well as the interactions among them. Following the SEIPS model (with core model components *in italics*), a NICU system could be defined as groups of *people* (e.g. infant patients, nurses, neonatologists, other clinical personnel, family members) interacting with *tools and technologies* (incubators, ventilators, feeding and medication delivery machines, physiological monitoring sensors and displays) to perform necessary *tasks* (controlling environmental conditions, monitoring and managing the patient's physiological state, promoting familial bonding) within the care *environment* (NICU physical space, layout of rooms and beds and nursing station, ambient lighting and sound levels, air quality), all under the context of larger *organizational conditions* (safety culture, team work among employees, policies regarding the involvement of family members in infant care). While the SEIPS model emphasizes patient safety as the systems-level property of interest, the analysis of our NICU system may instead emphasize the same goals as the biological system it approximates: the healthy growth and development of its infant patients.

NICU design efforts will often be limited to focusing on one or only a few of the many components that interact in complex ways to affect the growth and development of infant patients. In addition, time and budgetary constraints will likely dictate that the depth of system component analyses be far short of exhaustive. These limitations do not preclude a systems-oriented design approach, nor do they diminish its value. The spirit of this approach can almost always be incorporated into a design process by following three summary recommendations:

1. Judge the qualities of system components within the work context, rather than in isolation.
2. Recognize that changes to one component may have important implications for many other interacting components, and these implications may be difficult to foresee prior to implementing the changes. As much as possible, test in situ before fully committing to a design change.
3. Understand that many components have individual measures of quality, and sometimes design changes that are good for some components are bad for others. In these cases, what is important – and what should drive design considerations – is how changes impact the systems-level qualities of interest that are defined by the design goals.

References

Carayon, P., Schoofs Hundt, A., Karsh, B-T., Gurses, A.P., Alvarado, C.J., Smith, M., and Flatley Brennan, P. (2006). Work system design for patient safety: The SEIPS model. *Quality & Safety in Health Care, 15*(Suppl. 1), i50–i58.

Ulrich, R.S., Zimring, C., Zhu, X., DuBose, J., Seo, H-B., Choi, Y-S., Quan, X., and Joseph, A. (2008). A review of the research literature on evidence-based healthcare design. *Health Environments Research & Design Journal, 1*(3), 61–125.

Wickens C.D., Lee, J.D., Liu Y., and Gordon-Becker, S.E. (2004). *An Introduction to Human Factors Engineering* (2nd edn). Princeton, NJ: Prentice Hall.

4.7.2.6 External relationships

The NICU will often be directly adjacent to delivery rooms to allow for quick transfer of an infant in an emergency and to promote access by mothers. Due to the risk of abduction, many hospitals elect to situate the NICU in a location that allows for more controlled access. Proximity to surgery and specialized diagnostics is desired.

4.8 PICU and NICU examples

4.8.1 PICU/NICU Best Practice Research Project

One of the purposes of this book was to identify examples of PICUs and NICUs that might be of interest to design teams. Rather than limiting the study to those facilities that have been most effectively marketed, I developed criteria for determining notable pediatric and neonatal intensive care units using the following procedure. Initially an email was sent to individuals who had served on PICU and NICU standards committees to identify those facilities that they thought represented best practices. Subsequently, I looked for recipients of significant awards and recognition, including the Beacon Award for Excellence, *US News* Best Hospitals, the Vista Award, the Society of Critical Medicine, and the *Modern Health* magazine awards programs. In addition, projects showcased in journals such as *Healthcare Design* magazine and *World Health Design* were identified. This search resulted in a list of 33 PICUs and 59 NICUs. Clearly, not all of these facilities meet the criteria for best practice, but each of the facilities was identified as providing an example of a quality that might be useful to those wishing to design a new facility. They have been located geographically to aid those who are seeking sites to contact, research, or tour. The geographic distribution of these projects is shown in Figure 4.13.

4.8.2 Awards and recognitions

4.8.2.1 Beacon Award for Excellence

The Beacon Award for Excellence was created by the American Association of Critical-Care Nurses (AACN) "to recognize individual units that distinguish themselves by improving every facet of patient care" (AACN, n.d.). In 2010 the AACN updated its criteria for selection. The criteria address leadership, staffing, communication, knowledge management and best practices, evidence-based practice, and patient outcomes. While this award does not focus on the physical environment, good design provides the setting for achieving these goals. Up until 2012, recipients were limited to critical care units. Awards are given at the gold, silver, or bronze levels with a three-year designation. Figure 4.14 gives a list of facilities that provide pediatric and/or neonatal care and are currently Beacon Award for Excellence designees.

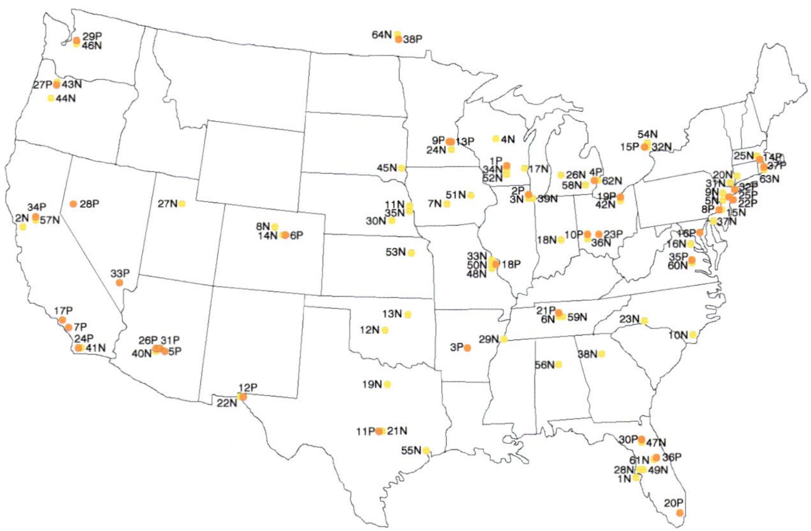

NICU list

1N All Children's Hospital, St Petersburg, FL
2N Alta Bates Summit Medical Center, Berkeley, San Francisco Bay Area, CA
3N Ann & Robert H. Lurie Children's Hospital of Chicago, Chicago, IL
4N Aspirus-Wausau Hospital, Wausau, WI
5N Atlantic Health Systems, Morristown, NJ
6N Baptist Hospital Beaman NICU, Nashville, TN
7N Blank Children's Hospital, Des Moines, IA
8N Boulder Community Foothills Hospital, Boulder, CO
9N Bristol Myers Squibb at Robert Wood Johnson University Hospital, New Brunswick, NJ
10N Cameron Women's and Children's New Hanover Regional Medical Center, Wilmington, NC
11N Children's Hospital & Medical Center, Omaha, NE
12N Children's Hospital at OU Medical Center, Oklahoma City, OK
13N Children's Hospital at Saint Francis, Tulsa, OK
14N Children's Hospital Colorado, Aurora, CO
15N Children's Hospital of Philadelphia (CHOP), Philadelphia, PA
16N Children's National Medical Center, Washington, DC
17N Columbia St. Mary's Hospital, Milwaukee, WI
18N Community Hospital North, Indianapolis, IN
19N Cook Children's Medical Center, Fort Worth, TX
20N Danbury Hospital Spratt NICU, Danbury, CT
21N Dell Children's Medical Center of Central.Texas, Austin, TX
22N El Paso Children's Hospital, El Paso, TX
23N Gaston Memorial Hospital, Gastonia, NC
24N Gillette Children's Specialty Healthcare, St. Paul, MN
25N Hasbro Children's Hospital, Providence, RI
26N Helen DeVos Children's Hospital, Grand Rapids, MI
27N Intermountain Medical Center, Salt Lake City, UT
28N Jennifer Leigh Muma NICU at Tampa General Hospital, Tampa, FL
29N Le Bonheur Children's Hospital, Memphis, TN
30N Lincoln Children's Hospital, Lincoln, NE
31N Maria Fareri Children's Hospital, Valhalla, NY
32N McMaster Children's Hospital, Hamilton, Ontario, Canada
33N Mercy Children's Hospital, Creve Coeur, MO
34N Meriter Hospital, Madison, WI
35N Methodist Women's Hospital, Omaha, NE
36N Miami Valley Hospital, Dayton, OH
37N Nemours/Alfred I. duPont Hospital for Children, Wilmington, DE
38N Northside Hospital Women's Center and Special Care Nursery, Atlanta, GA
39N Northwestern Memorial Hospital-Prentice Women's Hospital, Chicago, IL
40N Phoenix Children's Hospital, Phoenix, AZ
41N Rady Children's Hospital San Diego, San Diego, CA
42N Rainbow Babies & Children's Hospital, Cleveland, OH
43N Randall Children's Hospital at Legacy Emanuel, Portland, OR
44N Salem Hospital, Salem, OR
45N Sanford Children's Hospital, Sioux Falls, SD
46N Seattle Children's Hospital, Seattle, WA
47N Shands Hospital for Children at UF, Gainsville, FL
48N SSM Cardinal Glennon Children's Medical Center, St. Louis, MO
49N St. Joseph's Children's Hospital, Tampa, FL
50N St. Louis Children's Hospital, St. Louis, MO
51N St. Luke's Hospital, Cedar Rapids, IA
52N St. Mary's Hospital, Madison, WI
53N Stormont Vail Healthcare, Topeka, KS
54N Sunnybrook Health Sciences Women and Babies Program, Toronto, Ontario, Canada
55N Texas Children's Pavilion for Women, Houston, TX
56N UAB Women's & Infants Center, Birmingham, AL
57N UC Davis Children's Hospital, Sacramento, CA
58N University of Michigan C.S. Mott Children Hospital & Von Voigtlander Women's Hospital, Ann Arbor, MI
59N Vanderbilt University Medical Center, Nashville, TN
60N Virginia Commonwealth University Health System, Richmond, VA
61N Walt Disney Pavilion at Florida Hospital for Children, Orlando, FL
62N William Beaumont Hospital, Royal Oak, MI
63N Women & Infants Hospital of Rhode Island, Providence, RI
64N Women and Newborn Hospital, Health Sciences Centre Winnipeg, Winnipeg, Manitoba, Canada

PICU list

1P American Family Children's Hospital, Madison, WI
2P Ann & Robert H. Lurie Children's Hospital of Chicago, Chicago, IL
3P Arkansas Children's Hospital (Donald W. Reynold)s, Little Rock, AR
4P Beaumont Children's Hospital, Royal Oak, MI
5P Cardon Children's Medical Center, Mesa, AZ
6P Children's Hospital Colorado, Aurora, CO
7P Children's Hospital of Orange County/CHOC Children's, Orange, CA
8P Children's Hospital of Philadelphia (CHOP), Philadelphia, PA
9P Children's Hospitals and Clinics of Minnesota, St. Paul, MN
10P Dayton Children's Medical Center, Dayton, OH
11P Dell Children's Medical Center, Austin, TX
12P El Paso Children's Hospital, El Paso, TX
13P Gillette Children's Specialty Healthcare, St. Paul, MN
14P Hasbro Children's Hospital, Providence, RI
15P Hospital for Sick Children, Toronto, Ontario, Canada
16P Johns Hopkins Children's Center, Baltimore, MD
17P Mattel Children's Hospital UCLA, Los Angeles, CA
18P Mercy Children's Hospital, Creve Coeur, MO
19P Metrohealth Medical center, Clevelend, OH
20P Miami Children's Hospital, Miami, FL
21P Monroe Carell Jr. Children's Hospital at Vanderbilt, Nashville, TN
22P Mount Sinai Hospital, New York, NY
23P Nationwide Children's Hospital, Columbus, OH
24P Naval Medical Center San Diego (NMCSD), San Diego, CA
25P New York Presbyterian Morgan Stanley Children's Hospital, New York, NY
26P Phoenix Children's Hospital, Phoenix, AZ
27P Randall Children's Hospital at Legacy Emanuelttt, Portland, OR
28P Renown Children's Hospital, Reno, NV
29P Seattle Children's Hospital, Seattle, WA
30P Shands Hospital for Children at UF, Gainsville, FL
31P St. Joseph's Hospital and Medical Center, Phoenix, AZ
32P Steve and Alexandra Cohen Children's Medical Center of New York, New Hyde Park, NY
33P Sunrise Hospital & Medical Center, Las Vegas, NV
34P UC Davis Children's Hospital, Sacramento, CA
35P VCU Children's Hospital, Richmond, VA
36P Walt Disney Pavilion at Florida Hospital for Children, Orlando, FL
37P Women & Infants Hospital of Rhode Island, Providence, RI
38P Women and Newborn Hospital, Health Sciences Centre Winnipeg, Winnipeg, Manitoba, Canada

Figure 4.13: *Geographic location of PICUs and NICUs identified in the Best Practice Research Project*

Figure 4.14: *Current designees of the Beacon Award for Excellence (Source: AACN, n.d.)*

Hospital	*City*	*Designation*	*Designated until*
Children's Hospital of Alabama PICU	Birmingham, AL	Silver	January 2015
Children's Hospital Los Angeles PICU	Los Angeles, CA	Silver	April 2014
Children's Hospital Orange County PICU	Orange, CA	Gold	January 2015
Children's National Medical PICU	Washington, DC	Gold	January 2015
Children's National Medical NICU	Washington, DC	Silver	September 2014
Children's Healthcare of Atlanta CICU	Atlanta, GA	Gold	January 2016
Miami Children's Cardiac ICU	Miami, FL	Silver	September 2015
Miami Children's PICU	Miami, FL	Gold	January 2015
Miami Children's Cardiac PICU/NICU	Miami, FL	Gold	August 2015
Tampa General Hospital PICU	Tampa, FL	Silver	February 2016
Kosair Children's "Just for Kids" Critical Care	Louisville, KY	Silver	March 2015
Boston Children's Hospital NICU	Boston, MA	Gold	July 2014
Levine Children's Hendrick Center for Intensive Care	Charlotte, NC	Bronze	January 2016
Cincinnati Children's Medical Center PICU	Cincinnati, OH	Gold	June 2015
Randall Children's Hospital Legacy Emanuel PICU	Portland, OR	Gold	May 2015
La Bonheur Children's Cardiovascular ICU	Memphis, TN	Gold	September 2015
Covenant Health System PICU	Lubbock, TX	Silver	June 2015
Inova Fairfax Hospital PICU	Falls Church, VA	Gold	September 2015

4.8.2.2 US News and World Report

The selection process to determine the list of best hospitals for the *U.S. News and World Report* involves two sources: data regarding nurse staffing, low infection rates, and patient volume make up 75 percent of the score, while 25 percent of the score is the result of the recommendations of pediatric neonatologists who participated between 2010 and 2012 (*U.S. News and World Report*, 2013). Again, while these pediatric hospitals are not selected for their physical environment, the environment likely abets their success. Pediatric intensive care is not listed as a separate ranking category. The 2013 top ten hospitals for neonatology are listed in Figure 4.15.

Figure 4.15: *US News best neonatology children's hospitals (Source: U.S. News and World Report, 2013)*

Rank	*Hospital*	*City*	*U.S. News Score*
1	Cincinnati Children's Hospital	Cincinnati, OH	100.0/100
2	Texas Children's Hospital	Houston, TX	97.5/100
3	Boston Children's Hospital	Boston, MA	94.9/100
4	Children's Hospital of Philadelphia	Philadelphia, PA	94.7/100
5	Rainbow Babies an Children's Hospital	Cleveland, OH	91.4/100
6	Children's National Medical Center	Washington, DC	89.3/100
7	Children's Hospital Los Angeles	Los Angeles, CA	87.0/100
8	Monroe Carell Jr. Children's Hospital at Vanderbilt	Nashville, TN	84.7/100
9	Children's Hospital of Pittsburgh of UPMC	Pittsburg, PA	84.6/100
10	Johns Hopkins Children's Center	Baltimore, MD	80.9/100

Figure 4.16: *SCCM ICU Design Citation Award winners (Source: SCCM, 2013)*

PICU/NICU	*City*	*Date*
St. Elizabeth's Medical Center NICU	Boston, MA	1995
The Hospital for Sick Children PICU	Toronto, Ontario	1995
The Children's Medical Center NICU	Dayton, OH	1999
Children's Hospital and Regional Medical Center Pediatric and Infant Care Units	Seattle, WA	2002
Hamilton Health Science, McMaster Children's Hospital NICU	Hamilton, Ontario	2004
Arkansas Children's Hospital, Donald W. Reynolds PICU	Little Rock, AR	2005
Children's Medical Center of Dayton, Wallace Critical Care Complex	Dayton, OH	2007
Ann and Robert H. Lurie Children's Hospital of Chicago PICU	Chicago, IL	2013
Phoenix Children's Hospital PICU (honorable mention)	Phoenix, AZ	2013

4.8.2.3 Vista Awards

The American Society of Healthcare Engineering (ASHE) of the American Hospital Association (AHA) has sponsored the Vista Awards since 1993. The awards recognize excellence in healthcare design and construction initiatives (ASHE, n.d.). Three categories of awards are offered: new construction, renovation, and infrastructure. All types of healthcare facilities are eligible for this award. Since 2006 two NICUs have won this award, both in the renovation category: the Aspirus Wausau Hospital NICU in Wausau, Wisconsin renovation, in 2011, and the SSM Cardinal Glennon Children's Medical Center NICU and Surgery Addition, in St. Louis, Missouri, in 2009.

4.8.2.4 Society of Critical Care Medicine (SCCM) design citation

The ICU Design Citation, sponsored by the Society for Critical Care Medicine (SCCM) and the American Association of Critical-Care Nurses, and the American Institute of Architects Academy on Architecture for Health, is an award offered to a critical care unit that "combines functional ICU design with the humanitarian delivery of critical care" (SCCM, 2013). Criteria include a commitment to creating a healing environment, dedication to promoting security and safety, a commitment to efficiency, and attention to innovative, aesthetic, and creative design. Out of 27 recipients of the award or recipients of honorable mention, ten have been pediatric or neonatal facilities.

Since 1992, the pediatric/neonatal facilities listed in Figure 4.16 have won the award.

Cadenhead and Anderson (2009) noted trends among winners of the SCCM adult and pediatric ICU competition. The trends they identified were as follows:

- Larger units.
- All private rooms at about 250 square feet.
- A family zone in the patient room with amenities.
- Ceiling-mounted booms.

- A combination of centralized and decentralized units.
- Proximity to diagnostics and treatment.
- More administrative and education space on the unit.
- Distinct on-stage and off-stage circulation.
- Access to nature.

Examples of these award-winning and notable projects are shown throughout this book as illustrations of ideas raised in the text.

Chapter 5 provides a structured literature review of design research on PICUs and NICUs.

References

Ahmann, E., Abraham, M.R., and Johnson, B.H. (2003). *Changing the Concept of Families as Visitors: Supporting Family Presence and Participation*. Bethesda, MD: Institute for Family-centered Care.

Al-Samsam, R. H., and Cullen, P. (2005). Sleep and adverse environmental factors in sedated mechanically ventilated pediatric intensive care patients. *Pediatric Critical Care Medicine, 6*(5), 562–567.

Alves-Dunkerson, J.A., Hilsenrath, P.E., Cress, G.A., and Widness, J.A. (2002). Cost analysis of a neonatal point-of-care monitor. *American Journal of Clinical Pathology*, *117*(5), 809–818.

American Association of Critical-Care Nurses (AACN). (n.d.). Welcome to the Beacon Award for Excellence. Retrieved from aacn.org/wd/beaconapps/content/mainpage.pcms?menu=beaconapps

American Society of Healthcare Engineers (ASHE). (n.d.). Vista Awards. Retrieved from www.ashe.org/about/awards/vista/index.html

Anderson, P., and Weber, D. (June 24, 2012). NICU rapid design process. In *Association of Women's Health, Obstetric and Neonatal Nurses (AWHONN) Annual Convention*. Washington, DC. Retrieved from https://awhonn.confex.com/awhonn/2012/webprogram/Paper8600.html

Antonucci, R., Porcella, A., and Fanos, V. (2009). The infant incubator in the neonatal intensive care unit: Unresolved issues and future developments. *Journal of Perinatal Medicine*, *37*(6), 587–598.

Arnon, S., Shapsa, A., Forman, L., Regev, R., Bauer, S., Litmanovitz, I., and Dolfin, T. (2006). Live music is beneficial to preterm infants in the neonatal intensive care unit environment. *Birth, 33*(2), 131–136.

Bailey, E., and Timmons, S. (2005). Noise levels in PICU: An evaluative study. *Paediatric Nursing-Cardiff*, *17*(10), 22–26.

Bauer, P., Hoffmann, R.G., Bragg, D., and Scanlon, M.C. (2011). Perceptions of risk to patient safety in the pediatric ICU, a study of American pediatric intensivists. *Safety Science, 53*, 160–167.

Berry, L.L., Parker, D., Coile, R.C., Hamilton, D.K., O'Neill, D.D., and Sadler, B.L. (2004). The business case for better buildings. *Frontiers of Health Services Management*, *21*, 3–24.

Bilec, M.M., Ries, R.J., Needy, K.L., Gokhan, M., Phelps, A.F., Enache-Pommer, E., and Sheane, C.

(2009). Analysis of the design process of green children's hospitals: Focus on process modeling and lessons learned. *Journal of Green Building*, *4*(1), 121–134.

Blumberg, R., and Devlin, A.S. (2006). Design issues in hospitals: The adolescent client. *Environment and Behavior, 38*(3), 293–317.

Brown, S.L., Neese, R.M., Vinokur, A.D., and Smith, D.M. (2003). Providing social support may be more beneficial than receiving it: Results from a prospective study of mortality. *Political Science*, *14*(4), 320–327.

Browne, J. (2003). New perspectives on premature babies and their families. *Zero to Three*, *24*(2), 4–12.

Bruns, D.A., and Klein, S. (2005). An evaluation of family-centered care in a level III NICU. *Infants & Young Children*, *18*(3), 222–233.

Cadenhead, C., and Anderson, D. (2009). Critical care unit design, the winners and future trends: An investigative study. *World Health Design Journal, 2*(3), 72–77.

Carlson, B., Walsh, S., Wergin, T., Schwarzkopf, K., and Ecklund, S. (2006). Challenges in design and transition to a private room model in the neonatal intensive care unit. *Advances in Neonatal Care*, *6*(5), 271–280.

Carvalho, W.B., Pedreira, M.L.G., and de Aguiar, M.A.L. (2005). Noise level in a pediatric intensive care unit. *Jornal de Pediatria, 81*(6), 495–498.

Christensen, A.J., Dornink, R., Ehlers, S.L., and Schultz, S.K. (1999). Social environment and longevity in schizophrenia. *Psychosomatic Medicine, 61*, 141–145.

Cone, S.K., Short, S., and Gutcher, G. (2010). From "baby barn" to the "single family room designed NICU": A report of staff perceptions one year post occupancy. *Newborn and Infant Nursing Reviews*, *10*(2), 97–103.

Cooper Marcus, C., and Barnes, M. (eds). (1999). *Healing Gardens: Therapeutic Benefits and Design Recommendations*. Hoboken, NJ: John Wiley & Sons.

Cooper Marcus, C., and Sachs, N. (2013). *Therapeutic Landscapes: An Evidence-based Approach to Designing Healing Gardens and Restorative Outdoor Spaces.* Hoboken, NJ: John Wiley & Sons.

Corser, N.C. (1996). Sleep of 1-and 2-year-old children in intensive care. *Issues in Comprehensive Pediatric Nursing*, *19*(1), 17–31.

Coull, A., and Mare, G. (February 17, 2011). 201 inpatient unit – Neonatal intensive care unit/pediatric intensive care unit. Webinar presentation for the American Institute of Architects.

Cureton-Lane, R.A., and Fontaine, D.K. (1997). Sleep in the pediatric ICU: An empirical investigation. *American Journal of Critical Care*, *6*(1), 56–63.

Curry, Z.D., Shroyer, J.L., Staton, C.D., and Curry, D.J. (1996). Environmental assessment instrument development and usage for the analysis of adult and pediatric patient room design. *Journal of Family and Consumer Sciences, 88*(2), 53–58.

del Olmo, M.J., Garrido, C.R., and Tarrío, F.R. (2010). Music therapy in the PICU 0- to 6-month-old babies. *Music and Medicine*, *2*(3), 158–166.

Diaz, J. (2000). Brief history of ICU design. In D.K. Hamilton (ed.) *ICU 2010*. Houston, TX: Center for Innovation in Health Facilities.

Dick, K. (2011). *Lean implementation and pediatric intensive care unit bed availability analysis via simulation at the Winnipeg Children's Hospital.* Master's thesis. Retrieved from ProQuest Dissertation and Theses (MR84975).

Driscoll, S., Fleming, M., and Khilnani, P. (1993). Establishing a new pediatric intensive care unit. *Indian Journal of Pediatrics*, *60*(3), 331–339.

Eisen, S.L., Ulrich, R.S., Shepley, M.M., Varni, J.W., and Sherman, S. (2008). The stress-reducing effects of art in pediatric health care: Art preferences of healthy children and hospitalized children. *Journal of Child Health Care*, *12*(3), 173–190.

Enache-Pommer, E. (2008). *Lean and green healthcare facilities: Improving the delivery process in children's hospitals*. Master's thesis. Retrieved from http://etda.libraries.psu.edu/paper/8271/3555

Evans, R., and Madsen, B. (2005). Culture clash: Transitioning from the neonatal intensive care unit to the pediatric intensive care unit. *Newborn and Infant Nursing Reviews*, *5*(4), 188–193.

Feldman, R., Eidelman. A.I., Sirota. L., and Weller, A. (2002). Comparison of skin-to-skin (kangaroo) and traditional care: Parenting and preterm infant development. *Pediatrics, 110*(1), 16–26.

Ferris, T., and Shepley, M. (2012). A multidisciplinary human-centered approach to the design of incubation systems. In A.R. Andre (Chair), *Proceedings of the 2012 Symposium on Human Factors and Ergonomics in Health Care* (pp. 187–192). Santa Monica, CA: Human Factors and Ergonomics Society.

Frampton, S.B., and Charmel, P.A. (eds). (2008). *Putting Patients First: Best Practices in Patient-centered Care* (Vol. 33). San Francisco, CA: Jossey-Bass.

Frampton, S., Guastello, S., Brady, C., Hale, M., Horowitz, S., Bennett Smith, S., and Stone, S. (2008). *Patient-centered Care: Improvement Guide*. Derby, CT: Planetree, and Camden, ME: Picker Institute.

Gilad, E., and Arnon, S. (2010). The role of live music and singing as a stress-reducing modality in the neonatal intensive care unit environment. *Music and Medicine*, *2*(1), 18–22.

Gottlieb, M., and Dickeman, N. (2007). First do no harm: Environmental responsibility in the NICU. In J.D. Horbar, K. Leahy, and J. Handyside (eds) *NICQ 2007: Improvement in Action*. Vermont Oxford Network. Retrieved from http://pop.vtoxford.com/quality/ebook/NICQ_2007_Chapter_7.pdf

Griffin, T. (2006). Family-centered care in the NICU. *Journal of Perinatal and Neonatal Nursing, 20*(1), 98–102.

Grunden, N., and Hagood, C. (2012). *Lean-led Hospital Design: Creating the Efficient Hospital of the Future*. Boca Raton, FL: Productivity Press.

Gurascio-Howard, L., and Malloch, K. (2007). Centralized and decentralized nurse station design: An examination of caregiver communication, work activities, and technology. *Health Environments Reseach and Design Journal (HERD)*, *1*(1), 44–57.

Hartline, J.V. (2013). Rhythms, regulation, relationships, silence, sound, music noise. *Proceedings from the Physical and Developmental Environment of the High Risk Infant Conference*. Clearwater, FL: USF Health.

Henry Bowie, B., Hall, R.B., Faulkner, J., and Anderson, B. (2003). Single-room infant care: Future trends in special care nursery planning and design. *Neonatal Network: The Journal of Neonatal Nursing*, *22*(4), 27–34.

Jousselme, C., Vialet, R., Jouve, E., Lagier, P., Martin, C., and Michel, F. (2011). Efficacy and mode of action of a noise-sensor light alarm to decrease noise in the pediatric intensive care unit: A prospective, randomized study. *Pediatric Critical Care Medicine*, *12*(2), e69–e72.

Kaushal, R., Bates, D.W., Landrigan, C., McKenna, K. J., Clapp, M.D., Federico, F., and Goldmann, D.A. (2001). Medication errors and adverse drug events in pediatric inpatients. *JAMA: The Journal of the American Medical Association*, *285*(16), 2114–2120.

Kulkarni, A., Rybkowski, Z., and Smith, J. (July, 2012). Cost comparison of collaborative and IPD-like project delivery methods versus competitive non-collaborative project delivery methods. *Proceedings of the 20th Conference of the International Group for Lean*

Construction. San Diego, CA. Retrieved from http://www.iglc20.sdsu.edu/papers/wp-content/uploads/2012/07/79%20P%20076.pdf

Lawton, M.P., and Nahemow, L. (1973). Ecology and the aging process. In C. Eisdorfer and M.P. Lawton (eds) *Psychology of Adult Development and Aging* (pp. 657–668). Washington, DC: American Psychological Association.

Leibrock, C.A., and Harris, D. (2011). *Design Details for Health*. Hoboken, NJ: John Wiley & Sons.

Lobas, N.H., Armitstead, J.A., and Ivey, M.F. (1991). Expanding staff pharmacists' responsibilities to maintain pharmacy services in a neonatal intensive-care unit. *American Journal of Health-System Pharmacy*, *48*(8), 1708–1711.

Marshall-Baker, A. (2006). Human and environmental health: Sustainable design for the NICU. *Journal of perinatology*, *26*, S31–S33.

Marshall-Baker, A. (2011). Healthful environments for hospitalized infants. *Health Environments Research and Design Journal (HERD)*, *4*(2), 127–141.

McGrath, J.M. (2005). Single-room design in the NICU: Making it work for you. *The Journal of Perinatal and Neonatal Nursing*, *19*(3), 210–211.

Milford, C.A., Zapalo, B.J., and Davis, G. (2008). Transition to an individual-room NICU design: Process and outcome measures. *Neonatal Network, 27*(3), 299–305.

Miller, M.R., and Zhan, C. (2004). Pediatric patient safety in hospitals: A national picture in 2000. *Pediatrics, 113*(6), 1741–1746.

Montgomery, V.L. (2006). Analyzing human, nonhuman factors can improve patient safety. *AAP News*, *27*(6), 15.

Montgomery, V.L. (2007). Effect of fatigue, workload, and environment on patient safety in the pediatric intensive care unit. *Pediatric Critical Care Medicine*, *8*(2), S11–S16.

Morrison, W.E., Haas, E.C., Shaffner, D.H., Garrett, E.S., and Fackler, J.C. (2003). Noise, stress, and annoyance in a pediatric intensive care unit. *Critical Care Medicine*, *31*(1), 113–119.

Nelson, M. (2011). *Sustaining Lean in Healthcare: Developing and Engaging Physician Leadership*. Boca Raton, FL: CRC Press.

O'Brien, K., Bracht, M., Macdonell, K., McBride, T., Robson, K., O'Leary, L., and Lee, S.K. (2013). A pilot cohort analytic study of family integrated care in a Canadian neonatal intensive care unit. *BMC Pregnancy and Childbirth, 13*(supplement 1), S12. doi:10.1186/1471-2393-13-S1-S12

Ozcan, H. (2006). *Healing design: A holistic approach to social interaction in pediatric intensive care units in the United States and Turkey.* Doctoral dissertation. Retrieved from ProQuest Dissertations and Theses (3202268).

Pasha, S. (2011). *Usability of outdoor spaces in children's hospitals*. Doctoral dissertation. Abstract retrieved from ProQuest Dissertations and Theses (3471232).

Pasha, S. (in press). Barriers to garden visitation in children's hospital. *Health Environments Research and Design*.

Pate, M.F.D. (2012). It is easy being green: Greening the pediatric intensive care unit. *AACN Advanced Critical Care*, *23*(1), 18–23.

Pati, D., Cason, C., Harvey Jr, T.E., and Evans, J. (2010). An empirical examination of patient room handedness in acute medical-surgical settings. *Health Environments Research and Design Journal (HERD)*, *4*(1), 11–33.

Philbin, M.K. (2004). Planning the acoustic environment of a neonatal intensive care unit. *Clinics in Perinatolology, 31*(2), 331–352.

Powers, K.S., and Rubenstein, J.S. (1999). Family presence during invasive procedures in the pediatric intensive care unit: A prospective study. *Archives of Pediatrics and Adolescent Medicine*, *153*(9), 955–958.

Raju, T.K., Thornton, J., Kecskes, S., Perry, M., and Feldman, S. (1989). Medication errors in neonatal and paediatric intensive-care units. *The Lancet*, *334*(8659), 374–376.
Rosenberg, D.I., and Moss, M.M. (2004). Guidelines and levels of care for pediatric intensive care units. *Pediatrics*, *114*(4), 1114–1125.
Rybkowski, Z., Shepley, M., and Ballard, G. (2012). Target value design: Applications to newborn intensive care units. *Health Environments & Design Research*, *5*(4), 5–22.
Sadler, B.L., DuBose, J.R., and Zimring, C. (2008). The business case for building better pediatric facilities. In B.L. Sadler, and A. Joseph (eds) *Evidence for Innovation: Transforming Children's Health Through the Physical Environment* (pp. 96–115). Alexandria, VA: National Association of Children's Hospitals and Related Institutions.
Samra, H.A., McGrath, J.M., and Rollins, W. (2011). Patient safety in the NICU: A comprehensive review. *The Journal of Perinatal and Neonatal Nursing*, *25*(2), 123–132.
Scanlon, M.C., Mistry, K.P., and Jeffries, H.E. (2007). Determining pediatric intensive care unit quality indicators for measuring pediatric intensive care unit safety. *Pediatric Critical Care Medicine*, *8*(2), S3–S10.
Schieveld, J.N., Leroy, P.L., van Os, J., Nicolai, J., Vos, G.D., and Leentjens, A.F. (2007). Pediatric delirium in critical illness: phenomenology, clinical correlates and treatment response in 40 cases in the pediatric intensive care unit. *Intensive Care Medicine*, *33*(6), 1033–1040.
Shaffner, D.H. (2011). What does it take to get some peace and quiet in the pediatric, intensive care unit. *Pediatric Critical Care Medicine, 12*(2), 238–240.
Shepley, M. (2006). The role of positive distraction in neonatal intensive care settings. *Journal of Perinatology, 26*, S34–S37.
Smith, J., Bajo, K., and Hager, J. (2004). Planning a developmentally appropriate neonatal intensive care unit. *Clinics in Perinatology*, *31*(2), 313–322.
Smith, J.A., Hager, J., and Bajo, K. (2010). Making neonatal intensive care units more visually appealing. *Newborn and Infant Nursing Reviews*, *10*(2), 78–82.
Society for Critical Care Medicine (SCCM). (2013). ICU design citation. Retrieved from http://www.sccm.org/Membership/Awards/Pages/ICU-Design-Citation.aspx
Stevens, D.C., Khan, M.A., Munson, D.P., Reid, E.J., Helseth, C.C., and Buggy, J. (2007). The impact of architectural design upon the environmental sound and light exposure of neonates who require intensive care: An evaluation of the Boekelheide Neonatal Intensive Care Nursery. *Journal of Perinatology*, *27*, S20–S28.
Stone, P.W., Gupta, A., Loughrey, M., Della-Latta, P., Cimiotti, J., Larson, E., and Saiman, L. (2003). Attributable costs and length of stay of an extended-spectrum beta-lactamase-producing Klebsiella pneumoniae outbreak in a neonatal intensive care unit. *Infection Control and Hospital Epidemiology*, *24*(8), 601–606.
Talmi, A., and Harmon, R.J. (2003). Relationships between preterm infants and their parents: Disruption and development. *Zero to Three, 24*(2), 13–20.
Thomas, K.A., and Uran, A. (2007). How the NICU environment sounds to a preterm infant: Update. *MCN: The American Journal of Maternal/Child Nursing*, *32*(4), 250–253.
Tisdale, J.E. (1986). Justifying a pediatric critical-care satellite pharmacy by medication-error reporting. *American Journal of Health-System Pharmacy*, *43*(2), 368–371.
U.S. News and World Report. (June 14, 2012). Top ranked pediatric hospitals for neonatology. Retrieved from health.usnews.com/best-hospitals/pediatric-rankings/neonatal-care
Vandenberg, K.A. (2007). Individualized developmental care for high risk newborns in the NICU: A practice guideline. *Early Human Development*, *83*(7), 433–442.
Vats, A., Goin, K.H., Villarreal, M.C., Yilmaz, T., Fortenberry, J.D., and Keskinocak, P. (2012). The

impact of a lean rounding process in a pediatric intensive care unit. *Critical Care Medicine*, *40*(2), 608–617.
Watkins, N., Kennedy, M., Ducharme, M., and Padula, C. (2011). Same-handed and mirrored unit configurations: Is there a difference in patient and nurse outcomes? *Journal of Nursing Administration*, *41*(6), 273–279.
Wellman, J., Hagan, P., and Jeffries, H. (2010). *Leading the Lean Healthcare Journey: Driving Culture Change to Increase Value*. New York: Taylor & Francis.
White, R. (2004). Mothers' arms – the past and future of neonatal care? *Clinics in Perinatology*, *31*(2), 383–387.
White, R.D. (2006). Recommended standards for newborn ICU design. *Journal of Perinatology*, *26*, S2–S18.
White, R. (2011a). Design environment for developmental care. *Clinics in Perinatology, 38*(4), 745–749.
White, R. (2011b). The newborn intensive care unit environment of care: How we got here, where we're headed, and why. *Seminars in Perinatology, 35*(1), 2–7.
White R., and Newbold, P.A. (1995). Reinventing the newborn ICU. *The Healthcare Forum Journal, 38 (2)*, 30–33.
Whitelaw, A. (1990). Kangaroo baby care: Just a nice experience or an important advance for preterm infants? *Pediatrics*, *85*(4), 604–605.
Wrench, I.J., and Vyas, H.G. (1995). How to equip a paediatric intensive care unit. *Current Paediatrics*, *5*(1), 10–13.
Zborowsky, T., Bunker-Hellmich, L., Morelli, A., and O'Neill, M. (2010). Centralized vs. decentralized nursing stations: Effects on nurses' functional use of space and work environment. *Health Environments Research and Design*, *3*(4), 19–42.

Part Three: Research and guidelines on persons and the environment

PICU and NICU design research

5

The purpose of this chapter is to summarize the research relating to pediatric and neonatal intensive care environments in order to provide the reader with the best evidence to inform design decisions. The chapter begins with a summation of the meaning and role of evidence-based design (EBD). The subsequent section will describe the design research associated with each of several environmental components that apply to both PICUs and NICUs. The last two sections summarize research specific to each of these two settings.

5.1 Role of evidence-based design

The notion of EBD has been bandied about more than any other concept in healthcare design raised in the past 20 years. Both embraced and criticized, EBD has revolutionized the discussion around the development of medical facilities. EBD may be broadly defined as the creation and use of research and empirical evidence to support the design process. The definition of evidence-based design practice has been clearly articulated in several publications by Kirk Hamilton (e.g. Hamilton, 2003). EBD had its roots in the 1960s with the founding of the Environmental Design Research Association (EDRA). While researchers had been conducting studies on the impact of the physical environment upon human behavior for many years, this organization formalized the network of people interested in using research to inform the design process.

In the United States, much of the initial design research took place in educational settings. The Educational Facilities Laboratories (EFL), founded in 1958 by Harold Gores (Marks, 2009), was a generator and repository of design research data. Individuals associated with the EFL, such as Jonathan King, went on to found the Architectural Research Laboratory at the University of Michigan, at which several early studies involving healthcare settings took place. The full-scale mock-ups of the proposed patient rooms at the University of Michigan Hospital were among the most notable of these studies. The doctoral program at the University of Michigan at that time spawned such well-known healthcare design researchers as Roger Ulrich (Theory of Supportive Design), Stephen Verderber (*Healthcare Architecture in an Era of Radical Transformation*), and Janet Carpman (*Design that Cares*).

With regard to the application of EBD to the design of PICUs and NICUs, the literature is scant regarding the former and growing with regard to the latter. While conducting research for *Healthcare Environments for Children and their Families* (Shepley et al., 1998), we reviewed the articles addressed in the predecessor volume, *Child Health Care Facilities* (Olds et al., 1987). We found 277 articles on children's healthcare environments that reflected research, descriptive studies, guidelines, and literature reviews available up to 1987. Only 50 of these, however, involved substantive methods such as structured qualitative or quantitative research protocols

(18%). Thirty-two of the 277 addressed PICUs and NICUs (12%). For the subsequent decade, while writing *Healthcare Environments for Children and their Families*, we identified 59 research-based studies out of 190 (26%) published between 1987 and 1997; 72 of the 190 addressed PICUs and NICUs (38%) (see Figure 5.1).

More recently in NACHRI's *Evidence for Innovation: Transforming Children's Health through the Physical Environment* (2008), the authors were able to identify approximately 450 studies regarding children's facilities of which 320 met their inclusion criteria. No limits on the timeframe were indicated. Inclusion criteria consisted, among other things, of publication in a peer-reviewed journal, clearly defined environmental variables, and either an empirical study or in-depth literature review. Of this group, 223 were cited in *Evidence for Innovation*. Of those, 11 focused on PICUs (5%), 37 addressed NICUs (16%), and two focused on both settings, together representing a total of 22% of all studies.

The emphasis on NICUs is likely due to the following reasons:

- The similarities between PICUs and adult ICUs are stronger than the similarities between NICUs and adult ICUs, so research on adult ICUs has been thought to be adequate to be applied to the PICU setting.
- NICUs were historically small and in a single room, so the numbers of confounding independent variables were limited when conducting a study.
- NICU patients are making a transition from the womb to the extra-uterine environment, highlighting the role of the physical environment.
- The NICU population is considered frail.

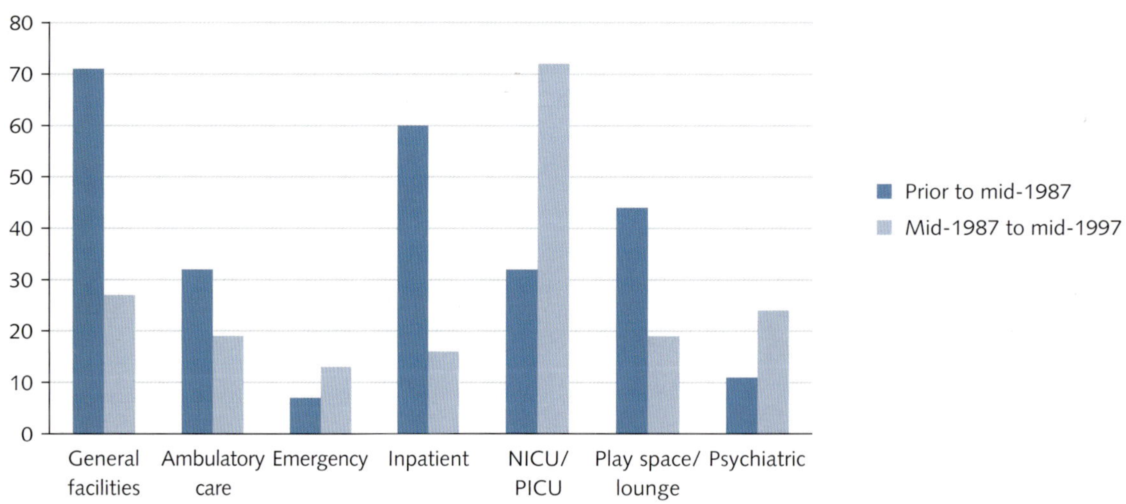

Figure 5.1: *Relative allocation of pediatric health design studies up to mid-1997 (Source: Derived from Shepley et al., 1998)*

5.2 Current EBD topics

Among the most salient topics in EBD are positive distraction in pursuit of stress reduction, environmental congruence, safety (infection control, fall prevention, medical error reduction), and the use of private rooms staff. Research associated with these subjects is described in the following sections.

5.2.1 *Positive distraction*

Positive distraction refers to the use of environmental experiences to detract from unpleasant and stressful thoughts. The underlying objective is to reduce stress, which will in turn enhance the immune system and thereby help in the healing process. Hospitals and healthcare environments have long been characterized as unpleasant, and designers have strived to reduce exposure to unpleasant experience.

In a previous article (Shepley, 2006), I stated that starting in the 1980s, research was initiated which, instead of focusing on reducing the negative aspects of the environment, redirected intention to reinforcement of positive experiences. These experiences were intended to allow the individual to project his or herself into the environment beyond the healthcare setting. Positive distraction allows "the individual to shift focus from negative foci within the health environment to the more restorative aspects of the non-medical world" (Shepley, 2006, p. S34).

The notion of positive distraction has been supported by the theories of multiple researchers including Jay Appleton (Prospect and Refuge Theory), and Stephen and Rachel Kaplan (Environmental Preference Theory). The gist of Appleton's theory is that the environment, particularly the natural environment, needs to provide a balance between stimulating experience and security. The Kaplans (1989), also interested in the role of nature, note that preference is related to our ability to learn from the environment. From an evolutionary perspective, learning is essential to survival. Environmental elements that can serve as positive distractions are nature, art, entertainment systems, music, and social interaction. The following description of positive distraction is drawn largely from Shepley (2006), "The role of positive distraction in neonatal intensive care unit settings."

5.2.1.1 Access to nature

As discussed above, there are several theories supporting the importance of access to nature. Stephen R. Kellert and Edward O. Wilson's work on the Biophilia Hypothesis (1993) is the most seminal. Biophilia refers to the innate affiliation of humans with other living organisms (Kellert and Wilson, 1993, p. 31). When this relationship is disrupted, as might be the case in healthcare settings, there can be negative psychological and emotional consequences.

Rachel and Stephen Kaplan (1989) elaborate on our fascination with nature in the context of the human inclination to acquire information and assert that we prefer environments which support such acquisition. Acquiring experience, particularly spatial information and information about the natural environment, is essential to our survival.

> From this perspective, then people not only are adroit in their use of information but crave it and continuously evaluate it. The evaluation of information is essential; effective functioning

> relies on sorting the good from the bad, the useful from the useless. Humans judge situations with such facility that they are often not aware of the act that such an evaluation is occurring.
>
> (Kaplan and Kaplan, 1989, p. 5)

Dr. Roger Ulrich is a strong proponent of the use of nature as a positive distraction. Apart from his well-known study suggesting that views from a hospital room window could positively impact patient outcomes (Ulrich, 1984), Parsons et al. (1998) found lower stress levels in subjects who viewed videos of a nature-dominated drive than those who viewed artifact-dominated drives. Ulrich and colleagues have also found that views of nature scenes were more effective in reducing stress than urban scenes after exposure to a stressful movie (Ulrich et al., 1991).

Numerous other researchers have addressed the importancc of nature with regard to healthcare environments. Seventy-five percent of workshop participants in a study by Anita Olds (1995) drew scenes of outdoor spaces and nature when they were asked to describe a place to go when they were ill. Cooper Marcus and Barnes (1995) found that people in hospitals went to hospital gardens to de-stress and reported positive mood changes when they were there. Interaction between animals and children in a healthcare setting is another means of associating with nature. Results from research have addressed reduced perception of pain (e.g. Sobo et al., 2006), and the provision of physiological and psychological benefits in pediatric populations (e.g. Urbanski and Lazenby, 2012).

The subject of windows is central to this discussion of positive distraction, as windows represent the interface between the presence of light – also essential to healing environments – and access to nature. Several researchers have found that windows have a positive impact on attentional fatigue (e.g. Sagha Zadeh, 2012). While it has been argued that windows may create additional expense during the construction phase, they also offer an operational cost saving through reductions in the need for electric lighting (Sagha Zadeh, 2012). More detailed information is available regarding appropriate windows. Stephen Verderber (1986) conducted research on hospital windows and found that they needed to be close and of significant size to be positively perceived. Walch et al. (2005) studied patient rooms on the sunny and non-sunny sides of buildings for cardiac patients and found shorter lengths of stay and lower mortality on the sunny side. Similar benefits from light were demonstrated by Beauchemin and Hays (1996), and Benedetti et al. (2001).

5.2.1.2 Art/color

In contemporary healthcare settings, the primary purpose of art is to uplift the experience of patients, staff, and families. In addition, art (painting, sculpture, etc.) serves to support wayfinding and to create a contextual link to the community in which it is located.

There has been some debate about which genre of art is most appropriate for healthcare settings. Ulrich and Lundén (1993) found that post-operative patients preferred realistic to abstract art; however, some argue that this response will be impacted by the particular nature of the abstract art in question, as well as the color palette. With regard to color, evidence suggests that anxious individuals prefer fewer saturated colors (Ireland et al., 1992). Art preferences may be personality related. Zuckerman et al. (1993) found that high sensation seekers tend to prefer abstract art. Due to the likelihood that patients in healthcare settings may be seeking less challenging environments, this may provide support for the notion that art should tend toward the more realistic. Researchers also believe that preference for abstract art may be the result of life experience; we know that architects and designers tend to prefer this genre, perhaps due to more exposure to modern art during their education.

5.2.1.3 Music

Several studies suggest the benefits of music for reducing stress. Researchers noted reduced self-reported stress levels in persons in surgery waiting areas where music was playing (Routhieaux and Tansik, 1997; Tansik and Routhieaux, 1999). In a literature review of 19 studies on the impact of music on pain and anxiety in children, Klassen et al. (2008) found that music was effective in reducing anxiety and pain during medical and dental procedures. The settings for the studies that were analyzed ranged from dental clinics to burn units. The authors noted that music may be particularly effective as an adjunct treatment to reduce pain in children with higher baseline pain or in the very young.

Researchers have not been able to confirm that a particular genre of music has more benefits than others. The literature on choice and control suggests that the ability to select one's own music is critical to the effectiveness of that music.

5.2.1.4 Entertainment

Entertainment systems in PICUs and NICUs are primarily for families and patients. Wrench and Vyas (1995) recommend the presence of televisions for parents, and toys and a playroom for siblings as a means of reducing anxiety. Access to computers is also recommended. While I was unable to find studies on the presence of television in PICUs, at least one research team (Guttentag et al., 1983) expressed concern about the amount of indiscriminate television viewing in acute care pediatric inpatient rooms.

5.2.2 *Safety*

Safety is a broad category involving infection control, fall prevention, and medical error reduction. Infection control is critical to avoiding the pervasive spread of nosocomial infections to other patients.

Fall prevention has been addressed by many researchers, primarily with adult inpatient populations. This being the case, Graf (2005) studied the falls of children to determine whether the adult scales were appropriate. In a study of 100 children who fell and 100 who did not, significant risk factors included length of stay, physical and occupational therapy, orthopedic diagnosis, use of seizure medication, and being IV/Heparin Lock free. In another study of tools for measuring the likelihood of falls, Razmus et al. (2006) concluded that episodes of disorientation and previous fall history were the best predictors.

Medication errors (typically, accidental distribution of inappropriate types or dosages of medications) are common on pediatric inpatient units (Kaushal et al., 2001). Several factors appear to contribute to medication errors, including noise, distractions, and light levels. Researchers have noted a specific link between light levels and wakefulness in nursing units (Sagha Zadeh, 2012). As most medication errors occur in dispensing, data on pharmacist behavior is of particular merit.

Studies suggest a relationship between distractions and pharmacist errors (Flynn et al., 1999), as well as light levels and pharmacist errors (Flynn et al., 1996).

5.2.2.1 Safety in PICUs

As with all inpatient facilities, infection control and medical errors are critical issues. Rice and Nelson (2005) summarized the need for safety in a PICU. Recommendations included improved communication, severity of diagnosis, mortality potential, catheter-related infections, unexpected endotracheal extubations, medication errors, and restraints. Sources of and statistics relating to adverse events (AEs) in pediatric intensive care are provided by Monroe et al. (2011) and Agarwal et al. (2011). Buckley et al. (2007) observed AEs and found 3.6 events per 100, which was comparable to other studies.

Several studies and reviews address infection control (e.g. Mello et al., 2009). Ben-Abraham et al. (2002) noted that PICU isolation rooms resulted in a reduction in the number of respiratory and urinary nosocomial infections (NIs), as well as a reduction in catheter infections. Deep and colleagues (2004) found that the rate of NIs was 27.3 percent, or 16.2 per 100 days, and Archibald et al. (1997) observed that NIs increased as a result of duration of PICU stay. Gupta et al. (2011) found that hospital-acquired infection (HAI) rates were 19.3/100, resulting in longer lengths of stay and higher mortality. Archibald and colleagues (1997) provide evidence that infections are negatively associated with the nursing hour-to-patient day ratio. Factors impacting risk have been found to be nutrition, Pediatric Risk of Mortality III-24 scores, post-operative care and invasive device use (Singh-Naz et al., 2000).

5.2.2.2 Safety in NICUs

One of the most comprehensive articles on safety in the NICU was written by Samra et al. (2011). These authors point out that medication errors are most common in premature babies, particularly those less than 30 weeks' gestational age and weighing less than 1,500 grams. Among the most frequent adverse events in the NICU include nosocomial infections (28%), catheter infiltrates (16%), intracranial hemorrhage and ischemia (10.5%), and accidental extubation (8%). Samra and colleagues identify the unique aspects of NICUs that contribute to potential risk as:

- The limited capacity to buffer the consequences of unintended medical treatment.
- Extended lengths of stay.
- The neonate's quickly evolving body size and use of off-label medications.
- The neonate's inability to directly communicate what he or she is experiencing.
- Lack of development of body systems that interferes with the absorption, metabolism, distribution, and excretion of drugs, resulting in greater likelihood of toxicity.

These issues, added to human factors such as lack of experience, inappropriate sense of security, fatigue, and, most importantly, lack of communication, are the most significant sources of error (Samra et al., 2011).

Regarding infection control, Johnson et al. (2010) found that MRSA was most common in very young children who had been in neonatal and pediatric intensive care. Larson et al. (2005)

examined the use of hand washing versus alcohol in an NICU and found the bacteria levels to be the same.

5.2.3 *Private rooms*

5.2.3.1 PICU private versus shared rooms

Several convincing studies suggest that private rooms reduce the frequency of HAI. However, Rose and Blythe (2008) conducted an extensive literature review on private versus shared pediatric rooms and, while normally supporting the use of private rooms, suggested cohorting as an alternative response in some cases due to the psychological importance of not being alone. Similarly, Morgan (2010) examined standard versus private pediatric patient room arrangements through a literature review, as well as surveys of professionals, children, and young people, and concluded that shared rooms should not be completely excluded.

This need for companionship may not be salient for PICUs as children in these units are frequently sedated and unable to interact with others. Based on the literature on adult rooms, most of the evidence for PICUs is that these should be private.

Recent research by Laura Poltronieri and colleagues set about exploring the impact of PICU private rooms on family behavior, staff patterns, and quality/safety measures. They found that with private rooms, the number of visitors and the durations of their visits were higher, nursing presence was higher, lengths of stay were shorter, and adverse events were fewer (Poltronieri and Schleien, 2010). This study is described in detail in the guest essay.

How PICU design impacts visitor behaviors, staff patterns, and quality/safety measures

Laura Poltronieri, AIA

The pediatric critical care unit is an extremely high-stress area in any children's hospital. New physical models of care, specifically private patient/family rooms, are being designed to address issues of family-focused care, patient/family visual and acoustic privacy, decreasing lengths of stay, and infection control. These emerging private room models often pose challenges to clinical staff who are used to working in more open environments.

Clinical staff members frequently express concerns that private rooms may compromise care or endanger their pediatric patients because of their perception of reduced staff visibility and greater distances to patients. Some staff members have suggested that design of these new family-focused units may lead to increases in unplanned extubation rates. Staff members also frequently express the opinion that open-cubicle curtained bays are the safest physical model in which to provide pediatric critical care, because they believe that staff members have greater visualization and awareness throughout the unit and can be at the bedside quicker when an emergency occurs. This research study set out to determine if these ideas about the relative safety of various physical models of PICU design were in fact true.

Study approach

Phase 1 of this study attempted to examine whether staff concerns for patient safety in private room models are warranted. This IRB approved research study systematically examined three pediatric intensive care units, all within the Morgan Stanley Children's Hospital of New York. The fact that all three PICUs, each with its distinct physical configuration, occur within one floor level of three interconnected buildings afforded a unique opportunity to compare safety data as well as visitor and nursing activity across all three models.

The specific research questions posed by the study included the following:

- Patient outcomes and unit safety
  - Do self-extubation rates differ between the three units?
  - Do medical errors and adverse event rates differ between the three units?
- Patient length of stay
  - Does acuity adjusted length of stay differ between the three units?
- Staffing patterns
  - Does percentage of nursing time at the bedside vary between the units?
- Family presence
  - Does the amount of on-unit and in-room family presence differ between the three units?

The three different physical configurations observed included the following:

1. 14-bed open unit with cubicle curtained bays; each bay approximately 155 NSF.
2. 13-bed unit with sliding glass fronts and glazed side walls with inter-connecting glass doors; each bay approximately 230 NSF.
3. 14-bed unit with sliding glass fronts and solid (opaque) side walls; each bay approximately 270 NSF.

A sample total of 8,416 on-site observation events, conducted during the course of seven days and four nights, included detailed activity mapping of patients, families, and staff on all three PICUs. The aggregate data generated from this environmental mapping process underwent thorough statistical analysis by an academic statistician.

Study subjects

The study subjects involved were 137 pediatric inpatients who were observed in their hospital rooms during 11 observation periods on seven calendar days in spring 2010. Their median age was 24 months with 32 percent under 12 months, an additional 31 percent aged 12–71 months, 20 percent aged 72–179 months, and 17 percent 180 months and older; 48 percent were female. In each of these observation periods, data was collected every 20 minutes, with a mean of 27.8 observations per child over multiple periods.

Since most subjects were observed for more than one period ($M = 2.30$ periods), the mean across all observations was calculated for each subject, and these means were used in all subsequent analyses. All variables were screened for violations of assumptions for GLM.

Almost every variable showed substantial skewness and/or kurtosis. We therefore used non-parametric statistics to analyze all variables. The age variable showed particularly severe skew, so subjects were divided into the four age bands described above; this variable was used in all subsequent analyses. A series of independent-samples median tests (the non-parametric equivalent to a one-way ANOVA) showed significant differences between PICU units on virtually all variables.

Additional study process and protocols

In addition, this in-depth research project used numerous multivariable research protocols in combination with one another to generate a comprehensive understanding of the impact which various PICU design features have on patients, family members, and staff. Phases 2 and 3 of the study included the following:

- Analysis of five-year historical patient outcome data, including lengths of stay, adverse medical event reporting systems data, and unplanned extubation rates.
- Thirty-one nursing questionnaire responses provided by nursing staff from the three units under observation.
- Eighty-two additional nursing questionnaires distributed among PICU nursing staff of three other children's hospitals.

Data analysis

Some of the most interesting findings from the study include the following:

- Family and visitor presence was significantly higher on the two units with private rooms versus the open-bay unit with cubicle curtains. This increased visitor presence included greater total number of visitors, greater number of visitors present at one time, as well as visitors present for longer periods of time. There were also fewer instances of patients with no visitors in these two private room units.
- Nursing presence at the bedside was greater in both private room models than in the open bay unit.
- The private room PICU with solid side walls had lower ALOS, accidental extubation rates, and adverse medical events reported than the other two units.
- Nursing presence at bedside was greater in both private room models than in the open-bay unit, with by far the greatest nursing presence occurring in the unit equipped with inroom charting computers. Nurses reported that with inroom computers family members often complain that they cannot readily find their nurse when they are charting in another patient room on the unit.
- In the private room unit with glass side walls, the interconnecting glass doors and side cubicle curtains were closed and drawn during 100 percent of all observations, which called into question the necessity and additional cost of these component items.
- Cubicle curtains were most likely to be open in the private room models, and more likely to be fully drawn in the open-bay unit. This finding challenges nursing staff's belief that patient visibility is greater in the open-bay unit.
- Nurses from all four children's hospitals reported that it is more important to see patients' monitors than to see the patients themselves.

- When away from the bedside nurses reported that it is more important to visualize their co-workers than it is to visualize their patients or patient monitors.
- Based on observation, during code events, team rounding, and end-of-life care as many as 20 people may be present at the bedside. The private room unit with 270 NSF per bed was the only one with room size that allowed for the entire rounding team to be present at the bedside at one time.
- ICU patients occupying rooms with window seats were more likely to get out of bed.
- According to questionnaire responses, "views to outdoors" and "quality of natural light" were highly ranked by nurses as "contributing to the quality of care."
- Other key unit attributes that nurses felt affected quality of patient care include the following:
  - Convenient location of hand hygiene stations.
  - Soothing interior ambience.
  - Size of patient care area around the bed.
  - Amount of storage space at bedside for supplies and equipment.
  - Charting medical record order entry system.
  - Relationship of nurse charting station to patients.
  - Relationship of additional nurse work areas to patients.
  - Distance from shared supply and equipment areas to patients.
  - Amount of proximal on-unit storage space for supplies and equipment.

Collaboration acknowledgment

Charles L. Schleien, MD, MBA, Clinical Sponsor, Research Co-investigator

Former Executive Vice Chairman, Department of Pediatrics

Professor of Pediatrics and Anesthesiology, Columbia University College of Physicians and Surgeons

New York-Presbyterian Morgan Stanley Children's Hospital

Jennifer Cromley, PhD, Assistant Professor, Temple University, Research Data Analyst

Project location

Morgan Stanley Children's Hospital of New York-Presbyterian

165th Street & Broadway, New York, NY 10032.

5.2.3.2 NICU single family versus open-bay rooms

Of all the topics that have been studied and discussed over the past decade regarding NICU design, the impact of single family rooms (SFRs) is undoubtedly the most common. One of the primary motivators behind these studies has been to encourage parental presence in the NICU, and researchers have shown that parents who stay on the unit are more involved with their children's care than those who stay elsewhere (Wigert, 2010).

Parental involvement improves NICU patient outcomes. For example, sleep is critical to the NICU baby's health (Colombo and De Bon, 2011), and Morgan et al. (2011) found a 176 percent increase in autonomic activity and an 86 percent decrease in quiet sleep when mother and child were separated, as opposed to engaging in skin-to-skin contact. Parent speech also impacts the occurrence and number of vocalizations in preterm infants (Caskey et al., 2011). Multiple authors have discussed the positive impact of single family versus open-bay NICU designs on parental interaction (e.g. Bowie et al., 2003; Brown and Taquino, 2001; McGrath, 2005; White, 2003, 2004, 2011).

Rather than describing in detail the content of each of the SFR versus open-bay studies, Figure 5.2 summarizes a representative sample. In addition, the comments of Dr. Robert White (see guest essay) provide a clear description of the status of this topic. Most research supports the use of SFRs with the exception of Pineda et al. (2013), who noted potential negative neurodevelopmental outcomes for SFR babies. However, the outcomes may be the result of leaving babies alone in private rooms rather than the SFRs themselves.

Figure 5.2: *Examples of research on NICU single family rooms*

Citation	*Outcome measures*	*Conclusions*
Carter, Carter, & Bennett (2008)	Length of stay, environmental stimuli, access to caregivers, access to information, personal privacy	The SFR is perceived by parents to offer an improved spacious environment that is less overstimulating for the infant and themselves. Access to staff, information, and overall support appears to be improved in spite of a larger overall floor area.
DiFiori & Schirripa (2013)	Infection, parental outcomes, parental satisfaction patient outcomes	SR mothers more likely to breast feed; parents visited longer and were more satisfied. Infection frequency unchanged.
Domanico, Davis, Coleman, & Davis (2011)	PEMR, mortality and nosocomial events, discharge weight, lengths and head circumferences, respiratory and nutritional parameters, breastfeeding success, noise level, illumination, air quality	Infants in the SFR unit had fewer apneic events, reduced nosocomial infections, and mortality. More mothers sustained mature milk lactation, and more infants were discharged breastfeeding.
Greer & Black (2013)	Length of stay, costs, walking behavior, parent satisfaction, family overnight, visitors	Families in SFR NICUs were more satisfied.
Harris, Shepley, White, Kolberg, & Harrell (2006)	Space allocations, construction costs, staff preferences and perceptions, and occupant behaviors	SFR NICU design provides solutions for increasing parent privacy and presence, supporting Health Insurance Portability and Accountability Act compliance, minimizing the number of undesirable beds, increasing staff satisfaction and reducing staff stress.
Oelrich (2003)	Patient outcomes, ALOS, communication, staffing, infection	Good communication was found in the SFR. There was an increase in nosocomial infections at one site which may have been due to carpet or increased acuity.

Citation	*Outcome measures*	*Conclusions*
Pineda et al. (2013)	Hemispheric asymmetry, cerebral maturation, language development	Infants in SFRs had a diminution of normal hemispheric asymmetry, lower amplitude EEG maturation, and lower language scores at 2 years.
Rosenblum (2005)	Weight, days requiring TPN, infections	The SFR demonstrated higher weight gain, fewer days before parental nutrition, and fewer HAIs.
Shepley, Harris, & White (2008)	Job Satisfaction Scale, Nurse Stress Scale, Satisfaction and perception of physical environment	SFR NICU design may increase staff satisfaction and reduce staff stress.
Shepley, Harris, White, & Steinberg (2008)	Behavioral observation of families	More frequent interactions were found in open-bay units, but longer interactions in SFRs. Recommended that open-bay units provide spaces for longer encounters, and that SFRs provide spaces that allow for spontaneous encounters.
Smith, Schoenbeck, & Clayton (2009)	staff perceptions and performance	Rankings of overall physical environment, patient care, job, technology, and off-the-job quality significantly improved in the SFR, but evaluations of patient care team interaction significantly declined. No meaningful changes from results were found up to 22 months afterwards.
Smithgall (2010)	HRV (heart rate variability), cardiac interbeat intervals, continuous electrocardiogram	The single private room encourages parental access to infants but does not impact maternal stress.
Stevens, Helseth, Khan, Munson, & Smith (2010)	Quality of employment, quality of work environment, quality of patient care, job quality in NICU, health and safety, safety and security, interaction with NICU team, interaction with technology, off-job quality of life, overall satisfaction	Staff perceptions of workplace quality were significantly higher in the SFR than the open-bay NICU. Exceptions were some aspects of health and safety, nature of interaction with NICU teams, and off-job quality of life.
Swanson, Peters & Lee (2012)	Teamwork, communication, development, facility, safety, and privacy	Advanced practitioners reported higher teamwork, but nurses did not. Nurse satisfaction initially higher in SFR, but declined.
Walsh, McCullough, & White (2006)	Observations of the nurses guided by a questionnaire identifying benefits, risks, and patient safety concerns	SFR is thought to be more effective for patient care and parent satisfaction compared to open bay. However, nurses believe success depends on sufficient staff, due to decreased patient visibility and longer distances. Large units present quality improvement, communication, and staff training challenges.

Securing the benefits of single family rooms

Robert White, MD

The transition to private rooms (perhaps more appropriately termed single family rooms) in the NICU has taken longer than in other areas of the hospital, for a variety of reasons. Administrators have been reluctant to give large expanses of real estate to a discipline formerly housed in a much smaller area, clinicians were reluctant to surrender the ability to have all their patients and colleagues within visual range, and valid questions lingered about the safety and value of private rooms in the NICU, where proven adult benefits such as a reduction in falls and improvement in patient satisfaction might not apply. To be sure, there are significant pros and cons to private rooms in the NICU. Proven benefits include increased family participation (Carter et al., 2008), presence (Carter et al., 2008; Pineda et al., 2012), and satisfaction (Stevens et al., 2011) with a concomitant improvement in infant length of stay (Ortenstrand et al., 2010), chronic lung disease (Orstenstrand et al., 2010), and apnea (Domanico et al., 2011). Babies may also benefit from a reduction in noise and risk of infection (Domanico et al., 2011). Caregivers generally consider private rooms beneficial to babies, families, and themselves (Smith et al., 2009; Stevens et al., 2010). Privacy for families is clearly improved, but this can be a double-edged sword, as both families (Pineda et al., 2012) and caregivers (Smith et al., 2009) can experience a sense of isolation and stress. This may even be true for babies, whose verbal development may be delayed in a private room setting if the family is not present most of the day.

Securing the benefits of private rooms while avoiding the hazards is both a design and operational challenge, one that has been successfully achieved in a number of pioneering NICUs. Two key elements of the design strategy are outlined below.

Design places and programs that encourage families and staff to gather

Collaboration is difficult in a NICU with private rooms arranged on either side of a long hallway with no central gathering area for staff or families (Smith et al., 2009). Identifying a small area at the end of the hallway with a window, comfortable seating, and liquid refreshments will allow families to meet casually near their babies' rooms without having to leave the unit. Perhaps they need to leave the room while the baby is having a procedure, but want to come right back when it is done. Or perhaps the baby is sleeping but they want to be nearby when he or she wakes up, or if the doctor comes by on rounds. Leaving the area to go to a family lounge or waiting room isn't nearly as attractive as having a place very near their baby's room.

For staff, "fly-by" or decentralized stations outside the rooms are convenient, but miss the fact that NICU nurses depend on team work – starting an IV, retaping an ET tube, orienting a new staff member – and the need for collaboration is an important medical need, and we learn from the social sciences an important psychological need as well. Ideally, private rooms would be arranged in clusters, or neighborhoods, that have "homes" (private rooms) for babies, "places of business" (nursing stations) for staff, and "parks" (general gathering areas) for both. For staffing purposes, these neighborhoods should be no fewer than eight beds, and preferably 10 to 12 beds so that a single nurse won't be responsible for the entire cluster when one of her colleagues has to leave the area (Walsh et al., 2006).

Provide options

Private rooms are not ideal for everyone. A family with twins or higher order multiples whose parents would like them to be in the same room is an obvious example. Babies whose parents rarely visit may be another example, especially when they are in cribs and could hear human voices from elsewhere in a multi-bed room but would be isolated with little verbal stimulus in a private room. Nils Bergman also points out that in many parts of Africa, being placed in a private room is the equivalent of solitary confinement – culturally, privacy is not always valued as highly as being part of a community, even during breast-feeding or similar activities that many Westerners would prefer to do in private.

The ideal unit design, then, provides options. Does the family prefer to stay in a private room with their baby(s)? There should be enough private and twin rooms with family space that supports their presence 24/7 to accommodate this. Likewise, there should be shared space for babies whose parents visit rarely and don't stay long when they do come, or babies whose parents would prefer to be in a room with a few other babies and families. Operationalizing this depends somewhat on the total bed number and on the configuration of the space available. In a hypothetical 40-bed unit, one might design two four-bed rooms for unrelated babies and the occasional higher order multiples, four twin rooms (this number will be very dependent on the unit's experience with twins – more in hospitals with an active infertility program, fewer in free-standing children's hospitals), and the remainder as private rooms.

One final option that should be considered, if permitted by the state's codes and certificate of need process, is to design some or all of the private rooms with enough space and headwall capacity for one critically ill infant which could also serve two intermediate infants in an overflow situation.

It is vitally important to recognize that private rooms by themselves are not the source of good neonatal outcomes. Extended, intimate human contact, especially with the parents and most especially with the mother, is crucial to optimal neonatal outcomes (White, 2011). Babies in a unit that is well designed, but where staff fail to fully encourage parental participation in care, will not experience their full potential.

References

Carter, B.S., Carter, A., and Bennett, S. (2008). Families' views upon experiencing change in the neonatal intensive care unit environment from the "baby barn" to the private room. *Journal of Perinatology, 28*, 827–829.

Domanico, R., Davis, D.K., Coleman, F., and Davies, B.O. (2011). Documenting the NICU design dilemma: Comparative patient progress in open-ward and single family room units. *Journal of Perinatology, 31*, 281–288.

Ortenstrand, A., Westrup, B., Brostrom, E.B., et al. (2010). The Stockholm neonatal family-centered care study: Effects on length of stay and infant morbidity. *Pediatrics, 125*, e278–e285.

Pineda, R.G., Stransky, K.E., Rogers, C., et al. (2012). The single-patient room in the NICU: Maternal and family effects. *Journal of Perinatology, 32*, 545–551.

Smith, T.J., Schoenbeck, K., and Clayton, S. (2009). Staff perceptions of work quality of a neonatal intensive care unit before and after transition from an open bay to a private room design. *Work, 33*, 211–227.

Stevens, D.C., Helseth, C.C., Khan, M.A., et al. (2010). Neonatal intensive care nursery staff perceive enhanced workplace quality with the single-family room design. *Journal of Perinatology, 30*, 352–358.

Stevens, D.C., Helseth, C.C., Khan, M.A., et al. (2011). A comparison of parent satisfaction in an open-bay and single-family room neonatal intensive care unit. *Health Environments Research and Design, 4*, 110–123.

Walsh, W.F., McCullough, K.L., and White, R.D. (2006). Nurses' perception of providing care in a single room newborn intensive care setting. *Advanced Neonatal Care, 6*, 261–270.

White, R.D. (2011). The NICU environment of care: How we got here, where we're headed, and why. *Seminars in Perinatology, 35*, 2–7.

5.3 Research on needs of PICU patients, families and staff

5.3.1 *Patient needs*

Regarding the specific needs of children, there is little information. Most researchers assume that they have similar requirements to those of adults; for example, the need to feel safe, the need for control (ability to manipulate the physical environment), access to visitors when desired, and the need for information. In one of few studies relating to pediatric intensive care, Karande et al. (2005) gathered input from children who had spent time in PICUs in India. The children made suggestions regarding increased comfort, and expressed a desire to not be exposed to procedures done on other children. This latter preference suggests the need for options for physical separation between children during procedures.

Another significant need of patients is to be able to rest. Berens (1999) conducted a literature review on the impact of noise and suggests that this could result in sleep disruption, hearing impairment, and stress in PICUs. Protocols recommended to control inappropriate noise levels include staff behavioral modification, changes in the environmental design, and the introduction of noise-canceling equipment.

In a broader study, including noise and other factors, Al-Samsam and Cullen (2005) examined sound level, staff interventions, and sleep in PICU children, and found that sound during the day is significantly louder than in the evenings, although the frequency of tactile encounters with staff remained the same. Patients wakened an average of 40 times per night and REMs were lower than a typical population of children. According to a pediatric patient interviewed in a study by Bishop (2008, p. 140),

> Although personally my main objection … is the fact that during the night and the early morning there's still light coming. … Noises. There's still noises of people around, they're really the main problems.

Regarding children's needs within the physical environment, one pre-/post-occupancy evaluation addressed pediatric acute care unit preferences. Shepley et al. (2012) compared a traditional room to a remodeled patient room that included more family space, more storage, variety in the ceiling design, entertainment and positive distractions, and large family areas. Using a facility evaluation checklist and the PedsQL survey instruments developed by Dr. James Varni, the researchers found that the new environment was rated more highly, but the differences in the PedsQL scores were insignificant.

5.3.1.1 Patient stress

Researchers generally agree that many adults experience disorientation and delirium after spending time in an intensive care unit. Ward-Begnoche (2007), and Silver et al. (2010) argue that this phenomenon also occurs in children in PICUs. According to these authors, after leaving the unit children report delusional experiences, which may be related to Post Traumatic Stress Disorder (PTSD).

In Rhonda Board's 2005 study, she contacted PICU graduates and asked open-ended questions about their experiences. The researchers calibrated the frequency of coping strategies and used drawings by children to evaluate stress levels. Board found that most children had some remembrance of their stay. Interactions with staff were thought of as good, but generally children did not like their PICU experience. Drawings did not demonstrate a high level of anxiety, in spite of the fact that coping strategies were few. One of Board's conclusions is that PICU patients be given opportunities for therapeutic play as a coping strategy.

Board notes that intubation reduces the opportunity to exercise coping techniques, so the potential exists that this group is particularly challenged. However, the negative experience of intubated children might not be critical if they are appropriately sedated and do not recall it (cf. Playfor et al., 2000).

5.3.1.2 Patient satisfaction

Karande et al. (2005) found relatively neutral responses when asking children about their PICU experience. In their study involving an Asian Indian population, 74 percent of the children had average impressions, 18 percent had negative impressions, and 16 percent had positive impressions. In terms of specific experiences, 52 percent of the children mentioned their impressions about the cleanliness of the environment, 64 percent remembered being afraid, 74 percent recalled being in pain, and 18 percent reported sleep disturbance. Playfor et al. (2000) interviewed children who had been discharged from a PICU in the UK and found that most of their recollections were neutral (60%) or positive (25%). Remembrance of pain was considerably lower – only 24 percent. According to this research team, those children who had been mechanically ventilated and sedated had little recollection of intubation. In summary, the evidence on pain in PICUs in developing countries suggests that proactive steps should be taken regarding pain management (Vidyasagar, 2005).

5.3.1.3 Examples of patient spaces in PICUs

Figures 5.3 to 5.10 are examples of patient spaces in PICUs in approximate chronological order. The location, design firm(s), and photo credit are provided. These examples are remarkable for the wide range in the design attributes, the family amenities, and room size.

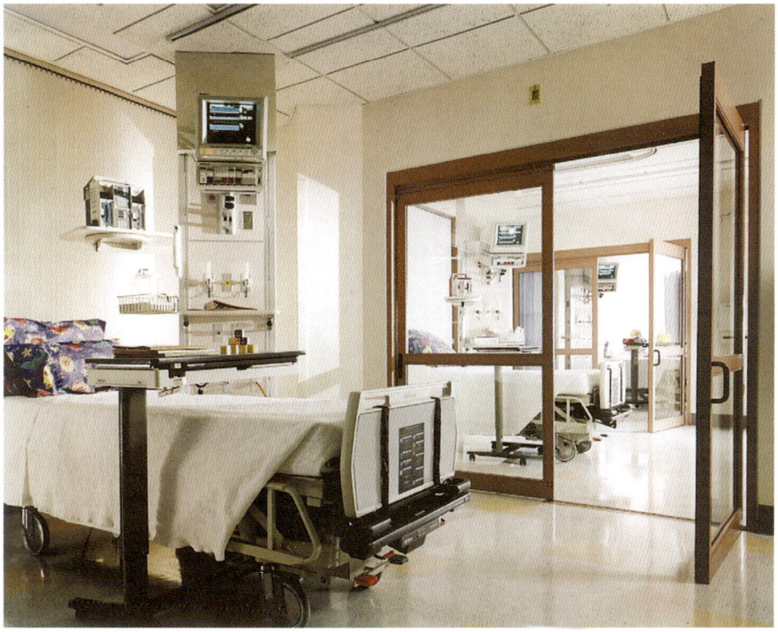

Figure 5.3: *Hasbro Children's Hospital PICU, Providence, RI (Architects: Shepley Bulfinch; Photo credit: Robert Miller)*

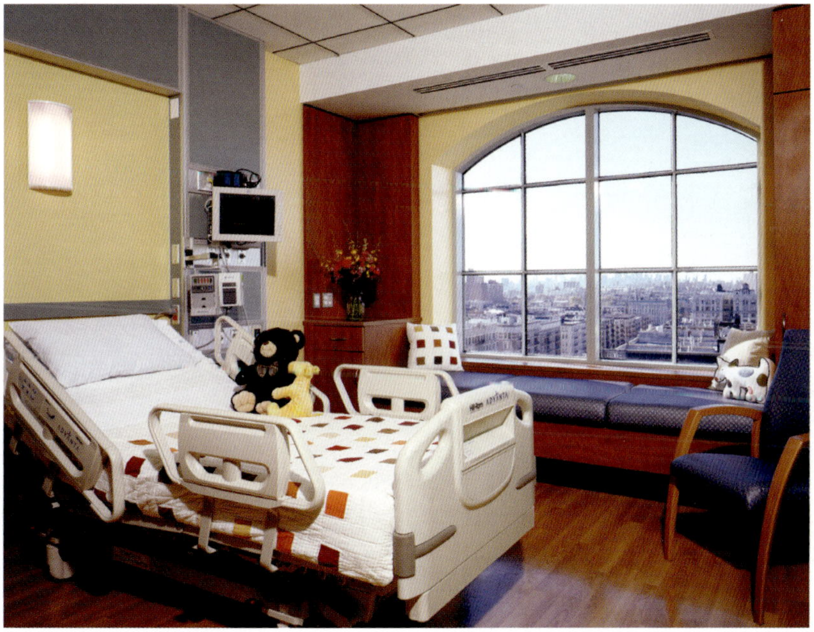

Figure 5.4: *New York-Presbyterian Morgan Stanley Children's Hospital PICU, New York, NY (Architects: Ewing Cole/Davis Brody Bond; Photo credit: Peter Paige Photography)*

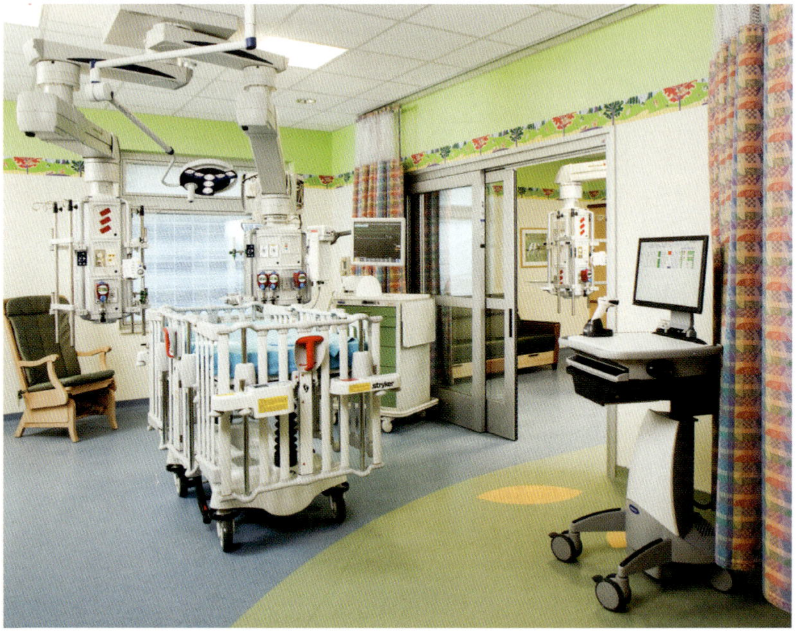

Figure 5.5: *Monroe Carell Jr. Children's Hospital at Vanderbilt PCCU, Nashville, TN (Architects: Earl Swensen Associates (ESa); Photo credit: Kyle Dreier/Courtesy of Esa)*

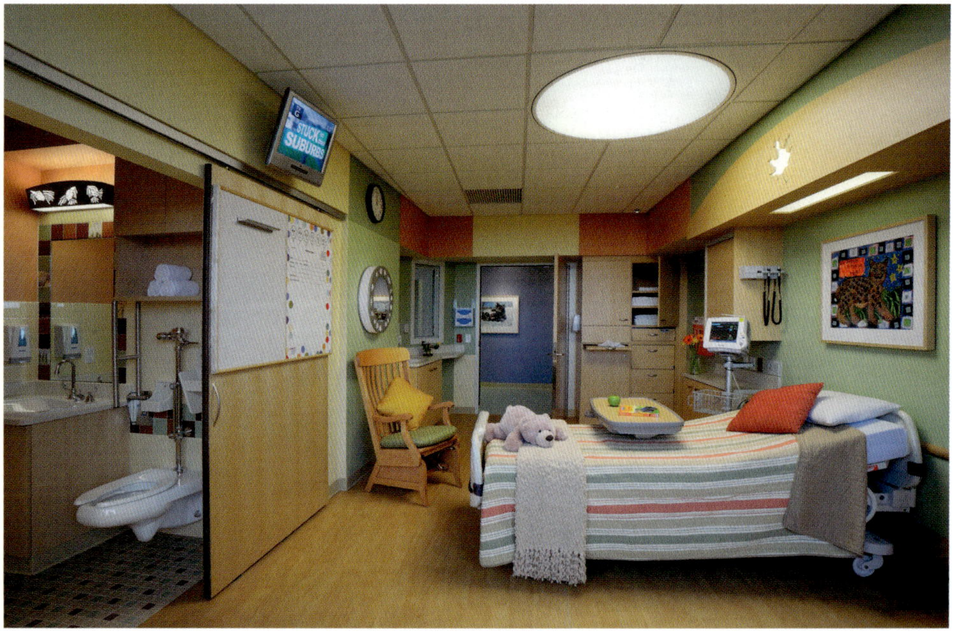

Figure 5.6: *American Family Children's Hospital PICU, Madison, WI (Architects: HDR; Photo credit: Ballogg Photography)*

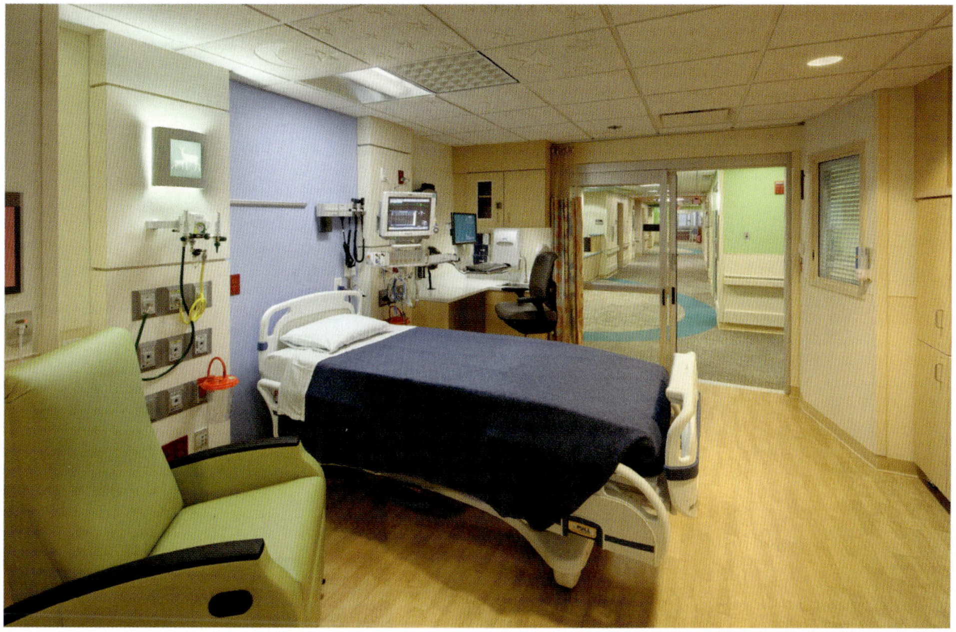

Figure 5.7: *Mercy Children's Hospital PICU, Creve Coeur, MO (Architects: Christner Inc.; Photo credit: Sam Fentress)*

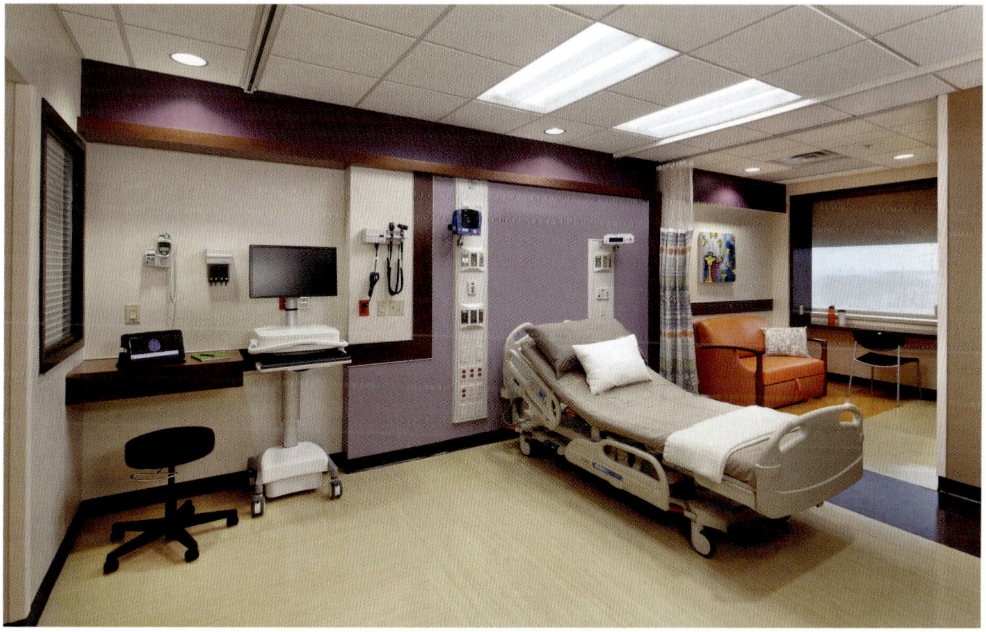

Figure 5.8: *Children's Hospitals and Clinics of Minnesota PICU, St. Paul, MN (Architects: HDR; Photo credit: Philip Prowse Photography)*

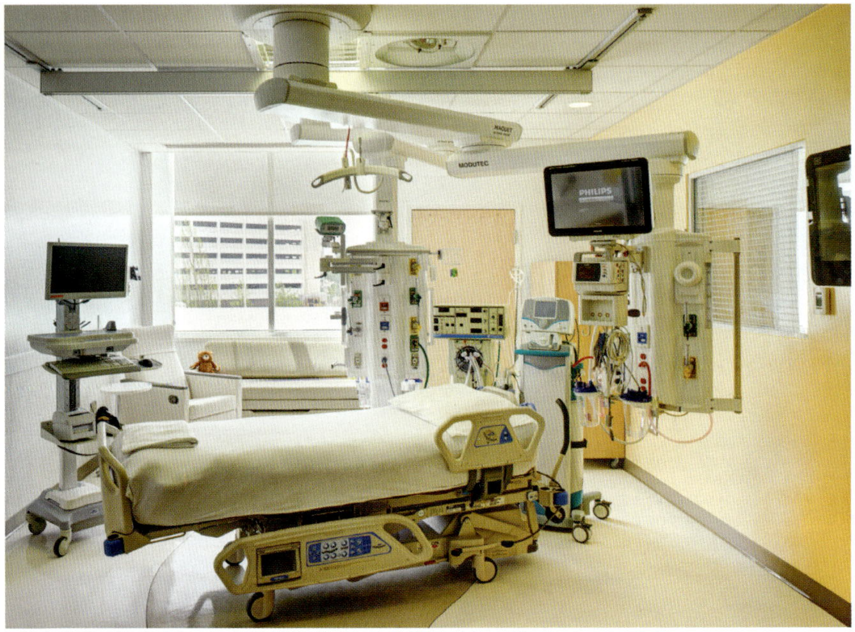

Figure 5.9: *Nationwide Children's Hospital PICU, Columbus, OH*
(Architects: FKP Architects;
Photo credit: Courtesy of FKP Architects)

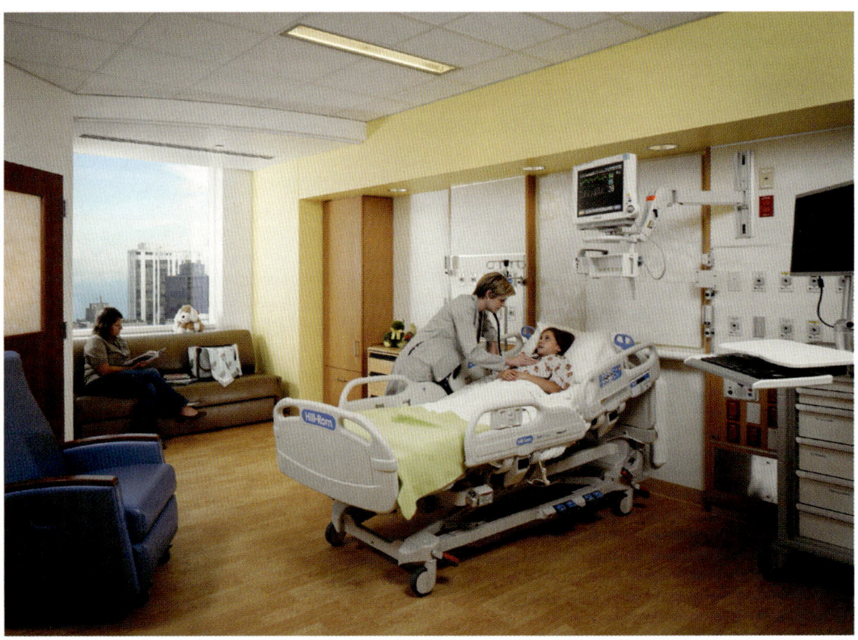

Figure 5.10: *Ann & Robert H. Lurie Children's Hospital of Chicago PICU, Chicago, IL*
(Architects: ZGF Architects LLP, Solomon Cordwell Buenz, Anderson Mikos Architects, Ltd.;
Photo credit: Nick Merrick © Hedrich Blessing)

5.3.2 Family needs

Although little has been written about patient needs in a PICU, there are a few studies that address pediatric family needs in an inpatient setting. The challenges to parents are multiple: difficulties in communication, a disconnect between the parental role at home and that in the hospital, and being placed in a high-stakes learning environment (Graham et al., 2009). The need for improved communication and greater parental participation are common topics in the literature (e.g. Latour et al., 2011).

Of the top 20 needs of families from a paper by Latour et al. (2008), the majority concern communication and information, in addition to knowing that the child is being treated for pain, and the ability to see him and her frequently. The theme of needing to be with the child has appeared in other studies (e.g. Heuer, 1993; Kasper and Nyamathi, 1988) as well as the need for information (Farrell and Frost, 1992). In a survey by Gold et al. (2006), the majority of PICU healthcare providers felt that family members would want to be present even during resuscitation (although this might make it more stressful for the physicians).

The Critical Care Family Needs Inventory (CCFNI) (Leske, 1991) has frequently been used to ascertain family needs. Using this tool, with modifications for pediatric application and demographic information, a study by Scott (1998) found strong similarities between family and staff perceptions of family needs. These needs included items that were similar to previous studies – information, assurance and proximity to the child. The research underlines the importance of incorporating parent contributions into a plan of care.

Lack of sleep is a common condition of parents of a child in the PICU and there is a clear need to make the inpatient units as peaceful and stress-free as possible. Stremler et al. (2008) asked parents via open-ended questions to discuss sources of sleep disruption. In addition to stress and modified sleep habits, parents identified the physical environment as challenging to sleep patterns. Using the PSS:PICU (Carter and Miles, 1989) tool, Smith et al. (2007) found that providing a bed in a patient PICU room resulted in lower stress levels.

5.3.2.1 Family stress

There are several studies that confirm the high stress levels of PICU parents, and evidence suggests that PICU parents suffer from PTSD (Balluffi et al., 2004). Needle et al. (2009) tested parental medical comprehension and anxiety in the first 24 hours after admission and found that 21 of 34 had higher state anxiety measures than those with generalized anxiety disorder. Mechanical ventilation of one's child was a significant predictor of high stress. One of the interesting outcomes of this research is that physicians did not recognize the high stress levels of families.

Uncertainty has been a dominant theme regarding this stress. Turner et al. (1990) determined through parent interviews that uncertainty is the consequence of conflicting information, ambiguity, and perceived inefficiency. Needle and colleagues (2009) noted that only 30 percent of families appeared to understand the medical issues, which suggests the need for enhanced communication between families and medical staff.

One means of reducing stress is to provide parents with the opportunity to help manage their child's condition. Parental presence may impact both the child's perception of pain and the level of comfort and confidence of the parent regarding the child's care. Rennick et al. (2011) conducted semi-structured interviews in response to the experience of mothers engaged in a "Touch and Talk" pain management intervention and found it to be effective.

5.3.2.2 Family satisfaction

Patient and family satisfaction impacts the patient base for a facility. Researchers have found a positive relationship between patient satisfaction and the financial viability of a hospital (see Figure 5.11). In research cited by Hall (2008) done by Press Ganey, hospitals were clustered into quartiles based on profitability. The least profitable hospitals were demonstrated to have the lowest satisfaction ratings. One researcher suggests that improving patient satisfaction in a Midwestern academic medical center resulted in additional revenues of $2.3 million (Garman et al., 2004). In the case of intensive care, even though the return to the hospital may not be for the use of critical care services, loyalty may result in the use of other hospital services.

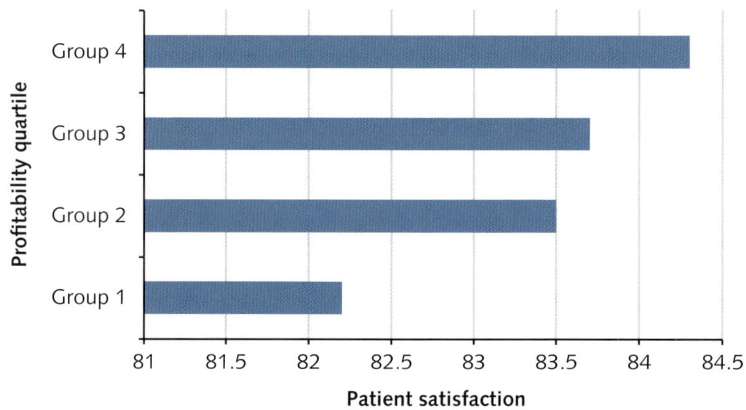

Figure 5.11: *Relationship between patient satisfaction and financial viability (Source: Derived from Hall, 2008)*

There are many activities that contribute to parental satisfaction, such as participating on medical rounds (Cameron et al., 2009), and the physical environment plays a significant role in supporting these events. Although not in a PICU setting, Sherman-Bien et al. (2011) conducted a study which demonstrated that satisfaction with the environment is a mediator between psychosocial functioning, and objective measures of the physical environment.

Issues relating to parental satisfaction have been addressed by architects worldwide. Guest authors Hallberg and Fröst describe similar objectives at the Neonatal ICU at the Karolinska Huddinge in their guest author essay.

5.3.2.3 Examples of family spaces in PICUs

Figures 5.12 to 5.18 are examples of family and shared spaces in PICUs in approximate chronological order. The location, design firm(s), and photo credit are provided. These spaces include circulation areas, lounges, sleep rooms, and areas outside nurses' stations.

Neonatal ICU at Karolinska Huddinge

Boubou Hallberg, MD, PhD

Peter Fröst, Architect, PhD, Professor

The reconstruction of the neonatal intensive care unit (NICU) at Karolinska University Hospital, Huddinge was conducted from 2007 to 2011. Neonatal care is a medical discipline that is progressing quickly and is constantly changing content. The old unit that needed to be replaced was finished only about 10 years ago. Since then, however, the numbers of beds and staff have increased significantly and the unit has moved from a Level II unit to a tertiary care unit and a regional center. The content of care changed in response to the more seriously ill infants in the department. Lack of space meant high stress for parents and problems with hospital-acquired multi-resistant bacteria (nosocomial infections). It also resulted in a poor working environment for staff in the old department.

The new neonatal ICU at Karolinska Huddinge is one of Europe's most modern neonatal units in operation. The department has 32 beds, including 12+2 for tertiary intensive care. Here, all newborns who need intensive care can have their parents living with them right next to the child's incubator 24/7. Avoiding separation of mother and child is a beacon of neonatal care at Karolinska University Hospital. Single rooms with shower and toilet for all families, large care surfaces, and the possibility of isolation are also built-in barriers to stop the spread of multi-resistant bacteria. The highest possible hygiene standard is a goal and the hospital has a zero vision for spreading infections. The department works both within Karolinska neonatal medicine and as part of a national network as a regional center. Activities such as systematic research, development, and quality work are steadily growing.

The process of designing the new neonatal unit has been unique and was performed using the Design Dialogue method. This is a design-driven approach for the early stages of building projects that is frequently used in healthcare planning in Sweden and has been developed by SWECO Architects. The work has been performed in close collaboration between architects, staff, and parents. Multi-professional innovation plays a crucial role. We worked in a series of interactive workshops where solutions and ideas were built jointly. Operation, care, and facilities developed in parallel. The space to which the project was initially predisposed was the same that the neonatal department used at that time. A first workshop identified goals and qualities of the project. The staff also made field trips to other new neonatal departments in Sweden and other countries. Studies and discussions of new research findings in neonatal family-centered care were implemented. In later workshops concrete proposals were built for solutions in support of the care process – both diagrammatic and room ideas. The architects transformed the solutions into layout proposals. During this work, it was discovered that the assigned area was not sufficient to meet the identified quality objectives. Hospital management then gave its permission to use more space. The proposal was thus developed. Various alternatives were evaluated using a scenario technique in combination with requirement analysis. A finished layout could then be selected. Since the renovation was done mainly in existing premises, implementation was carried out in two stages so that care could continue uninterrupted.

The department is a part of a large hospital complex and is situated on the seventh floor, accessed from the main communication corridor. There are two entrances to the department. A reception area and a large room where parents and relatives can stay and meet is connected to the "public" entrance. This is a "home-like" environment with a kitchen and comfortable furniture. The other entrance leads to the outpatient clinic and home care facilities. The department consists of several different parts and is organized following the child's process to leave the hospital to go home. The sickest infants are in the most interior and remote part of the NICU. The step-down unit with single rooms for the new family is situated closest to the entrance. Couplet care, where both the child and mother need hospital care, is provided at both Level III and Level II.

The NICU space is organized into four units with three patients each. Each patient has a private room that is open at one end for joint monitoring. A small room for parents with toilet and shower is connected to each patient room. In this way, no parent needs to be separated from his or her child. Mothers' beds are brought bedside to the incubator and care for the child is given skin to skin. In conjunction with the NICU facility is a nutritional lab and a pharmacy. Space is also available for private counseling of parents, education, and meditation.

The new design of the neonatal unit at Karolinska Huddinge is important to meet the needs of the family while at the same time maintaining the highest quality care, patient safety, and a good working environment. The families do not have to change department or staff when the infant's health status improves. When the child is better, there are step-down rooms on the same premises. Home healthcare also has its base within the new department. A vision of family-centered care with a coherent chain from intensive care to residential care at home has characterized the work.

5.3.3 Staff needs

5.3.3.1 Staff stress

Researchers have found that high stress levels and the challenges of caring for critically ill children and their families has an impact on job satisfaction, which in turn may influence retention (Bratt et al., 2000). While few studies focus specifically on pediatric critical care, multiple studies address the impact of stress on hospital staff and the resulting burn-out syndrome (e.g. Poncet et al., 2007). ICU physicians and nurses are reported to have more stressful jobs than the standard working population (Goodfellow et al., 1997). Self-perception of stress levels may be at variance with actual stress levels, however, as suggested by the following study.

Fischer et al. (2000) obtained cortisol samples of pediatric ICU (NICU and PICU) and intermediate care physicians and nurses to determine endocrine stress reactivity (see Figure 5.19). To control for confounding variables, data were gathered via questionnaires on experience, objective stress, workload, and emotional attitudes toward work. Stress levels among NICU and PICU physicians and nurses were significantly higher overall. Mean cortisol levels were lower in more experienced individuals, but only in individuals with more than eight years of experience, size, and frequency of reactions. Interestingly, a high proportion of individuals experienced endocrine reactions

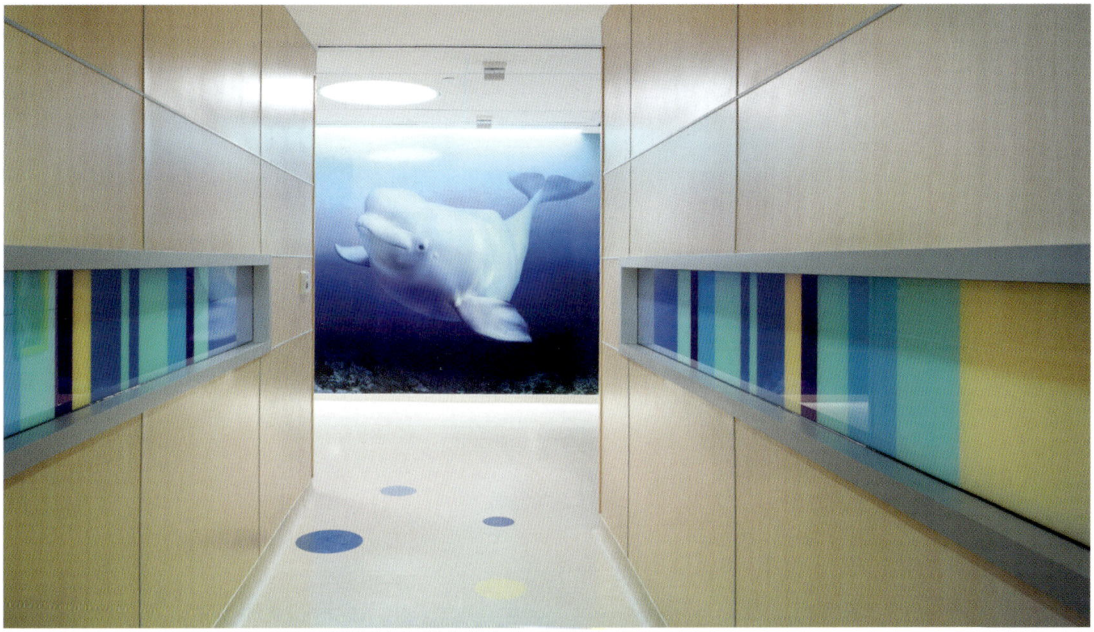

Figure 5.12: *Hospital for Sick Children Same Day Admit Unit, Toronto, Ontario, Canada (Architects: Zeidler Partnership Architects; Photo credit: Shai Gil)*

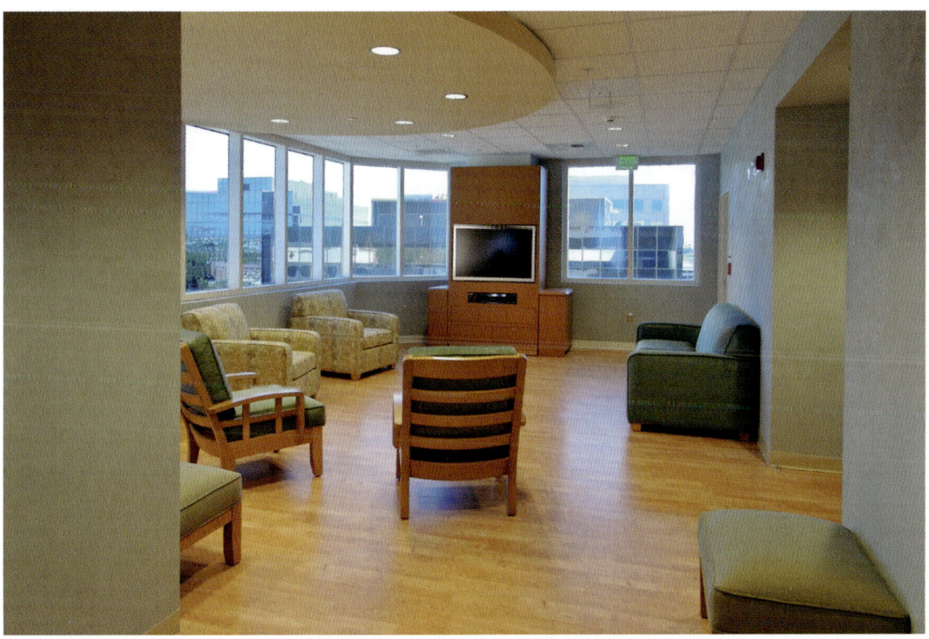

Figure 5.13: *Children's Hospital of Orange County PICU, Orange, CA (Architects: FKP Architects; Photo credit: Courtesy of FKP Architects)*

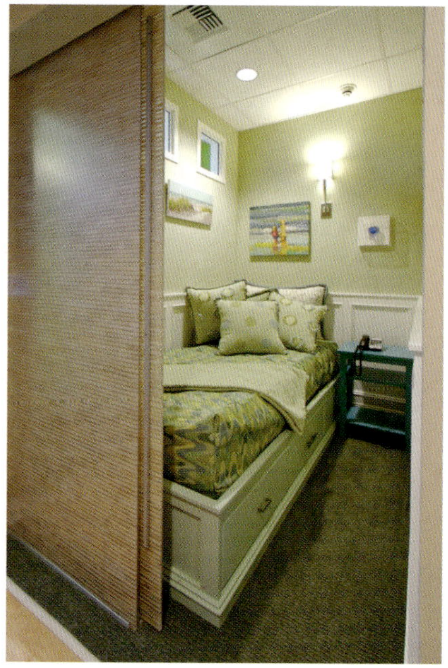

Figure 5.14: *Children's Hospital of Orange County PICU, Orange, CA (Architects: FKP Architects; Photo credit: Courtesy of FKP Architects)*

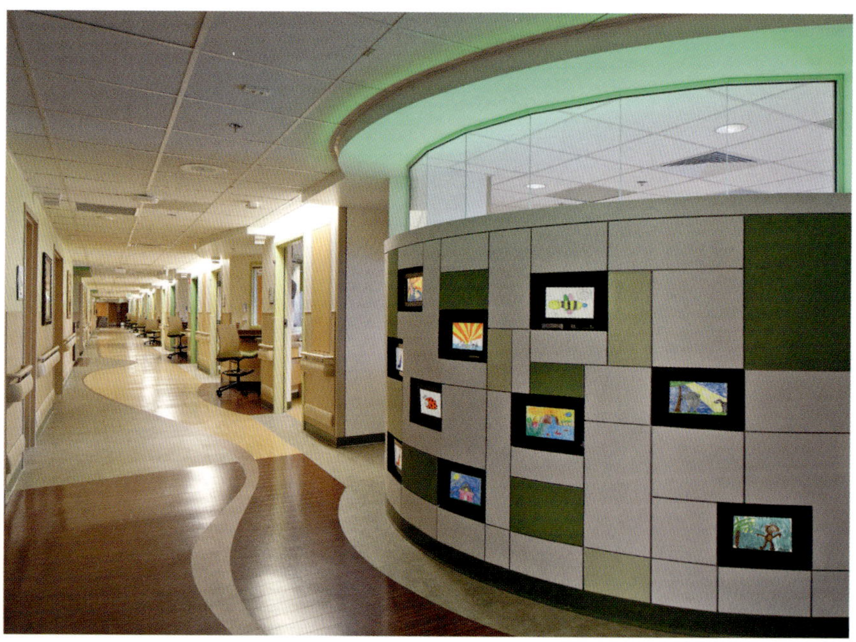

Figure 5.15: *Walt Disney Pavilion at Florida Hospital for Children PICU, Orlando, FL (Architects: Hunton Brady Architects; Photo credit: Ben Tanner)*

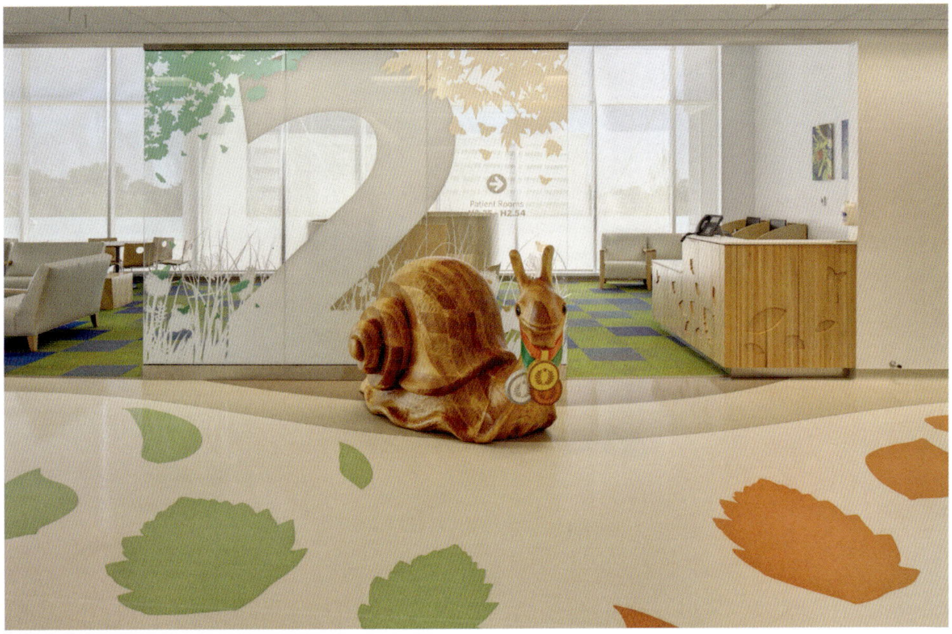

Figure 5.16: *Nationwide Children's Hospital PICU, Columbus, OH (Architects: FKP Architects; Photo credit: Courtesy of FKP Architects)*

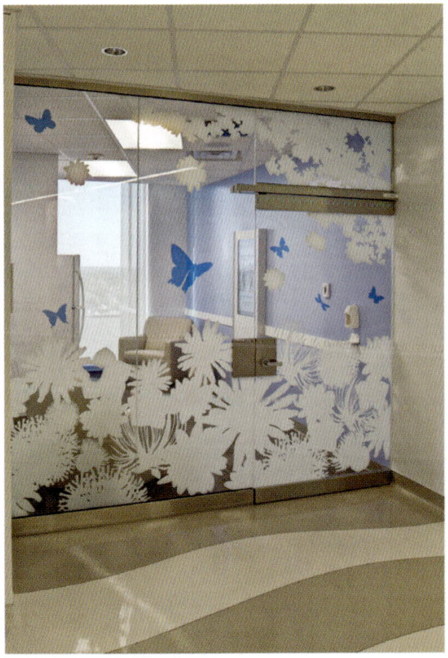

Figure 5.17: *Nationwide Children's Hospital PICU, Columbus, OH (Architects: FKP Architects; Photo credit: Courtesy of FKP Architects)*

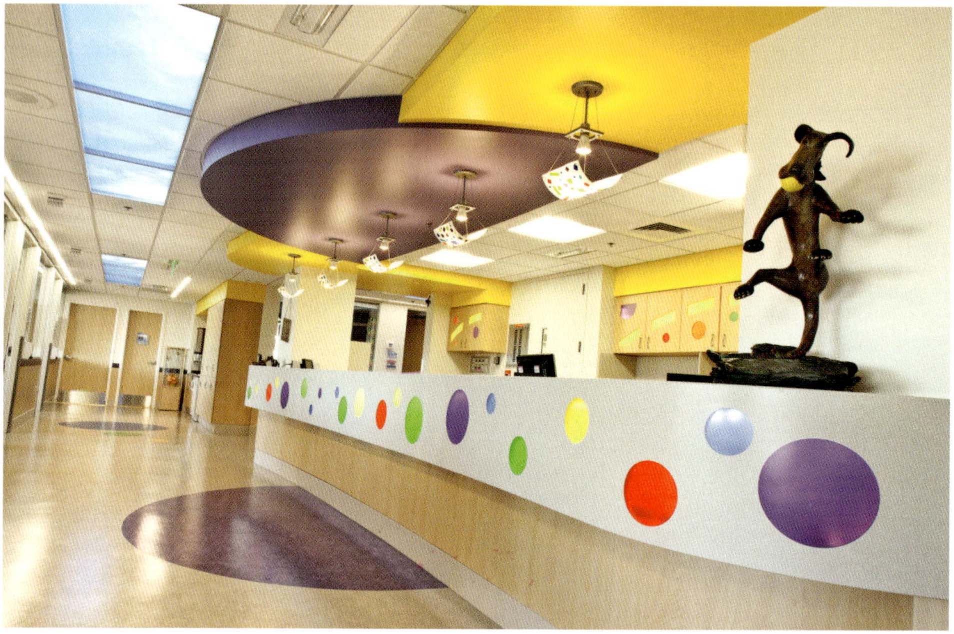

Figure 5.18: *Renown Children's Hospital PICU, Reno, NV (Architects: HMC Architects with interior design by Wilkoff Design Studio, LLC; Photo credit: HMC Architects with interior design by Wilkoff Design Studio, LLC)*

without conscious awareness of stress. Fischer et al. use repressed anxiety theory to explain this dissonance. The theory suggests that while fear can be hidden from the self, the biological representation cannot be controlled. As might be expected, the frequency of responses of both nurses and physicians was higher in less experienced staff. Figure 5.19 describes the activities evoking endocrine reactions in nursing staff. Data regarding physicians are also summarized in the Fischer et al. article.

In another study of PICUs/NICUs versus standard inpatient settings, Oehler and Davidson (1992), using the Maslach Burnout Inventory, found higher burn-out in critical care settings.

In addition to the stresses associated with work tasks, the physical environment has been found to contribute to stress. Morrison et al. (2003) measured noise levels in a PICU to determine whether they were correlated with nurse stress as measured by salivary amylase, questionnaires, and heart rate. Potential confounding variables were experience, coffee consumption, patient mortality risk, room assignment, and shift assignment. The most important environmental contributor to stress was sound. High sound levels were associated with tachycardia and evaluations of annoyance. Bailey and Timmons (2005) studied noise levels in the PICU and found that staff conversation was the most common source of noise.

5.3.3.2 Staff satisfaction

Although a few studies are available that discuss staff satisfaction as a result of operational protocols, surveys do not typically include environmental features. Ernst et al. (2004) studied

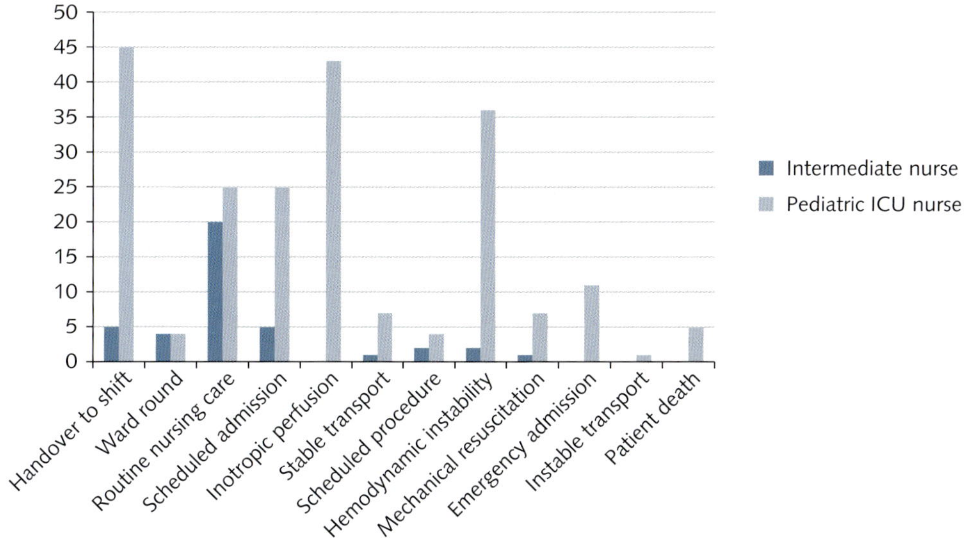

Figure 5.19: *Comparison of critical care and non-critical care cortisol events (Source: Derived from Fischer et al., 2000)*

nursing staff in a children's hospital, including three ICUs, and found that pay, sufficient time, confidence, and task assignment impacted satisfaction. The closest study I uncovered regarding satisfaction with the physical environment in inpatient units was by Tumulty et al. (1994), who found comfort to be a factor.

5.3.3.3 Examples of staff spaces in PICUs

Figures 5.20 to 5.31 are examples of staff spaces in PICUs in approximate chronological order. The location, design firm(s), and photo credit are provided. Staff spaces range from nurses' stations (centralized and decentralized) to lounges and nurse servers.

5.4 Research on needs of NICU patients, families and staff

5.4.1 *Infant needs*

One of the clear needs of an infant is a relationship with his or her parents. Morgan et al. (2011) found that maternal–neonate separation results in a 176 percent increase in autonomic activity and an 86 percent decrease in quiet sleep duration compared with the skin-to-skin contact.

Sleep is another significant need of infants. Sleep helps preterm newborns enhance clinical outcomes, achieve weight gain, improve oral feeding, and develop more substantive parent–infant relationships. Sleep is a key factor in the development of the brain. To protect sleep, Colombo and De Bon (2011) recommend reducing noise levels, creating periods of semi-darkness,

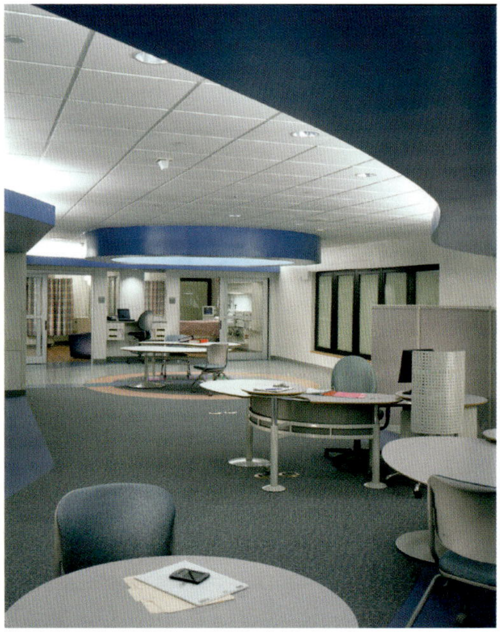

Figure 5.20: *Shands Hospital for Children at UF PICU, Gainesville, FL (Architects: Flad Architects; Photo credit: Courtesy of Flad Architects)*

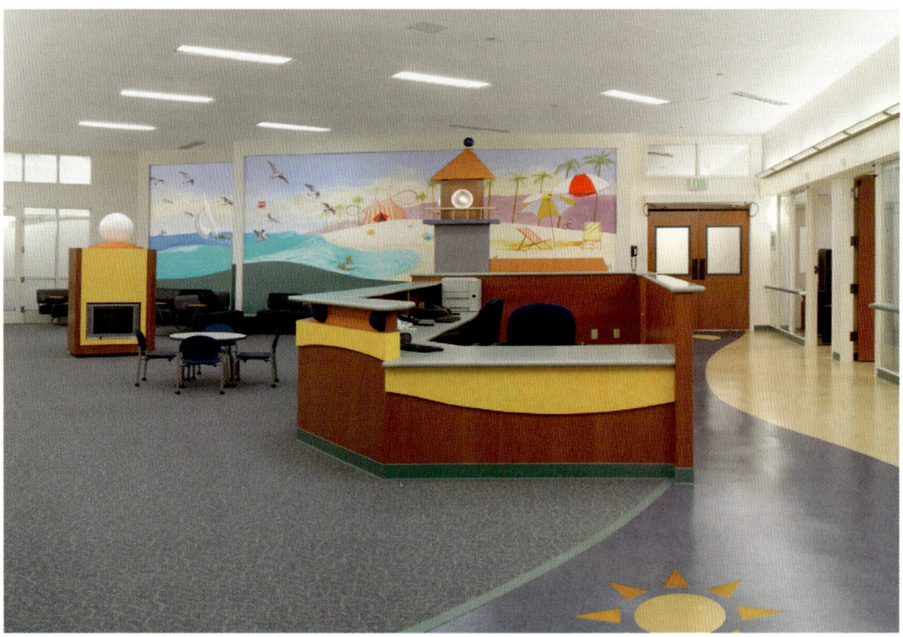

Figure 5.21: *Naval Medical Center San Diego PICU, San Diego, CA (Architects: Ravatt Albrecht & Associates)*

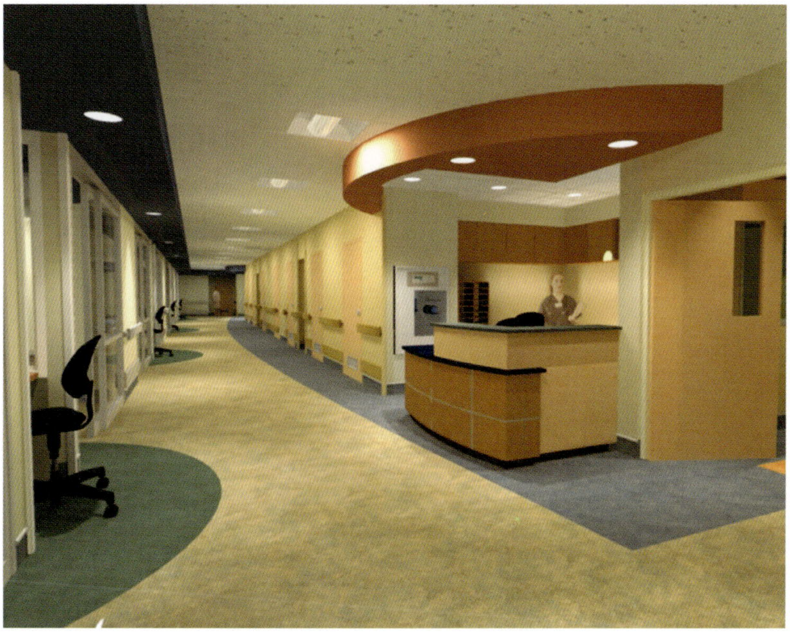

Figure 5.22: *Metrohealth Medical Center PICU, Cleveland, OH (Architects: DeWolff Partnership Architects, Cleveland, OH/Rochester, NY; Photo credit: Rendered by DeWolff Partnership Architects)*

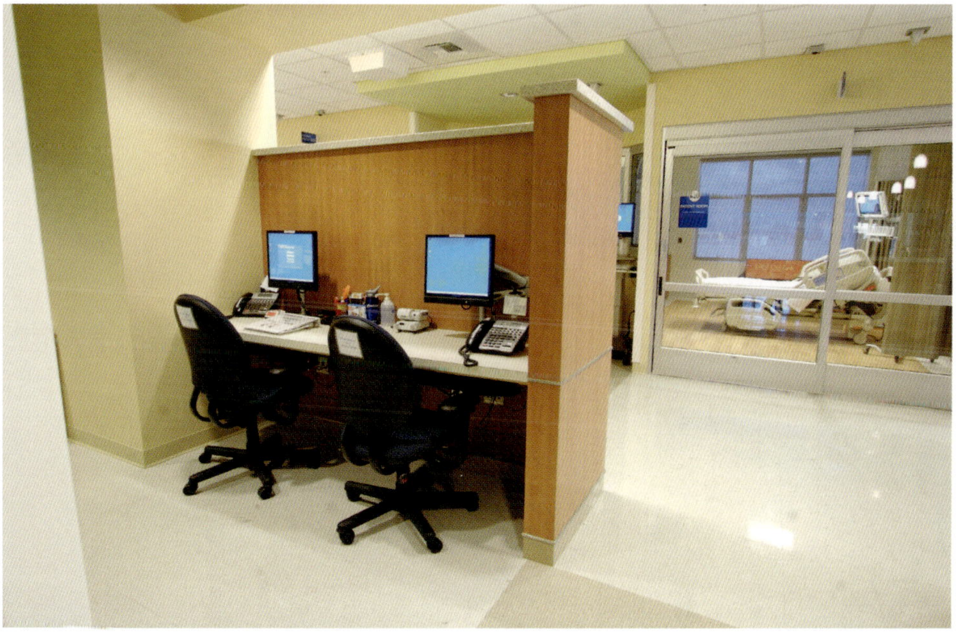

Figure 5.23: *Children's Hospital of Orange County PICU, Orange, CA (Architects: FKP Architects; Photo credit: Courtesy of FKP Architects)*

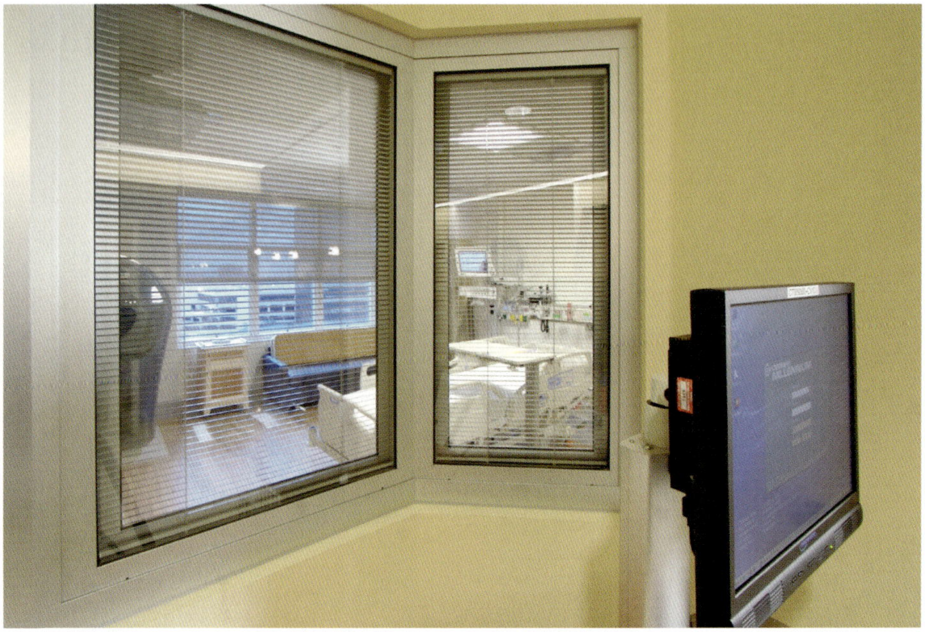

Figure 5.24: *Children's Hospital of Orange County PICU, Orange, CA (Architects: FKP Architects; Photo credit: Courtesy of FKP Architects)*

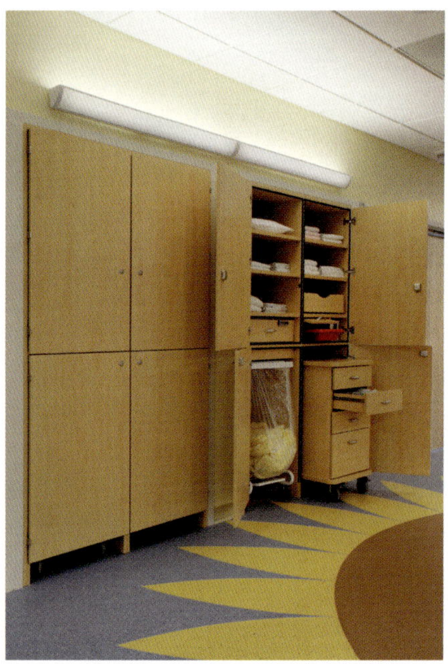

Figure 5.25: *American Family Children's Hospital PICU, Madison, WI (Architects: HDR; Photo credit: Ballogg Photography)*

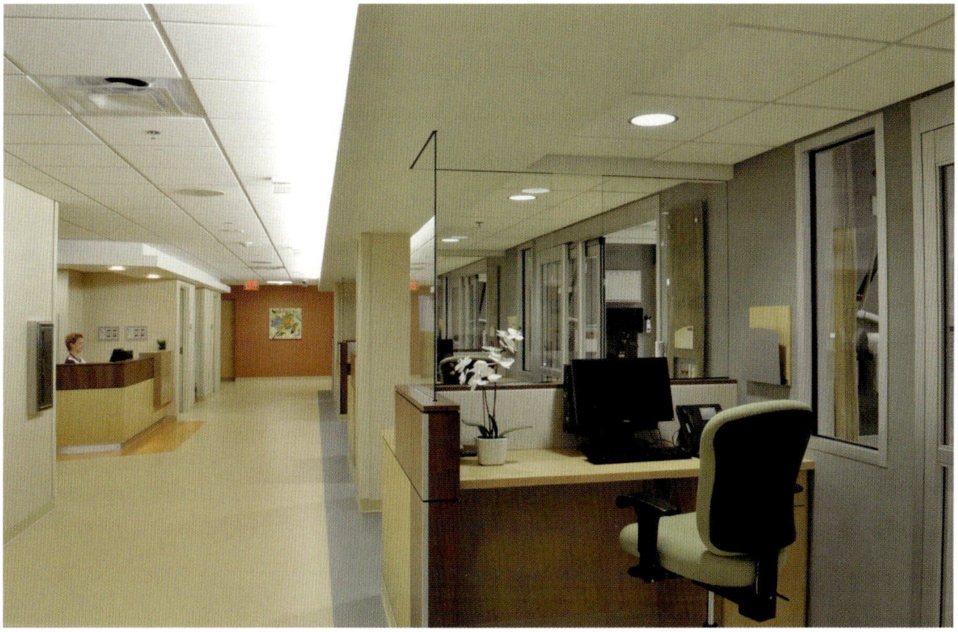

Figure 5.26: *Gillette Children's Specialty Healthcare PICU, St. Paul, MN (Architects: BWBR Architects, Inc.; Photo credit: Mark Baumhover, BWBR)*

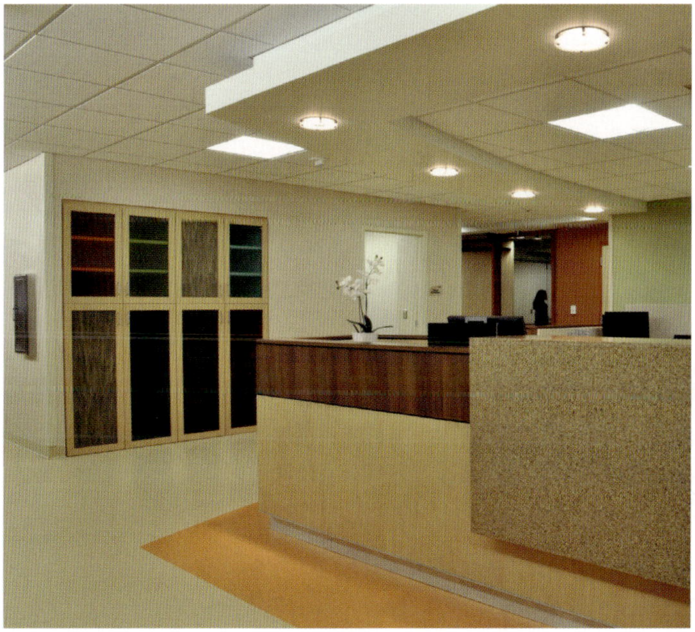

Figure 5.27: *Gillette Children's Specialty Healthcare PICU, St. Paul, MN (Architects: BWBR Architects, Inc.; Photo credit: Mark Baumhover, BWBR)*

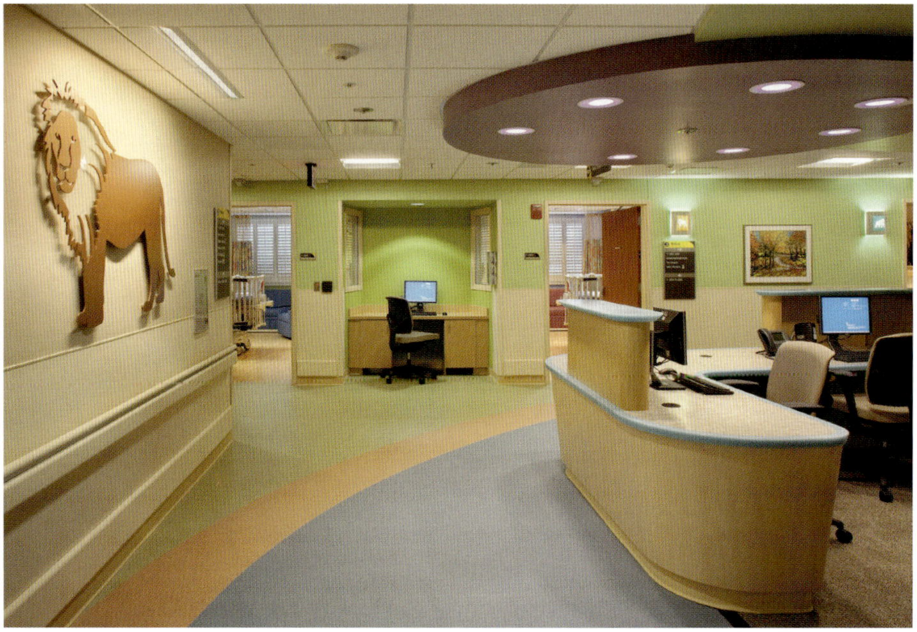

Figure 5.28: *Mercy Children's Hospital PICU, Creve Coeur, MO (Architects: Christner Inc.; Photo credit: Sam Fentress)*

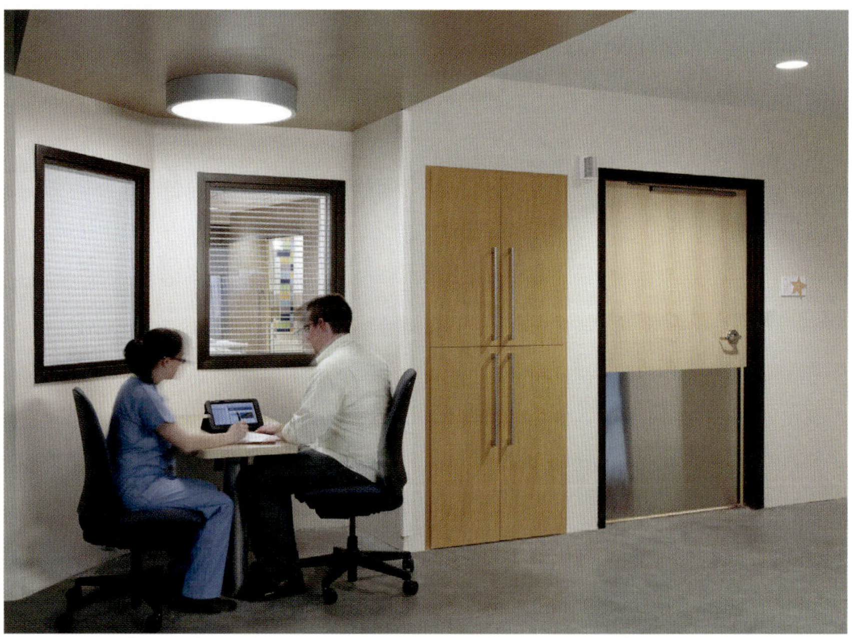

Figure 5.29: *Children's Hospitals and Clinics of Minnesota PICU, St. Paul, MN (Architects: HDR; Photo credit: Philip Prowse Photography)*

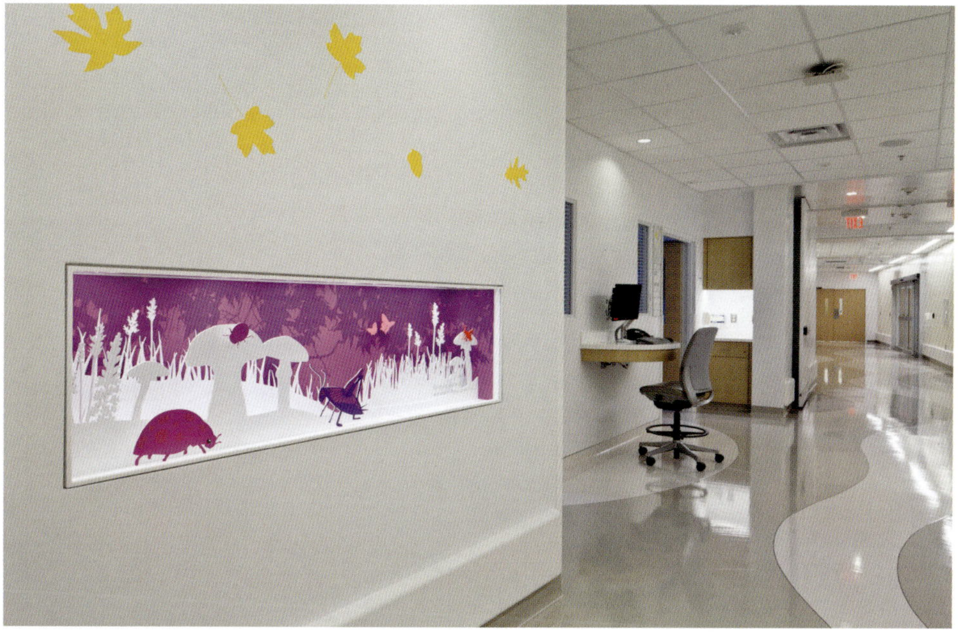

Figure 5.30: *Nationwide Children's Hospital PICU, Columbus, OH (Architects: FKP Architects; Photo credit: Courtesy of FKP Architects)*

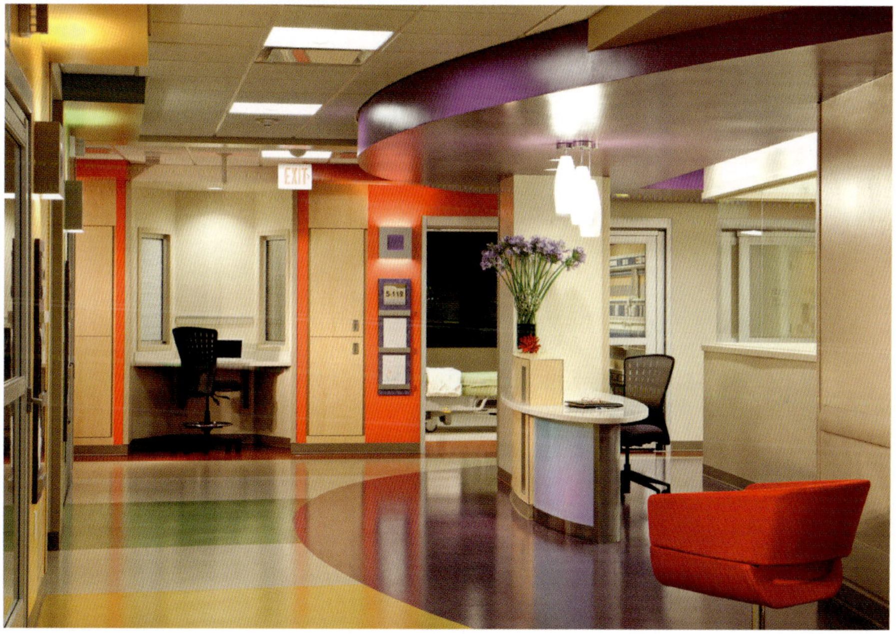

Figure 5.31: *Phoenix Children's Hospital PICU, Phoenix, AZ (Architects: HKS; Photo credit: HKS, Inc.)*

and protecting infants' faces from direct light. The presence of parents helps the baby feel more protected and allows him or her to relax.

Yamile Jackson discusses the role of brain-oriented care and family-centered care in the NICU in her guest author essay.

Advancing brain-oriented care in the NICU: challenges and opportunities

Yamile C. Jackson, CEO, PhD, PE, PMP

Parents often describe the NICU as a roller-coaster, and that was in fact our own experience. The five months in the NICU when my son Zachary was born in 2001 at 28 weeks and weighing 906 grams substantially changed my personal and professional life. I made a promise to him that his pain and struggle to survive were not going to be in vain. Zachary's story is a painful one, traumatic enough to be the inspiration of the TNT movie *14:Hours*, but it has a happy ending. Sadly, I truly believe that in 2001 I experienced an environment that was more centered in the family than what many families experience now in some hospitals.

I truly believe that Zachary beat all the odds and is alive and healthy today in large part because the staff empowered me and taught me how to be effectively involved. I kangarooed Zachary for five to seven hours of the 10 to 12 hours I spent in the NICU. I had to leave because there was no place for me to stay longer than that. The staff taught me how to become his "developmental specialist" so that I could continue his care at home following discharge. My appreciation goes to each and every staff member in all NICUs around the world and my mission is to help you offer developmental care that is centered in the family.

The Institute for Family-Centered Care (IFCC) lists the core concepts that help parents as: Dignity and Respect, Information Sharing, Participation, and Collaboration (AHA, 2004). "Family Participation" has as many interpretations as the number of NICUs and PICUs in the US; however, in all of them, newborns and their families need each other from birth and for the rest of their lives.

Since there are no standards, procedures, or scorecards that help a family or the staff determine the level of "participation of families" in a hospital, it is easy to understand why virtually all professionals give a positive response when asked if they practice family-centered care (FCC). Some even say they do so because they are open 24/7 or because they have single family rooms.

FCC is imperative in the NICU and PICU more so than in any other unit of the hospital because everything we do (or don't do) affects brain development and the lifetime of the baby, the family, and society at large. Working together with families will improve the babies' odds of enjoying as normal a life as possible.

It is not difficult to infer the level of family participation in an ICU: simply look around the unit. At any given time, what percentage of parents is present? For the time parents are present, what percentage of time do they spend holding the baby in skin to skin, or if they don't qualify for kangaroo care, they are by the bedside bonding, touching, talking, and reassuring the baby that he or she is not alone, abandoned, or in solitary confinement? Are parents confident about their ability to provide the best possible developmental care for their baby at the NICU and after discharge? Are fathers involved and encouraged to kangaroo their babies? Do parents feel hopeless and impotent or do they know how much they can help their babies and what kangaroo care can do so that they need to be present? Will they choose the same hospital if they have another baby? How have those numbers changed from last year/month?

> Family centered care is a philosophy of care that embraces a partnership between staff and families. Unrestricted parental presence in the NICU, parental involvement in infant caregiving, and open communication with parents are basic tenets of family centered care. By virtue of their continual presence and role in the NICU, nurses are in a unique position to support family centered care.
>
> (Griffin, 2006)

Don't stop after telling the parents the bad news – there is good news too.

Parents need and want to know how prematurity can affect their baby's life and what they can do to mitigate deficiencies and disabilities. Contrary to what I heard in the NICU in 2001 with Zachary, there is some evidence which suggests that apnea and bradycardia are not caused by the immaturity of the baby's system but by the poor environmental conditions we are providing in the NICU. Preemies do not "catch up" at 2.5 to 3 years old and many disabilities or deficiencies will not be known for years after discharge. Premature babies are not just tiny; they are at risk for a number of health concerns, including breathing difficulties, brain injury, eye disorder infection, bowel problems, and heart dysfunction. Some of these concerns are short term and others long term (Marlow, 2004).

One study found that at age 6, 22 percent of low birth weight children had at least one psychiatric disorder, with Attention Deficit Disorder and anxious disorders being the most common (Whitaker et al., 1997). More than half of babies who are born 10 weeks or more before their due date suffer brain damage (Volpe, 2000); and almost half of children who survive extremely preterm birth have neurologic and developmental disabilities (Peart, 2008). A study from the United Kingdom suggests that extremely preterm babies who survive to leave the hospital have about a 50:50 chance of being free of disability at age 2.5 (Wood et al., 2000).

However, the good news is that the evidence is bright when it comes to brain development and parental intervention. The baby's sleep is a basic physiological need. Sleep is very important for recovery, growth, brain development, learning, and memory. Moreover, disturbances in sleep can cause exhaustion, damage to the developing body, dysfunction of the immune system resulting in susceptibility to infection, and it can also cause serious stress and agitation (Bertelle et al., 2007; Graven, 2006).

I have spent 11 years helping babies sleep under the extreme conditions of the ICU and applying engineering, technology, ergonomics, and parental intervention (or its simulation) to the prevention of deficiencies commonly attributed to prematurity. Our goal is that every child can sleep, be comfortable and comforted on the bed or while being held so that the brain develops, she or he grows, experiences a safe and seamless inclusion into his or her family, and goes home enjoying the best possible quality of life for a lifetime.

There is evidence that babies sleep better in kangaroo care (Ludington-Hoe et al., 2006) and that cerebral oxygenation is improved during kangaroo care (Begum et al., 2008) and all the numerous benefits of kangaroo care for the baby. There is still the perception that kangaroo care (KC) is reserved for improving breast milk production or for underdeveloped countries that don't have access to equipment. Fortunately, it is recommended for babies in high-tech environments in NICUs in developed countries (Anderson et al., 2001), as it supports an infant's optimal adaptation to extra-uterine life, provides the optimal neurosensory environment for brain development, facilitates maternal–infant bonding and attachment, empowers the mother as primary caregiver, facilitates initiation of lactation and breast-feeding, and prepares for a successful discharge (Nyqvist et al., 2010).

Because preterm infants are susceptible to cerebral lesions due to immaturity, the effects of KC on cerebral hemodynamics ("blood movement") should be known. Cerebral oxygenation is an important parameter in cerebral hemodynamics (Begum et al., 2009).

It is my vision that parents and caregivers around the world support not only infant bonding and attachment to their parents, but also the child's sensory and brain development by minimizing the environmental stress of the neonatal and pediatric intensive care units.

References

American Hospital Association (AHA), Institute for Family-Centered Care. (2004). *Strategies for Leadership: Patient and Family-centered Care*. Chicago, IL, and Washington, D.C.: AHA. Retrieved from http://www.aha.org/aha/issues/Quality-and-Patient-Safety/strategies-patientcentered.html

Anderson, G.C., Dombrowski, M.A.S., and Swinth, J.Y. (2001). Kangaroo care: Not just for stable preemies anymore. *Reflections in Nursing Leadership, 2nd Quarter*, 32–34, 45.

Begum, E.A., Bonn, M., Ohtani, N., Yamashita, S., Tanaka, S., Yamamoto, H., Kawai, M., and Komada, Y. (2008). Cerebral oxygenation responses during kangaroo care in low birth weight infants. *BMC Pediatrics, 8*(1), 51–60.

Begum, E.A., Bonno, M., Ohtani, N., Yamashita, S., Tanaka, S., Yamamoto, H., Kawai, M., and Komada, Y. (2009). Cerebral oxygenation responses during kangaroo care in low birth weight infants. *Neonatal Intensive Care, 2*(2), 2–25.

Bertelle, V., Sevestre, A., Laou-Hap, K., Nagahapitiye, M.C., and Sizun, J. (2007). Sleep in the neonatal intensive care unit. *Journal of Perinatology and Neonatal Nursing, 21*(2), 140–148.

Graven, S. (2006). Sleep and brain development. *Clinics in Perinatology, 33*, 696–702.

Griffin, T. (2006). Family-centered care in the NICU. *Journal of Perinatal and Neonatal Nursing, 20*(1), 98–102.

Ludington-Hoe, S.M., Johnson, M., Morgan. K., Lewis, T., Gutman, J., Wilson, D., and Scher, M.S. (2006). Neurophysiologic assessment of neonatal sleep organization: Preliminary results of a randomized controlled trial of skin contact with preterm infants. *Pediatrics, 112*, e909–e923.

Marlow, N. (2004). Neurocognitive outcome after very preterm birth. *Archives of Disease in Childhood. Fetal and Neonatal Edition, 89*(3), F224--F228. doi:10.1136/adc.2002.019752

Nyqvist, K.H., Anderson, G.C., Bergman, N., Cattaneo, A., Charpak, N., Davanzo, R., Ewald, U.,

Ludington-Hoe, S., Mendoza, S., Pallas-Allonso, C., Pelaez, J.G., Sizun, J., and Widstrom, A-M. (2010). State of the art and recommendations. Kangaroo mother care: Application in a high-tech environment. *Acta Paediatrica, 99*(6), 812–819. doi:10.1111/j.1651-2227.2010.01794x, pp. 1–8.
Peart, K. (2008). Factors affecting survival, disability risk of extremely premature infants. Yale University. Retrieved from http://news.yale.edu/2008/04/28/factors-affecting-survival-disability-extremely-premature-infants-identified
Volpe, J.J. (2000). *Neurology of the Newborn*. Philadelphia, PA: WB Saunders.
Whitaker, A.H., Van Rossem, R., Feldman, J.F., Schonfeld, I.S., Pinto-Martin, J.A., Torre, C., Shaffer, D., and Paneth, N. (1997). Psychiatric outcomes in low-birth-weight children at age 6 years: Relation to neonatal cranial ultrasound abnormalities. *Archives of General Psychiatry, 54*(9), 847–856.
Wood, N.S., Marlow, N., Costeloe, K.., Gibson, S., and Wilkinson, A.R. (2000). *New England Journal of Medicine, 343*(6), 378–384.

5.4.1.1 Developmental care

Developmentally appropriate care is care that is customized to meet the needs of an infant at his or her specific age of physical maturation. The Synactive Theory of Development is a conceptual framework that describes the capabilities of the fetus and newborn. According to this theory (Vandenberg, 2007, p. 83),

> The infant's ability to regulate and control behavior emerges through continued interaction with the environment and is expressed through five systems: autonomic/physiology, motor, state, attention/interaction and self-regulation. In the healthy full term newborn the five subsystems are mature, integrated, synchronized and managed smoothly. The less mature, healthy or sick preterm newborn may be unable or partially able to manage environmental inputs, demonstrating over-reactive responses and poor tolerance from even minimal input.

According to Vandenberg, if medical staff are unable to interpret an infant's sensitivity levels and adjust care protocols, the infant will experience stress responses and lack of control. This idea of adjusting the level of the challenge of the environment to meet the competence of the individual is an exact reflection of Powell Lawton's Environment Competence/Press Theory (1974) discussed in Chapter 4.

Haumont discusses the Neonatal Individualized Developmental Care Assessment Program (NIDCAP) in this context in her guest author essay.

Moving away from the traditional NICU toward the early developmental care NICU

Dominique Haumont, MD

Perinatal mortality in very low birth weight infants has dramatically decreased during the past decades. However, 15 to 25 percent of these infants will show neurodevelopmental impairment later on. A recent meta-analysis showed that at school age those children scored around 10 points lower on cognitive tests compared to matched controls.

The aim of implementing early developmental care (EDC), a new field in neonatology, is to create an intervention program designed to provide support for optimal neurobehavioral development during this highly vulnerable period of brain growth. The theoretical framework, which underlies the approach, is supported by research in different scientific fields, including neuroscience, psychology, medicine, and nursing. EDC utilizes a range of medical and nursing interventions that aim to decrease the stress of preterm neonates in NICUs. The Neonatal Individualized Developmental Care Assessment Program (NIDCAP) is an integrated form of developmental care and appears to be the most comprehensive, holistic and family centered. NIDCAP addresses many aspects of what the preterm infant is experiencing. Reading the preterm infant's behavior and responding to the baby's stress signals, respecting sleep organization, diminishing pain, providing appropriate light and sound environment, and restoring the child–parent relationship are some of the factors that have an impact on outcome and which are addressed intensively when implementing the sophisticated and complex NIDCAP approach.

Changing the traditional NICU toward an EDC-NICU includes, most importantly, training nursing and medical staff, investing in their quality, and keeping parents in proximity to the infants. Introduction of EDC involves investment of time, energy, and financial resources. Success will depend on strong commitment of the medical, nursing, and hospital directors.

Traditional NICUs are typically designed for the administration of intensive care in the same way as adult intensive care. The developing aspect and the extreme vulnerability of the preterm infant, the need of the parental presence, and the duration of the stay have been totally neglected. Moving toward an EDC-NICU will push caregivers to struggle for space and new conceptual architectural driving trends. Major changes to achieve a developmental/healing environment consists in increasing infant care space, natural and individual lighting, decreasing noise, reflection on family-centered care, staff needs, and single rooms with rooming-in facilities. Developmental care could prove to be an important recent step in improving outcomes in extremely preterm neonates.

5.4.1.2 Music and maternal sounds

Researchers have studied the impact of music on infants in NICUs (e.g. Arnon et al., 2006; Cassidy and Standley, 1986; Standley and Moore, 1995). Standley (2002) conducted a meta-analysis of the impact of music therapy for premature babies and found a significant effect, not mediated by the infant's gestational age or birth weight.

Burke (2000) found that vibrotactile music did not promote sleep but did show evidence of reducing agitation and stress during medical interventions. Burke et al. (1995) also found a positive effect of music on the impact of medical interventions. Similarly, Butt and Kisilevsky (2000) suggest that music may help with the recovery from pain.

Standley and Moore (1995) conducted a study on exposure to music over several days. On the first day, the researchers reported high oxygen saturation levels, which decrease over subsequent days. They also found that babies had significantly depressed oxygen levels when the music was turned off.

One of the primary functions of music has been to mask inappropriate noise (Stewart and Schneider, 2000) or serve as a distraction, and this is a possible application to the NICU environment.

Another technique that has been used in NICUs is the incorporation of prenatal maternal sounds (voice and heartbeat) in the experience of newborns. Panagiotidis and Lahav (2010) found an incubator audio system to be safe and feasible. Doheny et al. (2012) found that preterm infants had a decreased risk of cardiorespiratory events when exposed to maternal sound stimulation as opposed to normal hospital sounds. The effect was significant in infants greater than 33 weeks' gestation, which suggested to the researchers that there is a specific therapeutic timeframe in which the maternal sounds are most effective.

5.4.1.3 Impact of lighting

There is a considerable body of research on appropriate lighting for newborn and premature infants. Dr. Stanley Graven provides an excellent description in his 2004 article of the neurosensory visual development of the fetus and newborn (Graves, 2004). This information serves as background when considering the design of the physical environment surrounding NICU infants.

As mentioned previously, the issue of appropriate light levels and acoustics is directly related to development care, as preterm birth interrupts the inter-uterine development of sensory systems. Inappropriate light and sound stressors have been found to impact sleep-awake phasing, self-regulatory behaviors, and other stress-indicating behaviors (Peng et al., 2009). Researchers note that the lighting needs of NICU infants are directly related to the gestational age and health status of the infant.

An early study (Giunta and Rath, 1969) suggested that high light levels might positively impact infant outcomes. These researchers exposed uncovered babies to constant light levels (90-foot candles) and compared them to those clothed in a 10-foot candle environment. The researcher found lower bilirubin levels (high levels are associated with jaundice) in the population that was exposed to the light. The exposed children in this study were not evaluated regarding the impact of the light levels on the development of their visual system; however, subsequent studies suggest that the light exposure does not negatively impact the retinopathy of prematurity (DiBiasie, 2006).

One of the most commonly discussed issues in lighting in NICUs is the role of circadian rhythms. Mirmiran and Ariagno (2000) note that circadian rhythms develop during the fetal period in response to maternal entraining; the day-night fetal heart rate rhythm is synchronized with the heart rate, rest-activity, cortisol, body temperature, and melatonin of the mother. The presence of these rhythms in young preterm infants should be supported in the care of the premature infant, although this should be done with an awareness of the negative implications of over-stimulation. Intense variations in light levels, for example, would not be appropriate for low gestational-age infants. Brandon et al. (2002) found that cycled light had short-term advantages over long periods of near-darkness. Those infants experiencing cycled light demonstrated greater weight gains. There were no statistical differences between ventilator days, auditory loss, length of stay, and retinopathy.

According to Frank et al. (1991), the most common lighting problem is strong overhead lighting, as is used in open-bay settings. Others have indicated the difficulty associated with lack of ability to reduce light levels or raise light levels when necessary for specific tests, a particular problem in an open-bay setting. For example, light levels may need to be reduced to very low levels to support equipment used in the assessment of pneumothorax (Beeram, 2013).

More detailed information on other research related to light in the NICU is provided in the guest essay by Yilin Song.

Lighting in the NICU

Yilin Song, M. Arch, PhD in Architecture candidate

Lighting is one of the most important environmental factors in NICU design. Lighting influences the outcomes of infants, the experience of families, and the behavior of healthcare professionals. However, the actual effect of lighting, especially of daylight, is a complicated topic and that needs significant exploration.

Infants and caregivers have different lighting needs. For babies, their needs may vary by gestational age and health condition. Babies sleep for most of the day before they are 1 year old (White, 2004). Meanwhile, considering their underdeveloped visual systems, the primary principle of lighting design in NICUs is to eliminate excessive direct light on infants, and to provide an appropriate sleeping environment (Bowen, 2009; White, 2006). From the perspective of caregivers, they observe patients day and night, detect infants' skin coloration, measure their heart and respiration rates, and write down or input electrical medical records near the bedside. While the dim lighting seems appropriate for the infants in the NICU, it is a quite difficult work environment for caregivers to maintain alertness and fulfill tasks and healthcare responsibilities (White, 2005). Staff require bright lighting to improve their work efficiency and effectiveness, and therefore ensure patient safety.

Both electric lighting and daylight have advantages and disadvantages. With good planning and control, electric lighting can provide the required lighting levels for any space at any time. However, people who stay in electric lighting environments for a long time may become disoriented; their circadian rhythms are disrupted, especially for nurses and staff who work night shifts (Stevens and Rea, 2001).

In contrast, daylight is a more natural and sustainable approach; the lighting levels change in response to time, dates, and weather. Both patients and caregivers can experience the diurnal cycle, which may have positive influences on their physical and spiritual conditions.

We all know that natural light benefits people's circadian rhythms. Figueiro et al. (2006) mentioned that babies "receive light/dark signal information through maternal time-of-day cues (e.g., hormones and activity)" before birth (p. S24). Mann et al. (1986) compared day–night cycled light with continuous lights, while Brandon and colleagues (2002) studied the influence of near-darkness to cycled light on preterm infants. Both of their studies found significantly more weight gain in the group of infants in a day–night cycled light environment (Floyd, 2005). Other related research illustrates that infant patients with cycled lighting had fewer days on ventilators, improved motor coordination, and earlier initiation of oral feedings. Lower light levels in NICUs reduce infant respiratory instability; decrease their heart and respiratory rates and activity levels; and reduce time spent on mechanical ventilation and oxygen support (Bowen, 2009).

In addition to the biological need for natural light in human beings, views of nature are important. Previous studies offer evidence that providing views of nature may decrease staff stress and increase their satisfaction (Ulrich et al., 2008). In the Recommended Standards for Newborn ICU Design developed, the authors suggest having at least one source of daylight visible from the NICU room instead of requiring direct access to daylight. The reason behind it is the psychological benefit of windows to caregivers and patient families (White, 2006).

The main challenge of daylight is the difficulty of constantly maintaining and controlling the required levels of lighting. In the NICU the most critical issue is to prevent excess lighting exposure to infants. The design of the environment and medical protocols must avoid direct light into infants' eyes by shielding the incubator with a cover; lowering indirect lighting during the night, and permitting infants to sleep while maintaining staff work (Floyd, 2005; Bowen, 2009). We need to explore more effective ways during both the design process and the caring practices.

References

Bowen, L. (2009). The effects of light on the neonate. *FANNP News, 20*(4), 1, 4–5.

Brandon, D.H., Holditch-Davis, D., and Belyea, M. (2002). Preterm infants born at less than 31 weeks' gestation have improved growth in cycled light compared with continuous near darkness. *Journal of Pediatrics, 140*, 192–198.

Figueiro, M.G., Appleman, K., Bullough, J.D., & Rea, M.S. (2006). A discussion of recommended standards for lighting in the newborn intensive care unit. *Journal of Perinatology, 26*, S19–S26.

Floyd, A.M.D. (2005). Challenging designs of neonatal intensive care units. *Critical Care Nurse, 25*, 59–66.

Mann, N.P., Haddow, R., Stokes, L., Goodley, S., and Rutter, N. (1986). The development of ultradian and circadian rhythms in premature babies maintained in constant conditions. *Early Human Development, 27*(1–2), 33–152.

Stevens, R.G., and Rea, M.S. (2001). Lighting in the built environment: Potential role of circadian disruption in endocrine disruption and breast cancer. *Cancer Causes Control, 12*(3), 279–287.

Ulrich, R.S., Zimring, C., Zhu, X., DuBose, J., et al. (2008). A review of the research literature on evidence-based healthcare design. *Health Environments Research and Design Journal, 1*(3), 101–165.

White, R.D. (October 18, 2004). Lighting – Practical applications in the newborn ICU. Retrieved from http://www.pediatrix.com/documents/lighting_prac.pdf

White, R.D. (2005). The physical environment of the neonatal intensive care unit – Implications for premature newborns and their care-givers. *Business Briefing: US Pediatric Care 2005*, 13–15. Retrieved from http://www.touchbriefings.com/pdf/1268/White.pdf

White, R.D. (2006). Recommended standards for newborn ICU design. *Journal of Perinatology, 26*, S2–S18.

5.4.1.4 Acoustics

The inappropriateness and possible negative impact on health outcomes of unnecessary noise on NICU children is clear. Excessive noise has been found to negatively impact the premature infant by increasing blood pressure, heart rate, and respiratory rate, and decreasing oxygen saturation (Bremmer et al., 2003). Noise levels have been found to be greater in Level III than in Level II NICUs (Levy et al., 2003).

A discussion of the acoustical needs for infants is informed by the literature survey provided by Stanley Graven (2000). The following 10 of his 16 conclusions are of particular interest to the acoustical design of neonatal environments:

1. The human fetus is sufficiently developed at 23 to 25 weeks for sound to produce physiologic effects.
2. The human fetus has the ability to discriminate voices and develop auditory memory regarding speech and music.
3. Prenatal exposure of the fetus to maternal speech may impact subsequent language development.
4. The sequence of the senses is thought to be touch, movement, chemosensory (e.g. olfactory), auditory, and then visual, regardless of whether the birth is premature.
5. Intense low-frequency sound *in utero* can damage hair cells of the cochlea.
6. The auditory system is sufficiently developed by 30 to 32 weeks to support auditory learning.
7. The *in utero* sound experience is impacted by the maternal tissues which attenuate frequencies >250 Hz.
8. Continuous sound >60 dB has been associated with hearing damage.
9. Noise >50 dB has been associated with sleep disturbance.
10. Preterm infants may be subject to learning problems later in life.

Researchers have noted that sound levels in ICUs frequently exceed recommended standards (e.g. Larson, 2010; Thomas and Uran, 2007; Vandenberg, 2007). Vandenberg (2007) recommends that sound levels should not exceed 50 dB and transient sounds should not exceed 70 dB. In a study of a NICU in Canada, Kent et al. (2002) noted that noise levels inside an incubator (61 dB) were higher than the levels outside (58 dB). The areas associated with staff activity occasionally measured 120 dB. Saunders (1995) found that covering the incubator was an effective way of reducing noise.

One of the expectations of the benefits of SFRs is their potential ability to control noise. Liu (2011) compared SFRs to open-bay units and found SFRs to be quieter except when high-frequency ventilation was used.

According to Frank et al. (1991), the biggest contributors to acoustical problems are large rooms, space limitations, overcrowding, and staff conversation. Issues with regard to staff conversation have also been identified by Bremmer et al. (2003). Slevin et al. (2000) identified the variety of sources as shown in Figure 5.32. According to this study, reductions in light, noise, and activities have been associated with reduced diastolic blood pressure, arterial pressure, and infant movements – typically desirable outcomes (Slevin et al., 2000). In spite of efforts to reduce noise levels in NICUs, researchers have had difficulty achieving appropriate standards (Byers et al., 2006). One solution – the inclusion of foam in an incubator – decreased the noise level by an average of 3.27dB (Johnson, 2001).

Thear and Wittmann-Price (2006) measured the impact of a series of protocol and environmental modifications on noise levels including a noise indicator when sound levels exceeded 60 dBs, an hour of quiet three times a day, changes in nurse schedules, instructions to parents and memos to ancillary staff about the importance of noise control, and door replacement. Noise reductions were achieved and continued to be effective three, six, and twelve months later.

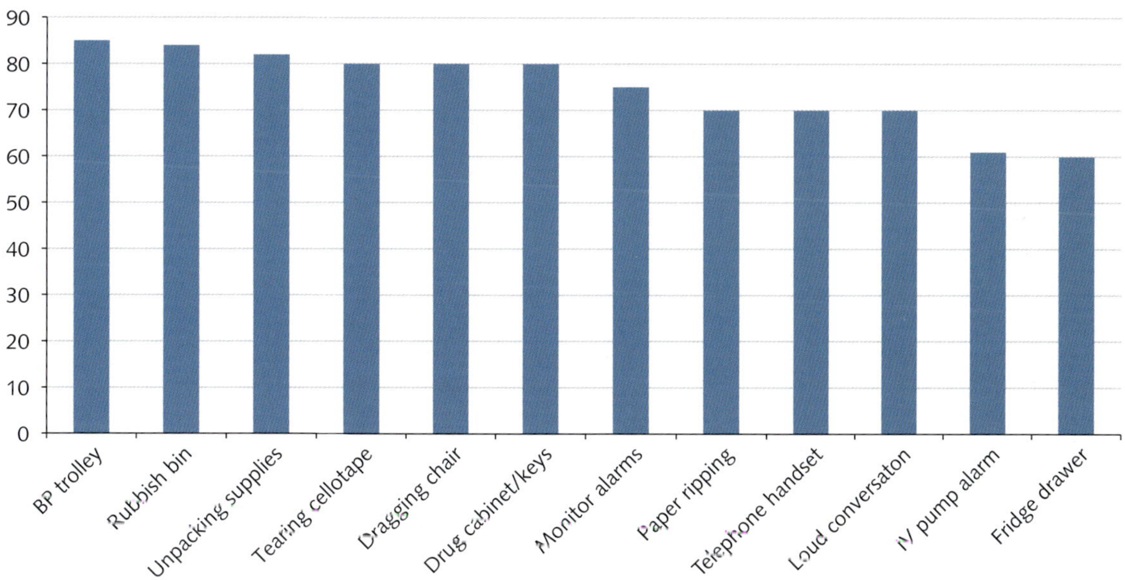

Figure 5.32: *Noise sources and dB levels in NICU (Source: Derived from Slevin et al., 2000)*

Gray and Philbin (2004) provide an in-depth summary of the effects of the NICU environment on the auditory attention and hearing of infants, noting the difficulties preterm infants face with regard to the challenges of a chaotic environment (as well as the difficulties faced by NICU adults). According to these researchers, the differences between the acoustical experience of a third-trimester fetus and a preterm baby are as follows:

- Fluid conducted versus air conducted.
- Mostly low frequencies versus all audible frequencies.
- Quiet to moderately loud versus loud to extremely loud.
- Narrow ranges of patterned signals with a moderately competing background versus a wide range of unpatterned signals competing with a loud background.

- Multiple repetitive patterns versus few or no patterns.
- Signals associated with circadian rhythms versus no circadian rhythms.

According to Gray and Philbin (2004, p. 257),

> We assume that an acoustic environment similar to that of the third trimester fetus would be most advantageous to the preterm infant's physiologic and behavioral stability as well as long-term outcome … it seems prudent at least to eliminate the acoustic sources of stress or disorganization known to be associated with noise. Many developmental challenges associated with intensive care are very difficult to alleviate: pain, handling, separation from expected physiologic supports and regulation of the mother's body. However, the acoustic environment can be managed purposefully through design and construction of the physical space and equipment and by conscious action on the part of adults using the space.

One of the primary reasons for providing single family rooms is their potential for developmentally appropriate acoustical control. Philbin makes the important point that providing a single family room in and of itself does not mean that acoustical control has been achieved (see Philbin, guest essay).

Noise and single room design: correction/prevention and an interesting alternative

M. Kathleen Philbin, RN, PhD

The pendulum swings

NICU staff have worked in impossibly crowded, multiple-bed rooms for so many years that, once in view, the single infant/parent room became a force of its own. Room size became an institutional goal and bragging right. NICUs with plenty of space had it all. Others with limited space had single rooms at a price: no parent lounge, a staff lounge too small for the staff, meeting rooms on another floor, etc. Others with meager space had crowded cubicles for rooms, curtains for the fourth wall, noise, and unhappy parents and staff alike.

Hallway deflections

The single-room NICU is often arranged along a lengthy hallway with patient rooms on one side (for daylight) and staff spaces on the other. The hallway is in constant use. The staff of one, new, jaw-droppingly beautiful NICU say the noise is unbearable and worse than the old NICU. The hallway has standard hospital ceiling panels, a thin laminate floor, and spectacular walls – all of them reflective. It is absolutely straight and very long, with pockets on the side for staff work and an open Level II nursery just off one end. The noise affects everyone. A sound wave can travel the full length without interruption, deflect from the end wall, travel back, deflect from that end wall, and on and on. Waves moving at an angle are deflected into the hallway by every surface. The movement of a stool at a workstation measured 88 dBA about 5 feet from the source. Snapping shut the clasp of a small plastic box was 98 dBA at one end of the hallway and 89 dBA at the other. Having recently spent a fortune, administration is not interested in mitigation.

Recruitment

Single rooms themselves can be noisy. This seems illogical for a large room with four walls, a door, and two people, even if all the surfaces are hard. Indeed, the room is very quiet when activities are quiet and few. However, the quietness and reflective surfaces can operate together to cause a moderately loud sound to be perceived as jarring and louder than indicated by a sound level meter. The perception of greater loudness is due to the contrast with the usual quietness and is a function of hearing called recruitment (Green, 1976, pp. 322–324). In this room normal activity becomes a constant, jarring noise.

Acoustical glare

Sound in some single rooms may be perceived as unpleasant, even if not loud. Leo Beranek writes, "If the sidewalls ... or surfaces ... are positioned to produce early sound reflections [as they would be in a small room with hard surfaces], the sound from them may take on a brittle, hard, or harsh quality, analogous to optical glare" (Beranek, 2004, p. 31).

Mitigation

Each of these problems can be mitigated by maximum surface absorption. The ceiling is a large plane where highly absorbent ceiling panels can reduce sound more than any other surface treatment. Some can absorb 100 percent of the sound reaching them, while hospital grade panels absorb about 50 percent. The cost difference between the two is small and the acoustic difference is dramatic.

Acoustic treatment of the floor is usually the second most effective and practical means of sound reduction. Some sheet flooring has multiple options for cushioning layers with some options able to prevent sound originating on the floor. This flooring has a durable surface, comes in many colors and patterns, resists staining, does not need waxing, cushions joints for long periods of standing, and *reduces* sound by 20 percent. Hospitals use such flooring routinely in operating rooms. Again, the difference when walking between this and standard laminate on cement is immediate and dramatic.

Jogs in a hallway lower sound levels by adding deflecting surfaces that interrupt long reverberation distances. Non-90-degree angles where planes intersect also interrupt reverberation by adding more deflections than 90-degree angles.

Beyond noise and quiet

Planning a new NICU is an opportunity to go beyond noise prevention and create a specific sound quality such as warmth, or definition/clarity, or intimacy, or listener envelopment (Beranek, 2004, pp. 31–32). Consultation to achieve a specific sound quality need not be expensive if work with the room acoustics specialist starts with initial planning.

The multiple-bed room: space and privacy

Multiple-bed rooms use space efficiently and have many advantages for nursing assignments and patient care. However, staff tend to oppose them out of concern for noise and for parent and staff privacy. Multiple-bed rooms can be as quiet as any other. Attractive individual (not assigned) parent spaces can be built near the unit. Substantial, movable screens can provide visual privacy for family and staff. Speech privacy is also possible. "Speech privacy" means that one person, a specified distance from others in conversation, can hear voices and but not specific words. Designing for specific speech privacy requirements is a common function of acoustical engineering.

A single room also has speech privacy but speech and personal isolation as well. Most mothers in a single room would not use the call bell for something small but worrying; they would sit with their anxiety. In a multiple-bed room, by contrast, a nurse is likely to be nearby and available to "take a look." Above all, the advantage of a multiple-bed room is that parents can go home knowing their baby is with a nurse and not in a room alone.

The myths

The following, quite mistaken beliefs are strongly held by some involved in NICU design.

1. "Sound floats up, a characteristic that makes a very high ceiling a good means of sound attenuation."
2. "Sound in a three-wall room will be caught by a 2" lip on a 15" fur-down across the top of the absent "fourth" wall. All sound in the room goes up to that lip area and stays there, keeping it from going into the hall."
3. "Between-bed curtains are effective sound barriers."
4. A large piece of equipment in the middle of a room or a picture on a wall will "break up" sound and lower sound levels.

References

Beranek, L. (2004). *Concert Halls and Opera Houses: Music, Acoustics, and Architecture*. New York: Springer-Verlag.

Green, D.M. (1976). *An Introduction to Hearing*. Hillsdale, NJ: Lawrence Erlbaum Associates.

5.4.1.5 Climate

Researchers have documented the thermal comfort needs of infants. As one example, Salihoğlu et al. (2011) recommend a temperature of 22 to 26 degrees Centigrade (71.6 to 78.8 degrees Fahrenheit) and relative humidity of 30 to 60 percent. Thomas et al. (2010) found that NICU climate conditions vary by season, a situation that should be acknowledged to keep the indoor environment stable. The researchers' thermal analysis indicated seasonal temperature differences, with specific regard to humidity and evaporative temperature. Thomas and colleagues point out that room temperature is only one measure of room climate. Consideration must be given to evaporative, air, and radiant temperatures, as well as humidity. Evaporative temperature is of concern because premature skin is very permeable and highly susceptible to heat and fluid loss (Thomas et al., 2010).

Sherman et al. (2006b) note that the younger the gestational age of a baby, the less fat and glycogen has been stored for heat production. In addition, the body surface area-to-weight ratio is lower than most adults, which, along with skin permeability, promotes rapid heat loss or gain and water loss. Incubators and radiant warmer beds are the primary devices for keeping infants warm.

5.4.1.6 Examples of infant spaces in NICUs

Figures 5.33 to 5.45 are examples of infant spaces in NICUs in approximate chronological order. The location, design firm(s), and photo credit are provided. The examples reflect the wide range of options and transitions that have taken place over time.

5.4.2 Family needs

Family-centered care has been a trend in neonatal intensive care and is becoming an increasingly important factor when designing the NICU. Recent research suggests that proactive, family-integrated care has a positive impact on family and baby outcomes (O'Brien et al., 2013). When considering how to encourage families to stay with infant patients and participate in the care of infants, the perceptions and feelings of NICU families must be explored. A more thorough understanding of family needs will result in a more family-friendly environment. One very important need emerged in research conducted by Moore et al. (2003). Case studies of 11 units that supported family-centered care to varying degrees revealed the need for families to have unlimited access to their child. Saunders et al. (2003) conducted a before-and-after study of the impact of family-centered care protocols on outcomes but found no differences in clinical outcomes over a two-year period. However, surveys of staff and parents were not included in this study.

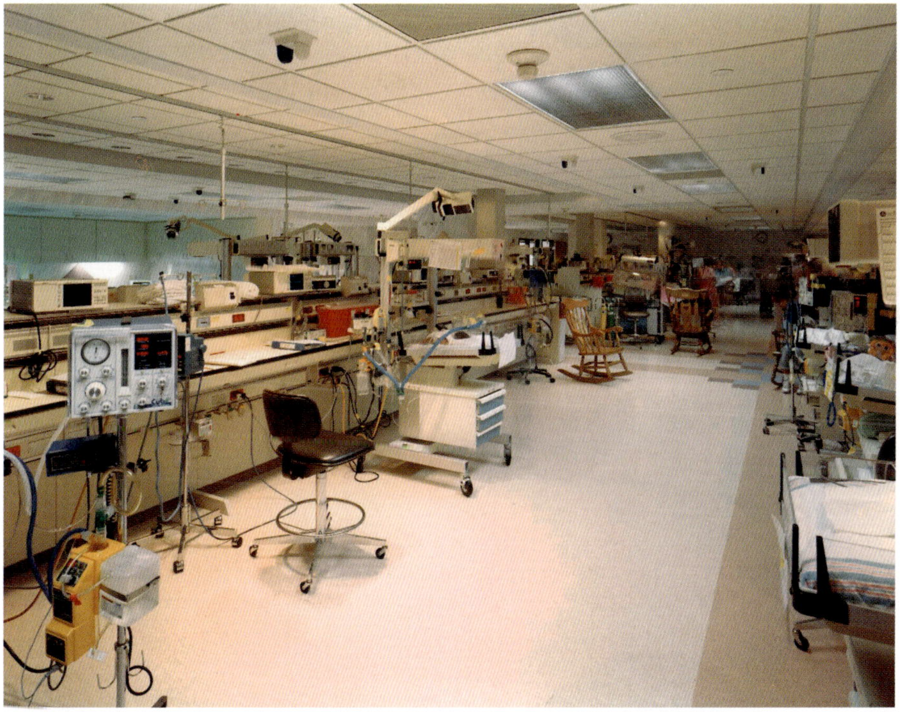

Figure 5.33: *Shands Hospital for Children at UF NICU, Gainesville, FL, 1988 (Architects: Flad Architects; Photo credit: Courtesy of Flad Architects)*

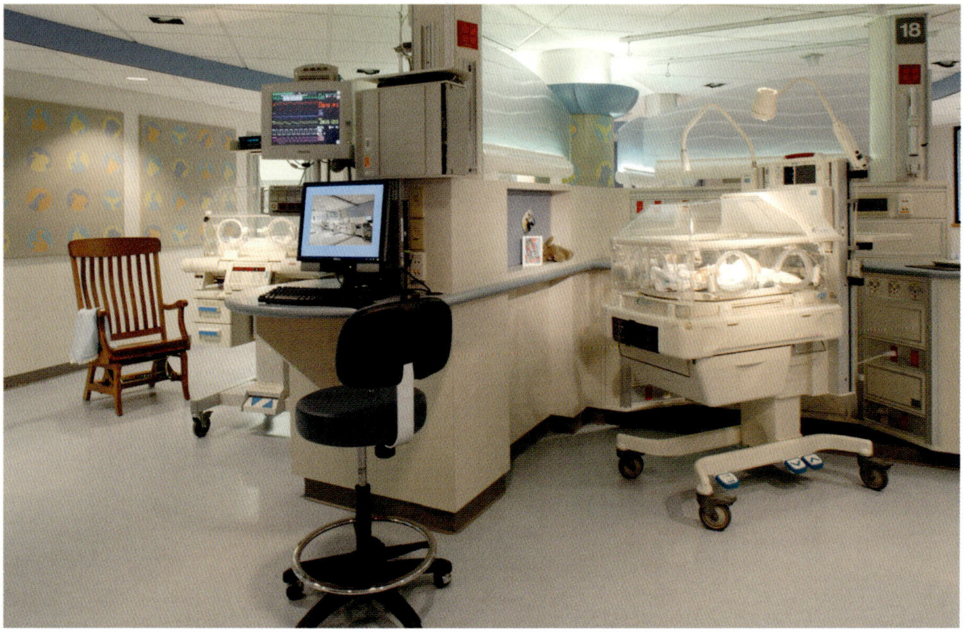

Figure 5.34: *Shands Hospital for Children at UF NICU, Gainesville, FL, 2004 (Architects: Flad Architects; Photo credit: Nei Rashba)*

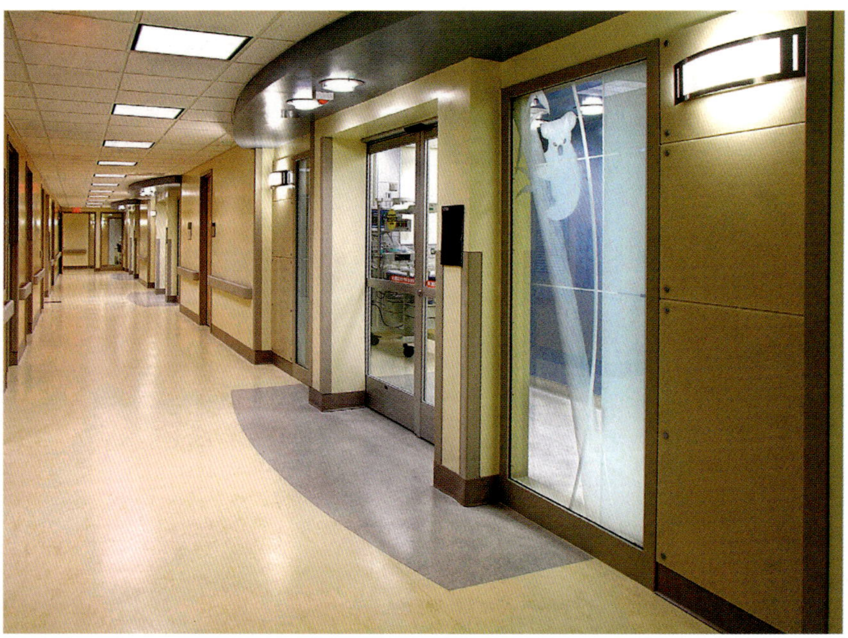

Figure 5.35: *UC Davis Children's Hospital NICU, Sacramento, CA (Architects: Stantec; Photo credit: Dean J. Birinyi, ASMP)*

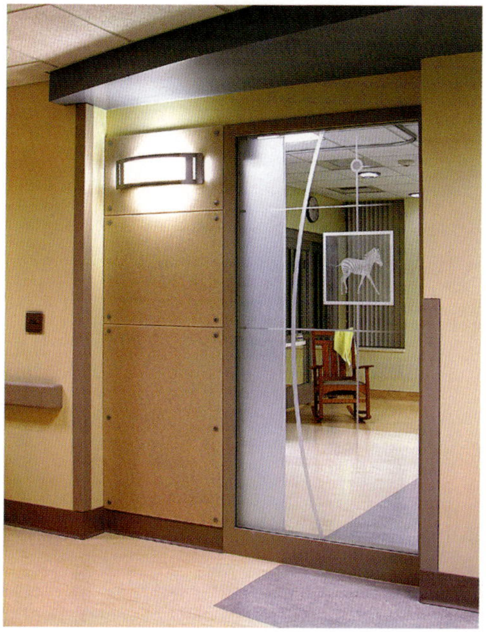

Figure 5.36: *UC Davis Children's Hospital NICU, Sacramento, CA (Architects: Stantec; Photo credit: Dean J. Birinyi, ASMP)*

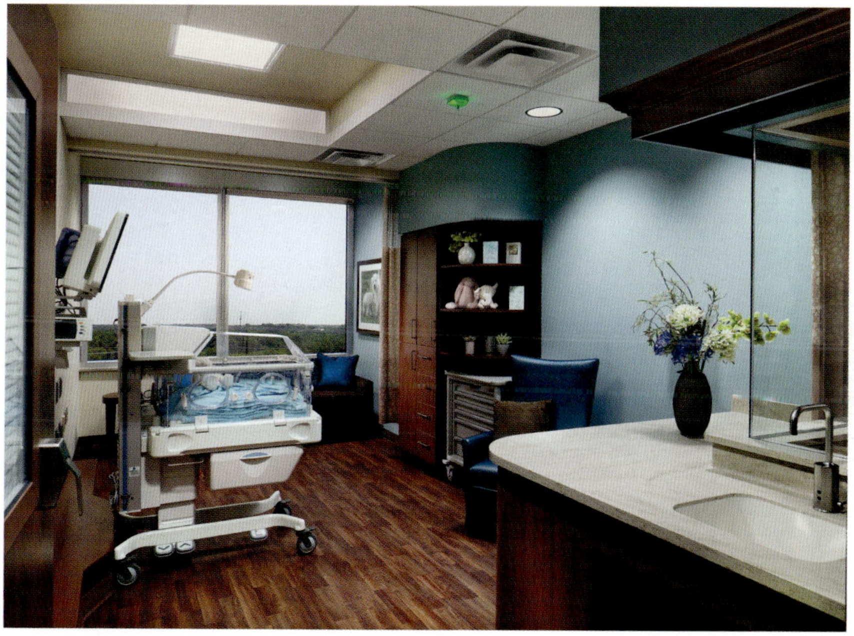

Figure 5.37: *Community Hospital North NICU, Indianapolis, IN (Architects: RTKL Associates; Photo credit: Jeffrey Totaro)*

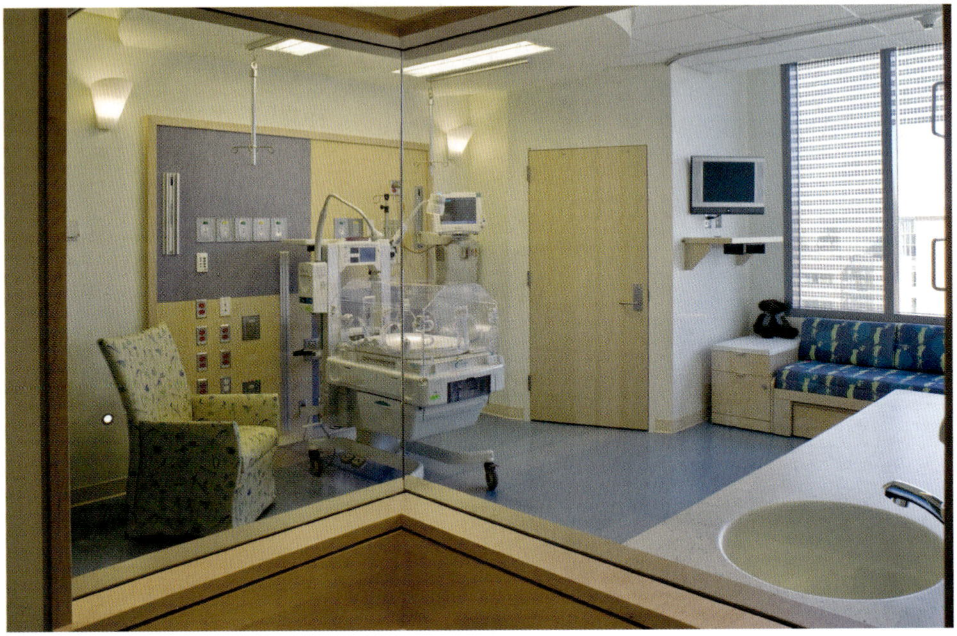

Figure 5.38: *Children's Hospital Colorado NICU, Aurora, CO (Architects: ZGF Architects LLP; Photo credit: Courtesy of ZGF Architects LLP; Eckert & Eckert Photography)*

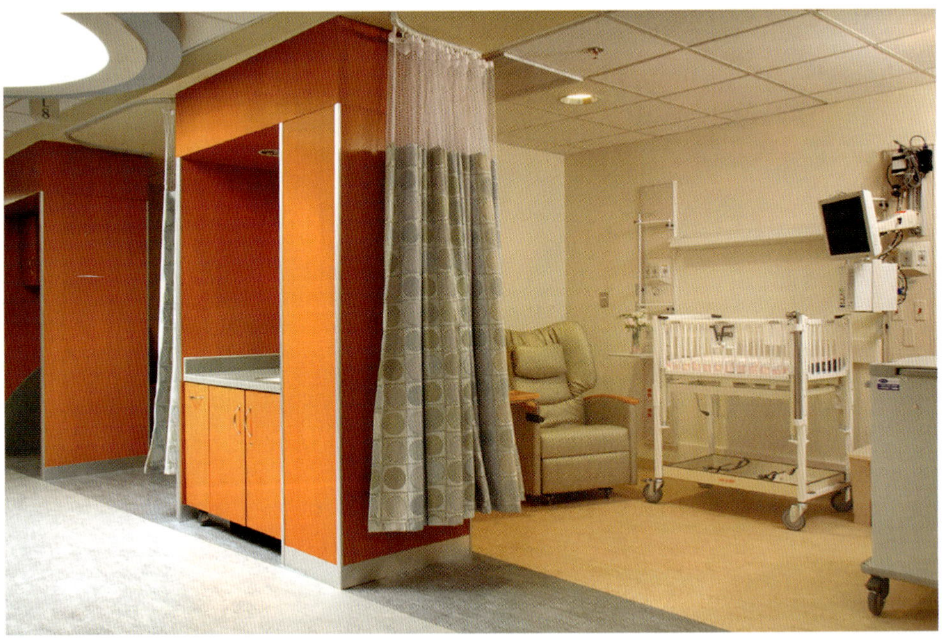

Figure 5.39: *Northside Hospital Women's Center and Special Care Nursery NICU, Atlanta, GA (Architects: Howell Rusk Dodson; Photo credit: Dave Dawson Photography)*

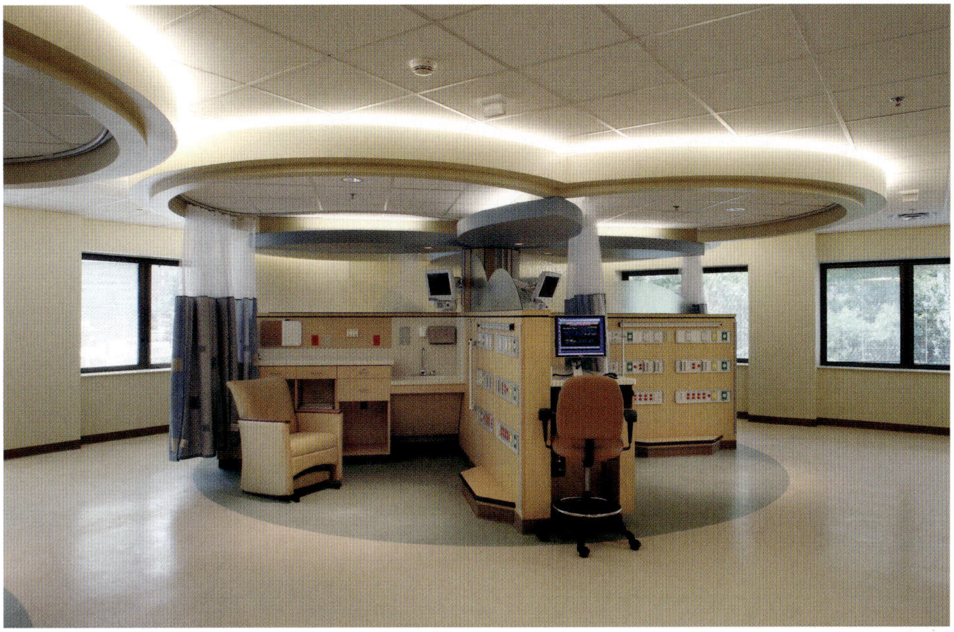

Figure 5.40: *Baptist Hospital Beaman NICU, Nashville, TN (Architects: Thomas, Miller & Partners; Photo credit: Courtesy of Thomas, Miller & Partners)*

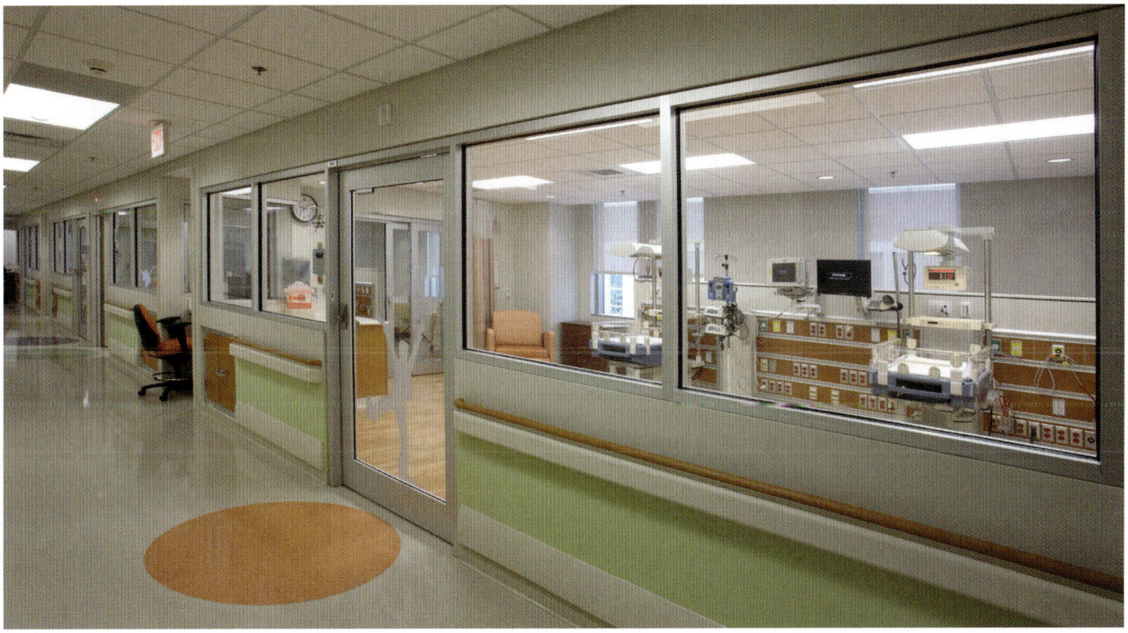

Figure 5.41: *Le Bonheur Children's Hospital NICU, Memphis, TN (Architects: FKP Architects; Photo credit: Courtesy of FKP Architects)*

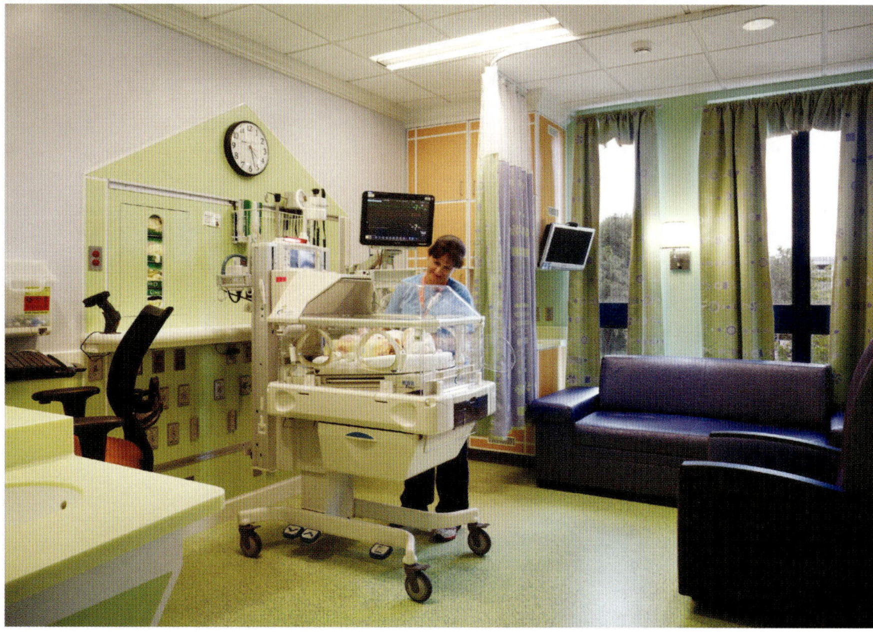

Figure 5.42: *Cook Children's Medical Center NICU, Fort Worth, TX (Architects: FKP Architects; Photo credit: Courtesy of FKP Architects)*

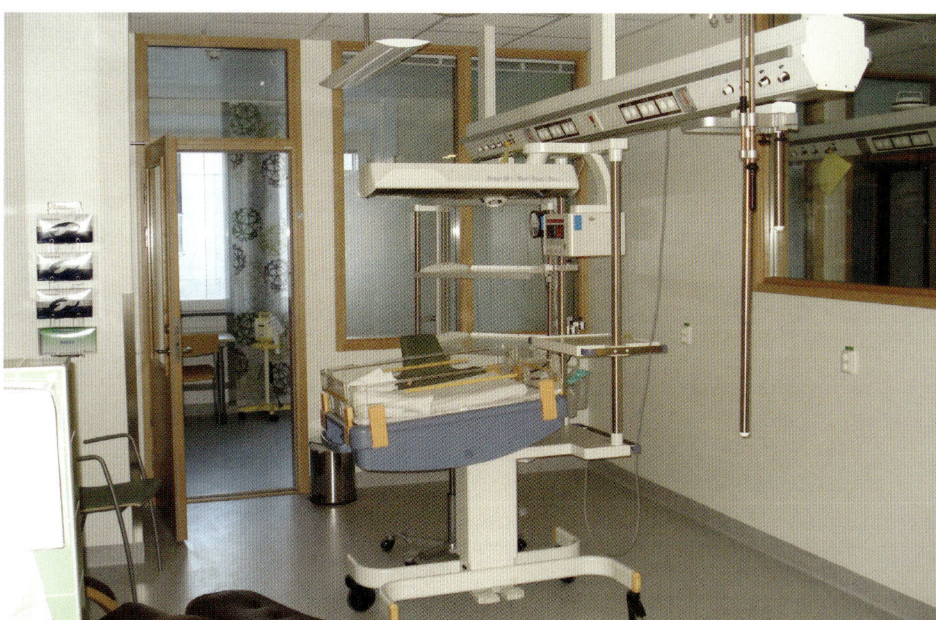

Figure 5.43: *Karolinska University Hospital NICU, Huddinge, Sweden (Architects: Sweco Architects SA Photo credit: Sandra Hegestam)*

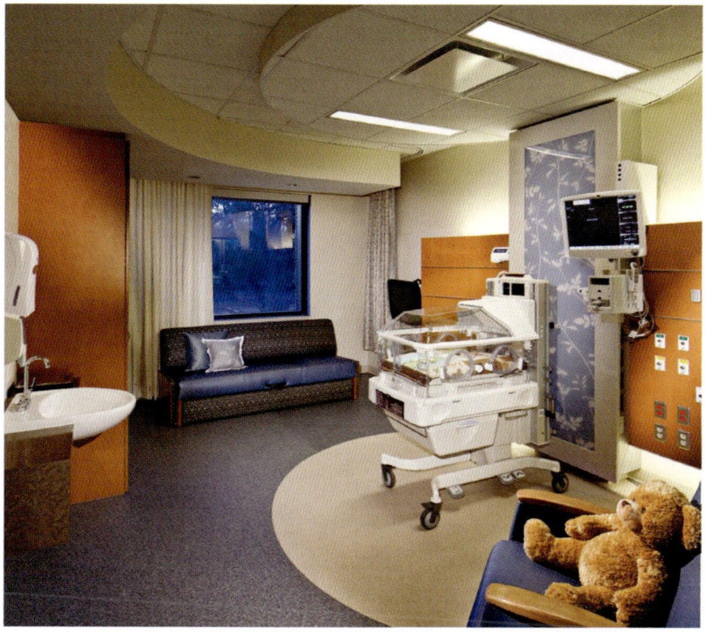

Figure 5.44: *St. Joseph's Hospital NICU, Tampa, FL*
(Architects: HKS;
Photo credit: HKS, Inc.)

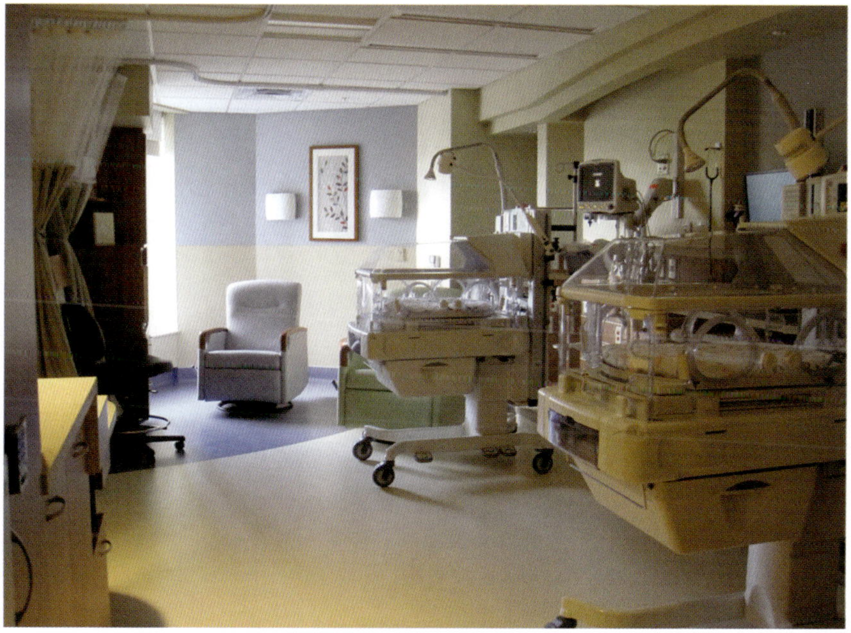

Figure 5.45: *St. Mary's Hospital NICU, Madison, WI*
(Architects: Flad Architects;
Photo credit: Courtesy of Flad Architects)

Expanded visitation hours and the ability to stay on the unit is an expressed need of families. Travel time and costs likely limit how much parents visit their children, as does the parents' need to care for siblings and attend to work demands. Using a questionnaire, Giacoia et al. (1985) found that parents who were not local to the region visited and called less often, and typically had lower incomes. Lewis et al. (1991) studied the patterns of visiting and relationship of visiting to post-NICU activities. The researchers noticed that the number of NICU visits decreased from day 2 to day 12 and then stabilized through day 21. Children whose parents did not live together, had intraventricular hemorrhages, or who were not first-born were visited least.

Thus, enough space for sleeping and for sibling care surface are two important needs of the families of NICU patients. In the article "Mothers' arms – the past and future locus of neonatal care?," White (2004) states that parents in NICUs perceive these factors, as well as the layout of equipment, presence of a telephone, access to the internet, and the presence of workspace at the bedside, as more important than privacy.

In another study on the needs of parents in family-centered care, researchers highlighted the need to enlarge space at the infant's bedside (Bruns and Klein, 2005). In a study at Copenhagen University, interviews with parents indicated the need for smaller rooms (fewer babies per room) and sleeping accommodation near the baby (Beck et al., 2009). The case study by Bunker-Hellmich (1987) suggests that there may be a relationship between the congested overlapping use of space in the unit and staff opposition to visiting.

The needs of fathers and mothers in NICUs may differ. According to Fegran et al. (2008b), fathers viewed the NICU birth as a shock but were prepared for immediate involvement. Mothers felt the need to regain a relationship with the child. One of the mothers in Huber's NICU interview study stated,

> It took about three weeks to realize ... I'm my baby's mother and he's my child. I have a say in what his care is gonna be and how he is gonna progress...I should be involved in that. It took me three weeks to really feel like I have my legs to stand on.
>
> (Huber, 1998, p. 68)

The relationship between families and their babies is important; however, Talmi and Harmon (2003) note that the NICU environment may disrupt parent–infant relationships, and the task-oriented NICU environment may overlook relationship development. To help build relationships, the hospital may use psycho-educational intervention, offer mental health services, link families with parent-to-parent support groups, train staff, promote developmentally appropriate caregiving, highlight meaningful moments, and offer a program of monitoring, assessment, and support.

Depending on the demographic characteristics of the family member, the degree and type of support may vary. For example, with regard to family Income, Sargent (2009) found a significant relationship between lower incomes and the need for support.

Debra Harris, who is a design researcher and also had the personal experience of having her baby in a NICU, describes this experience from both perspectives in her guest author essay.

The life and times of the NICU: parent experience and quality of care

Debra Harris, PhD

The reasons an infant ends up in the neonatal intensive care unit (NICU) vary, as does the parent's experience. My daughter was delivered six weeks early with an emergency C-section because I was suffering from HELLP Syndrome. HELLP Syndrome is a group of symptoms that include hemolysis (the breakdown of red blood cells), elevated liver enzymes, and low platelet count. Fortunately, my daughter was born fully developed and only needed monitoring; she was in NICU not because of her own limitations but because of mine. She was there for safekeeping while I recovered. I did not see her for the first four days of her life, except for the moments after the C-section before she was carried off to be examined and placed under the watchful eye of the NICU nurse. I was reliant on that nurse and the others who watched over and took special care of my daughter when I could not. The care and understanding shown to me by the healthcare staff was personal, professional, and exceptional.

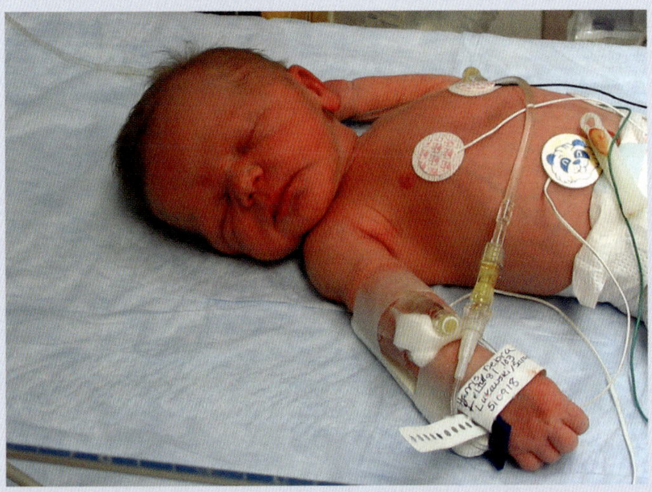

Figure 1: *Author's daughter in NICU*

Every parent's experience in NICU is different and distinctly their own. As a researcher focusing on environmental impacts, I have conducted studies that included many NICUs – open bays, single family rooms (SFR), and combination units. I have had the opportunity to observe parents in this setting and have seen incidents where parents claim ownership of their space and the unit; I have also seen incidents where the exhaustion, worry and stress overwhelm the parent due to their concern for their infant's health and well-being. The parents' experience is shaped by their infant's health status, the quality of care received, and the NICU environment.

Recently, I had an exchange with an administrator who stated that if they needed to transfer a patient out of one of their hospitals that has a SFR NICU to another hospital that has an open-bay NICU, the parents did not want to make the transfer; however, if a transfer was required from the open-bay to the SFR unit, then the parents were happy to make that transition. While this communication was purely anecdotal, evidence indicates that parents in SFR units have more interactions with their infants and longer (although fewer) conversations with other parents in the unit. SFRs provide parents with more privacy with their infant; and, comparable to the open-bay unit, community support through interactions with other parents (Harris et al., 2006; Shepley et al., 2008).

On another day with another administrator, I observed parents who were with their child in a single family room and had just received the news that they would be going home after the weekend. It had been a long road for these parents and their excitement was contagious. Even though they had a private room, they knew many of the healthcare staff and even the administrator I was with that day. Clearly, the SFR unit team had provided quality care and communication. One of the things that I think I will always remember about that day was when the new mother came up to the administrator and gave him a hug with a big smile on her face. She was radiant. For the administrator, he was genuinely happy, but it was clear to me that he was an integral part of that healthcare team. He knew every nook and cranny of that unit and knew those parents by name.

In today's healthcare climate, providing quality of care has expanded to include healthcare services, communication, and the impact of the environment, as posited by the Centers for Medicare and Medicaid Services (CMS) with the implementation of the Hospital Consumer Assessment of Healthcare Providers and Systems (HCAHPS). Basically, HCAHPS is a series of measures including a patient satisfaction survey that CMS will use to score a hospital to determine reimbursement rates, creating a pay-for-performance system. Environmental design elements in healthcare planning may influence factors that contribute to a hospital's HCAHPS score and, ultimately, the bottom line. Attributes of NICU design that focus on patient (parent) satisfaction; staff work effectiveness, communication and retention; and patient outcomes such as length of stay, patient transfers, and hospital-acquired illness and injuries will contribute to the assessment. Particular questions in the patient satisfaction survey address cleanliness and noise levels.

While the HCAHPS scores are focused on the whole hospital and not specifically the NICU, many of the survey questions are related to patient-centered care design, the basis of the single family room NICU. The evidence from NICU studies that indicate the relationship between the environmental and occupant outcomes provides insight for identifying meaningful measures that influence the patient, family and caregiver experience. While the evidence of NICU studies has shown positive outcomes for patients, families and staff, tying the outcomes to performance and the bottom line presents the next challenge – a challenge to quantify the environmental design impacts on quality of care.

References

Harris, D.D., Shepley, M.M., White, R.D., Kolberg, K.J.S., and Harrell, J.W. (2006). The impact of single family room design on patients and caregivers: Executive summary. *Journal of Perinatology, 26*, S38-S48. doi: 10.1038/sj.jp.7211583

Shepley, M., Harris, D.D., and White, R. (2008). Open-bay and single-family room neonatal intensive care units. *Environment and Behavior, 40*(2), 249–268.

5.4.2.1 Family stress

> [Y]ou could tell she was really hurting. [Crying] You can't take away any of the pain or anything. You just have to watch her go through it. You can't touch her, you can't hold her. It is just hard not to be able to do anything to help.
>
> (NICU parent, Huber, 1998, p. 50)

There are multiple sources of stress in the NICU, but as a number of researchers have discovered, the environment can be a contributing factor in reducing or increasing stress. Gale et al.'s study in the UK (2004) found that most parents identify their infants' pain as a primary source of psychological stress. Parents may not be prepared for their baby's pain or the impact of painful procedures. There might be a mismatch between parent and staff perceptions of infant pain, and the family member's inability to fulfill the parental protective role. Staff support, involvement in parenting in the NICU, and information resources that help parents may help alleviate stress.

Lee and Hsu (2012) conducted a study using wrist actigraphy (devices located on the wrist that record activity), sleep deprivation indices, sleep diaries, and quality-of-life assessment on first-time mothers in NICUs. The majority of the subjects were stressed, fatigued, and depressed. Lack of sleep was significantly associated with these variables as well as poor mental and physical quality of life.

Active participation in the care of one's baby has been reported as a means of reducing parental stress. This notion derives from reports that a sense of efficaciousness will enhance feelings of control. Related to this topic, the Stockholm Neonatal Family-Centered Care Study (Mörelius et al., 2012) examined the impact of the caregiving relationship between parents and preterm infants in NICUs as a means of reducing stress. This study used salivary cortisol testing of infants and their mothers before and after changing the baby's diaper at discharge. While there was no change in the cortisol levels in the before-and-after family-centered intervention (pre- and post-diaper change), there was a correlation between the stress status of infants and mothers in the two conditions.

Understandably, the families and parents of NICU patients experience high levels of stress, regardless of the environment. Smithgall (2010) found that mothers of the infant patients suffer high stress levels whether they are situated in the open-bay rooms or in single family rooms. However, the physical environment may mitigate some of the sources of stress by supporting sleep and normalization activities.

5.4.2.2 Family satisfaction

Parent gender and length of stay appear to influence satisfaction. With particular regard to gender, Tsironi et al. (2011) found that men were less satisfied, as indicated in a survey, but their ability to access the infant was curtailed by protocol in the sites associated with this study. Other studies, where fathers had more access, found them to more highly rate their experience (e.g. Mitchell-Dicenso et al., 1996), from which we might conclude that satisfaction may be strongly linked to protocols impacting access to one's child. In the Mitchell-Dicenso study, satisfaction was not related to other variables such as marital status, acuity, parent age, parent education, or family income.

The Mitchell-Dicenso study described above was focused on the development of a tool to evaluate the satisfaction of parents in a NICU. Subjects were given a broad questionnaire to identify factors that most impacted dissatisfaction and that were perceived as most important. Many of the items in the distilled questionnaire related to communication. Due to the evident importance of communication as a need of families, several researchers have examined family satisfaction with this activity. Again, fathers and mothers may have different experiences with regard to communication. In a study by Jones et al. (2007), fathers found ineffective communication to be more about strategies for obtaining information while mothers were more concerned about being treated as equal partners. Reid et al. (2007) did not find differences between mothers and fathers, but did identify an increase in the negative evaluation of communication over time in the NICU.

The relationship between a nurse and parent is complicated due to the need for closeness between these individuals, while enabling the nurse to maintain a level of professionalism (Fegran et al., 2008a). Overall experience in the NICU, however, has been associated with the quality of the relationship between nurses and parents.

5.4.2.3 Examples of family spaces in NICUs

Figures 5.46 to 5.63 are examples of family spaces in NICUs in approximate chronological order. The location, design firm(s), and photo credit are provided. A variety of spaces are shown, including patient room areas and general waiting spaces.

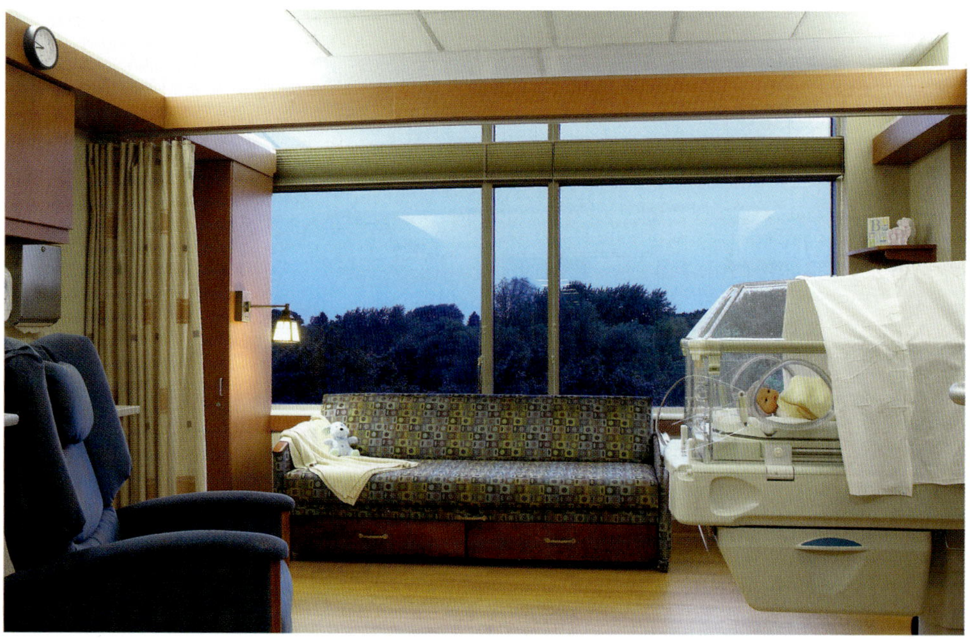

Figure 5.46: *Sanford Children's Hospital NICU, Sioux Falls, SD (Architects: Ellerbe Becket (AECOM); Photo credit: George Heinrich/Heinrich Photography)*

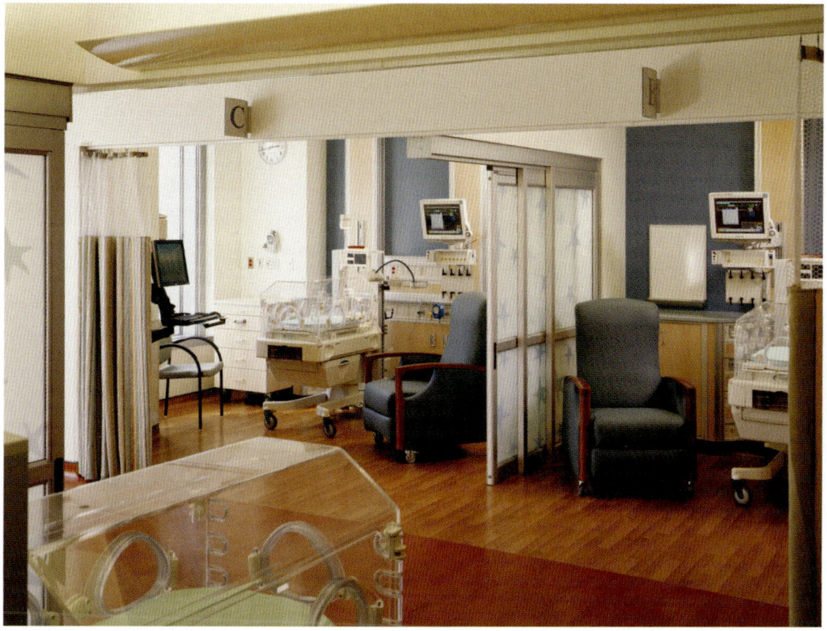

Figure 5.47: *Northwestern Memorial Hospital-Prentice Women's Hospital NICU, Chicago, IL (Architects: VOA+Cannon Design Collaborative; Photo credit: Nick Merrick © Hedrich Blessing)*

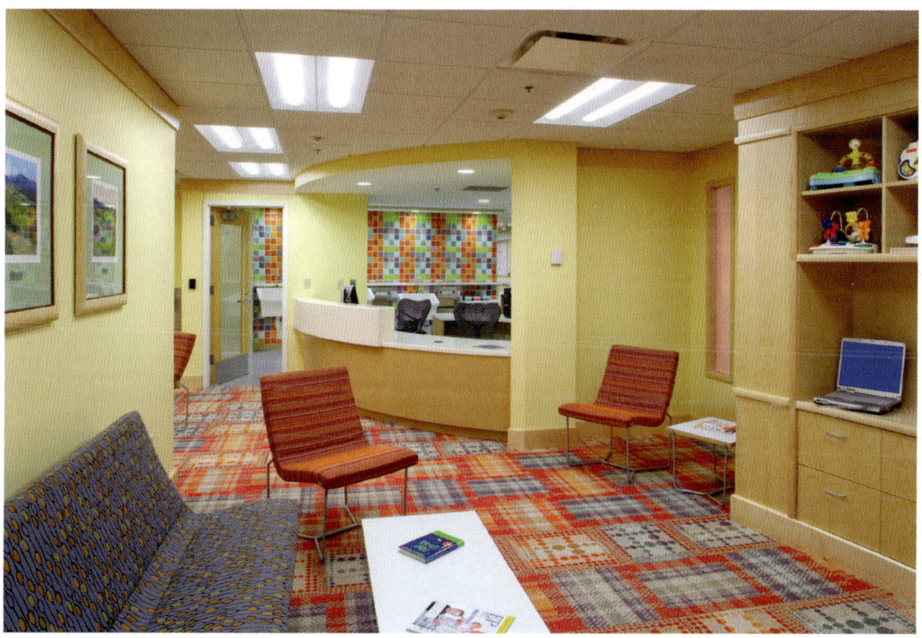

Figure 5.48: *SSM Cardinal Glennon Children's Medical Center NICU, St. Louis, MO (Architects: Christner Inc.; Photo credit: Sam Fentress)*

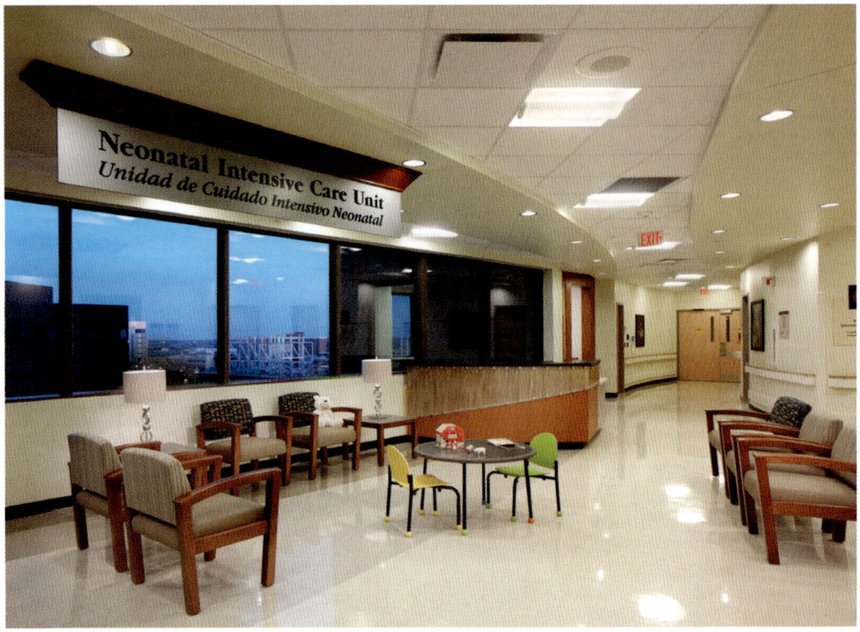

Figure 5.49: *Virginia Commonwealth University Health System NICU, Richmond, VA (Architects: HKS; Photo credit: Ed LaCasse)*

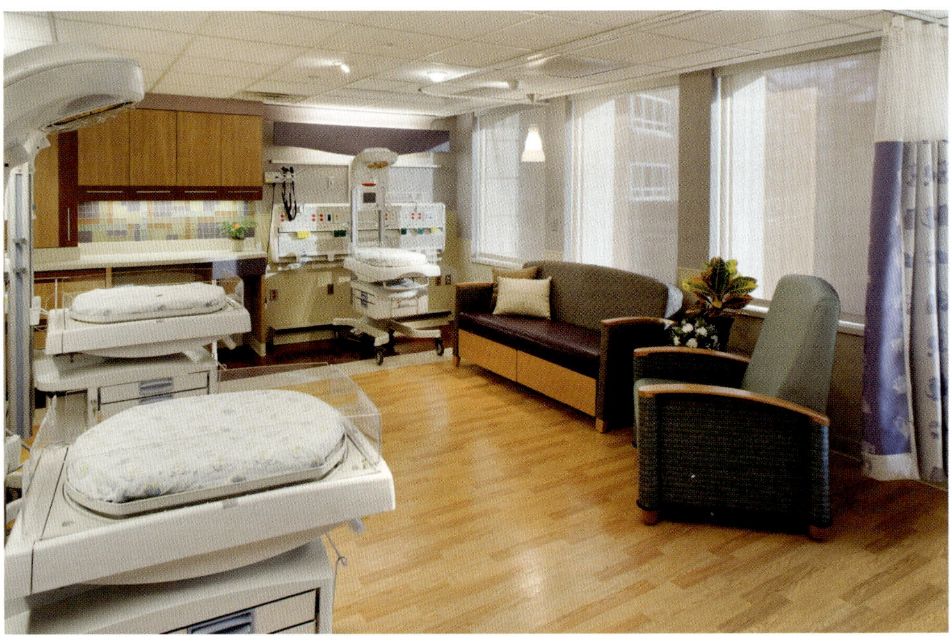

Figure 5.50: *Atlantic Health Systems NICU, Morristown, NJ (Architects: Buckl Architects; Photo credit: Courtesy of www.gregbenson.com)*

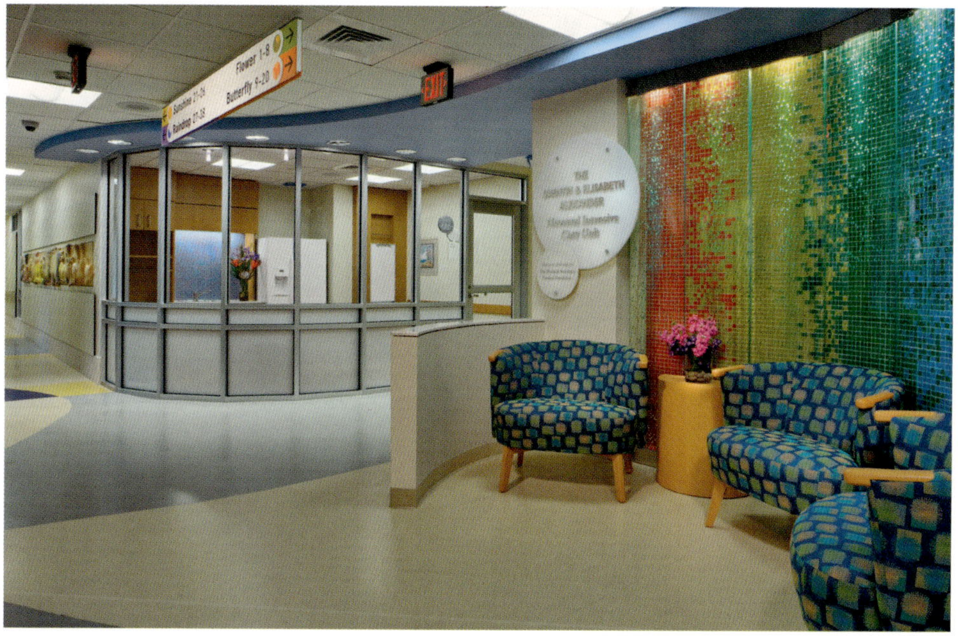

Figure 5.51: *Rainbow Babies and Children's Hospital NICU, Cleveland, OH (Architects: Parkin Architects Ltd in association with Array Architects; Photo credit: Scott Pease)*

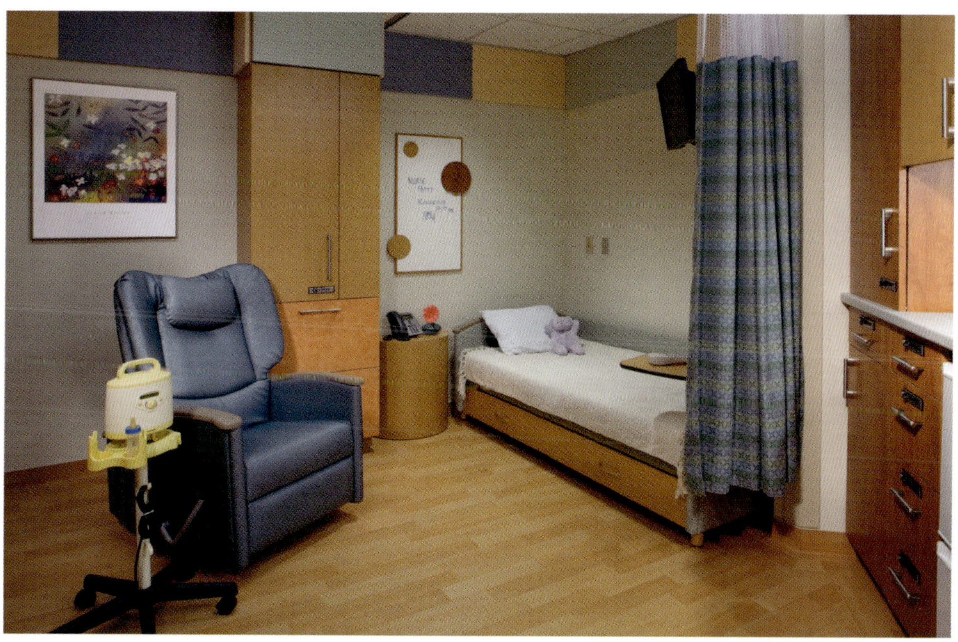

Figure 5.52: *Rainbow Babies and Children's Hospital NICU, Cleveland, OH (Architects: Parkin Architects Ltd in association with Array Architects; Photo credit: Scott Pease)*

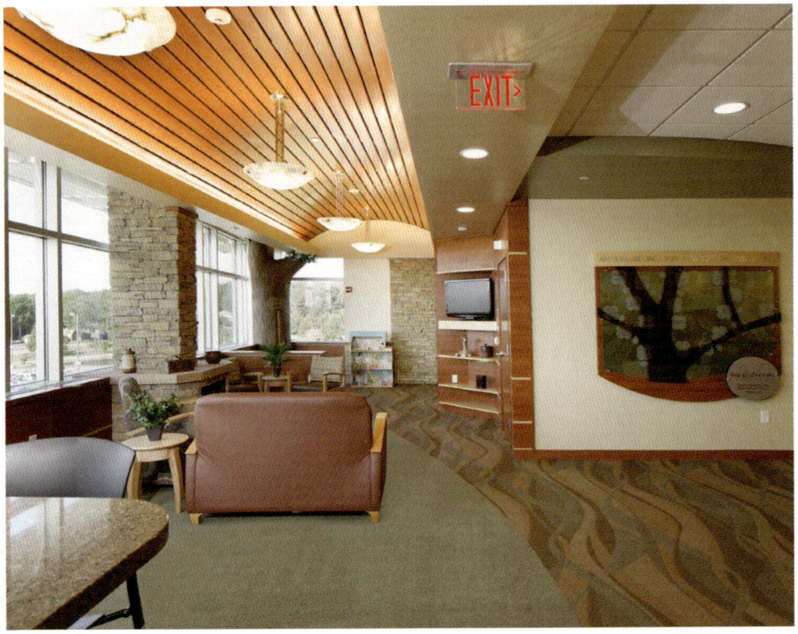

Figure 5.53: *Aspirus Wausau Hospital NICU, Wausau, WI (Architects: Plunkett Raysich Architects, LLP; Photo credit: Weston Imaging)*

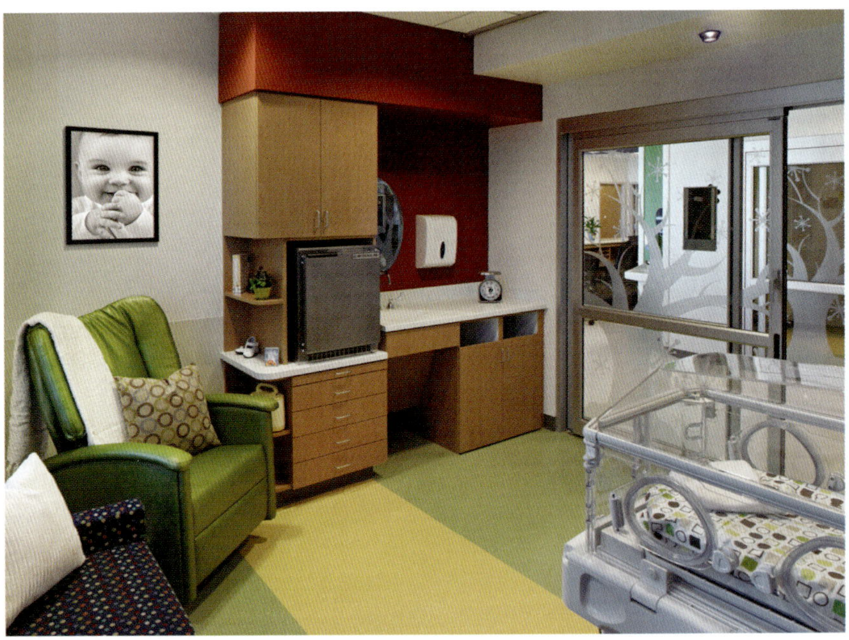

Figure 5.54: *Children's Hospital at St. Francis NICU, Tulsa, OK (Architects: Page Southerland Page, LLP; Photo credit: John W. Davis, DVDesign Group)*

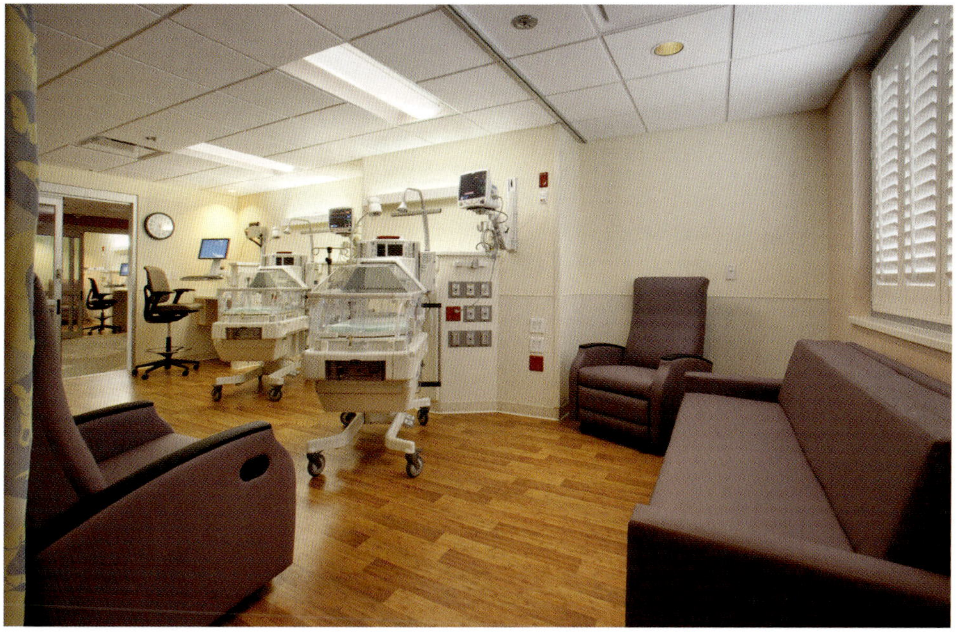

Figure 5.55: *Mercy Children's Hospital NICU, Creve Coeur, MO (Architects: Christner Inc.; Photo credit: Sam Fentress)*

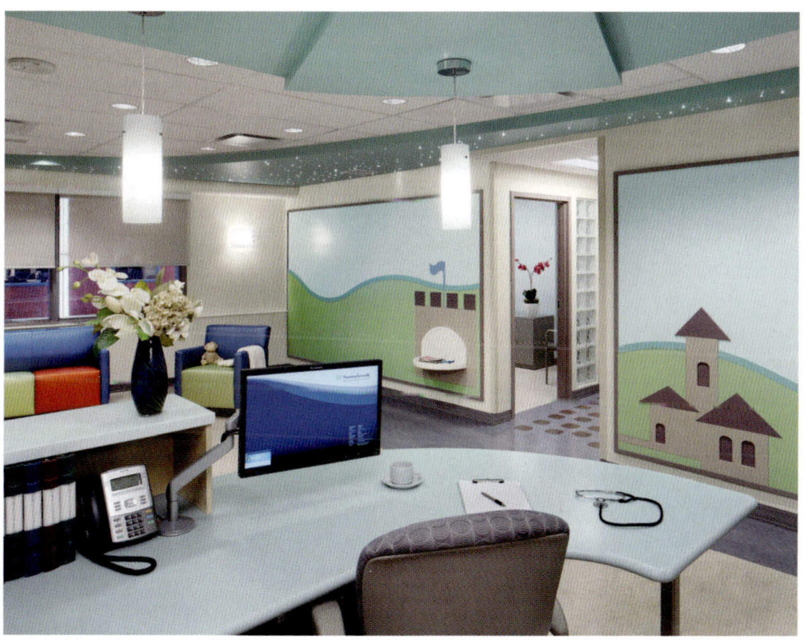

Figure 5.56: *Sunnybrook Health Sciences Women and Babies Program NICU, Toronto, Ontario, Canada (Architects: Parkin Architects Ltd in association with HDR Architects; Photo credit: Richard Johnson Photography)*

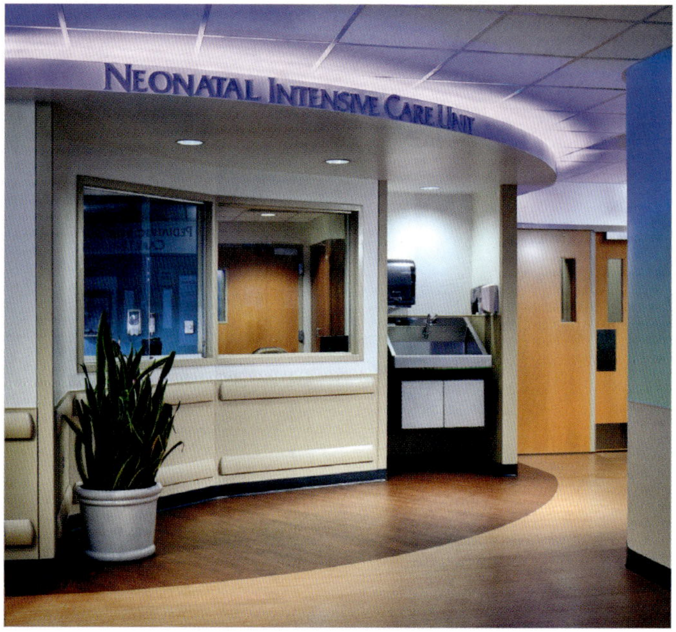

Figure 5.57: *Walt Disney Pavilion NICU at Florida Hospital for Children, Orlando, FL (Architects: HuntonBrady Architects; Photo credit: Joseph Lapeyra)*

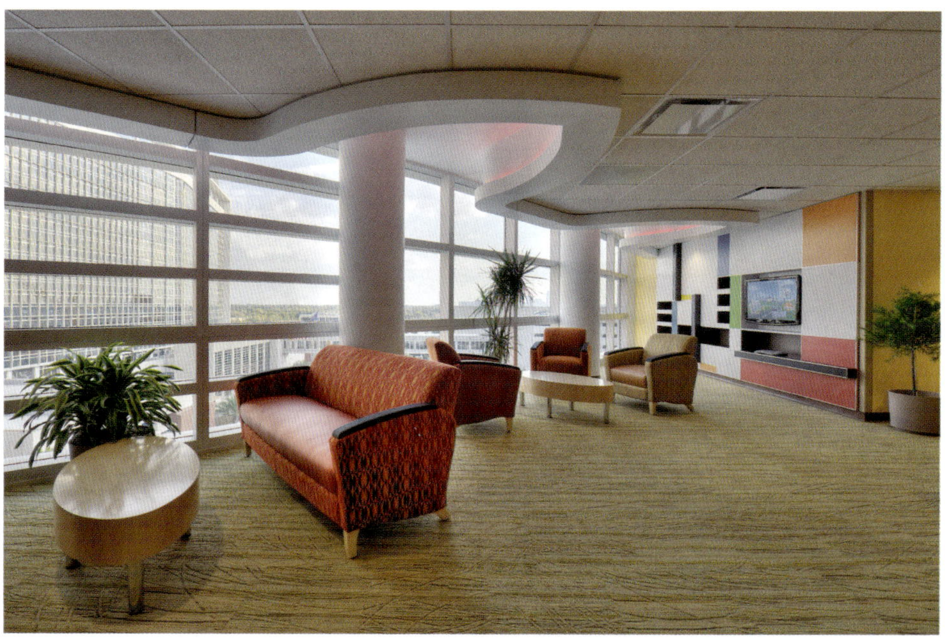

Figure 5.58: *Walt Disney Pavilion NICU at Florida Hospital for Children, Orlando, FL (Architects: HuntonBrady Architects; Photo credit: Ben Tanner)*

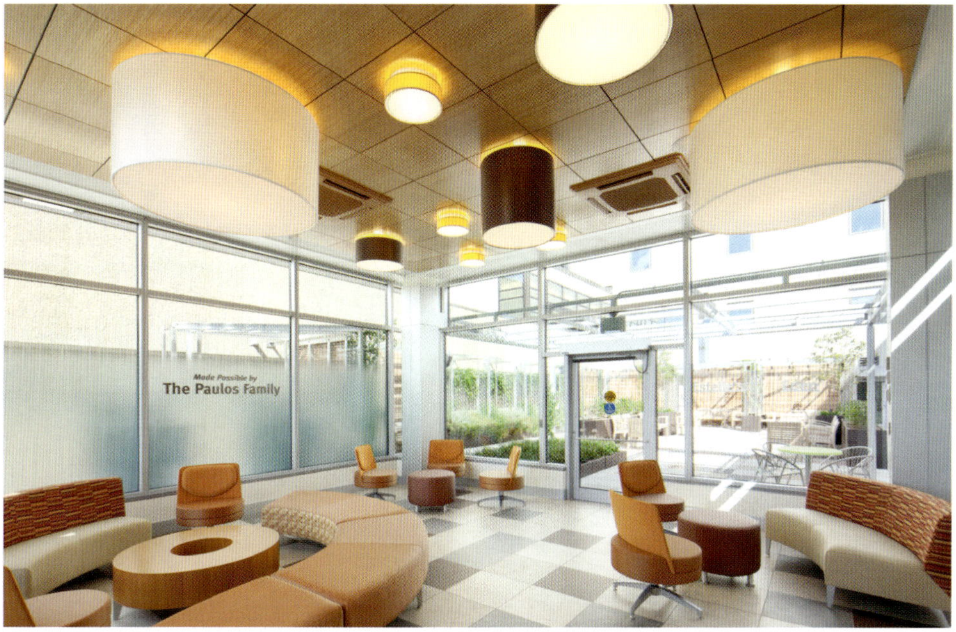

Figure 5.59: *Danbury Hospital Spratt NICU, Danbury, CT (Architects: Perkins Eastman; Photo credit: Sarah Mechling/Perkins Eastman)*

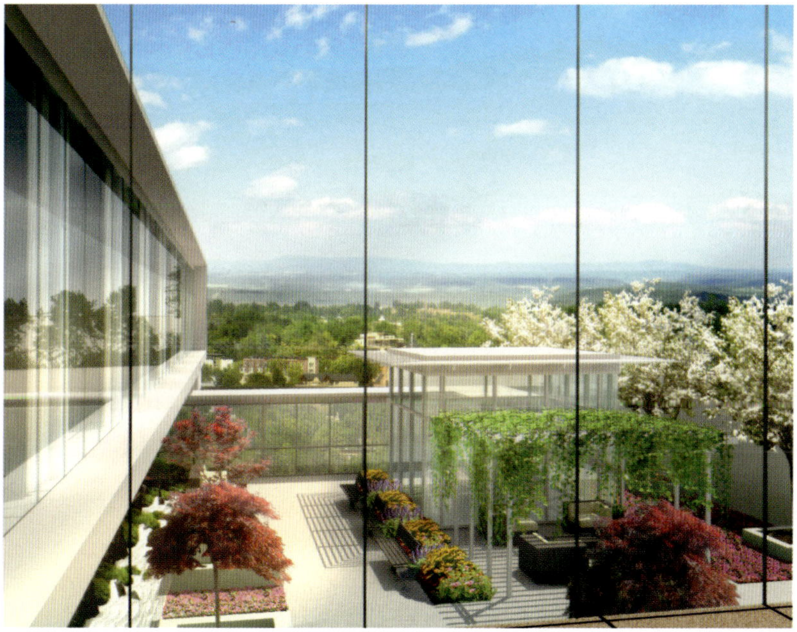

Figure 5.60: *Danbury Hospital Spratt NICU, Danbury, CT (Architects: Perkins Eastman; Photo credit: Sarah Mechling/Perkins Eastman)*

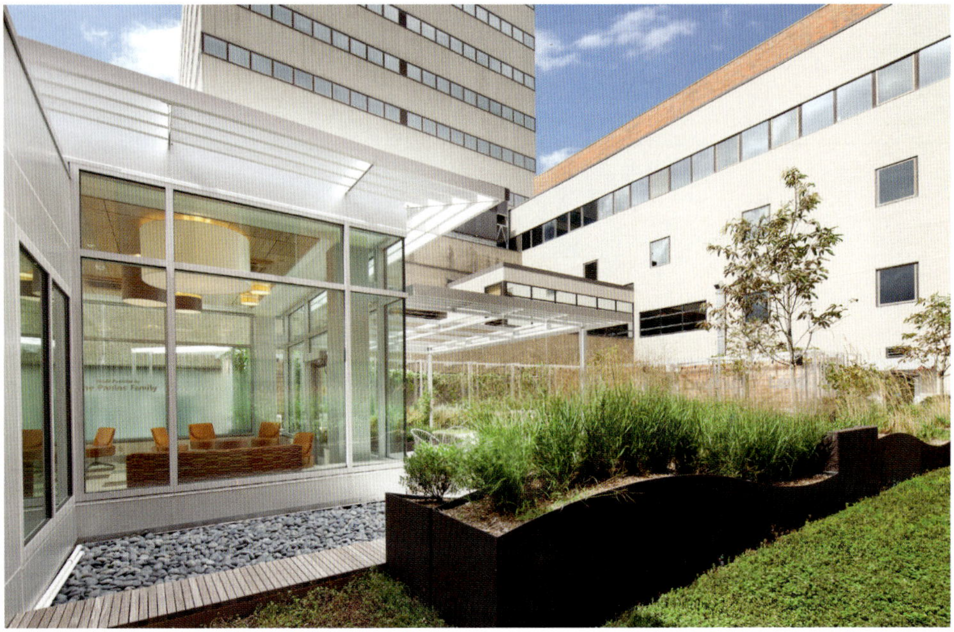

Figure 5.61: *Danbury Hospital Spratt NICU, Danbury, CT (Architects: Perkins Eastman; Photo credit: Sarah Mechling/Perkins Eastman)*

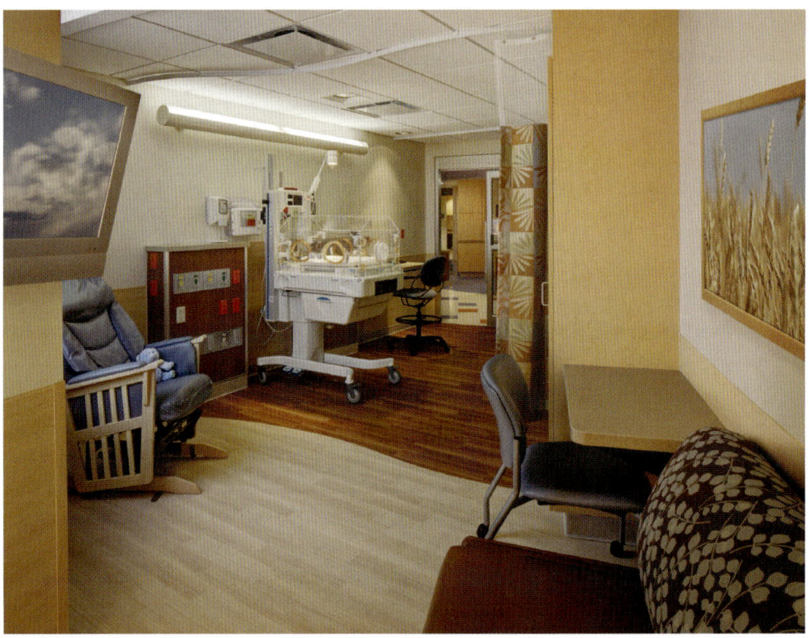

Figure 5.62: *Columbia St. Mary's Hospital NICU, Milwaukee, WI (Architects: Plunkett Raysich Architects, LLP; Photo credit: Tricia Shay Photography)*

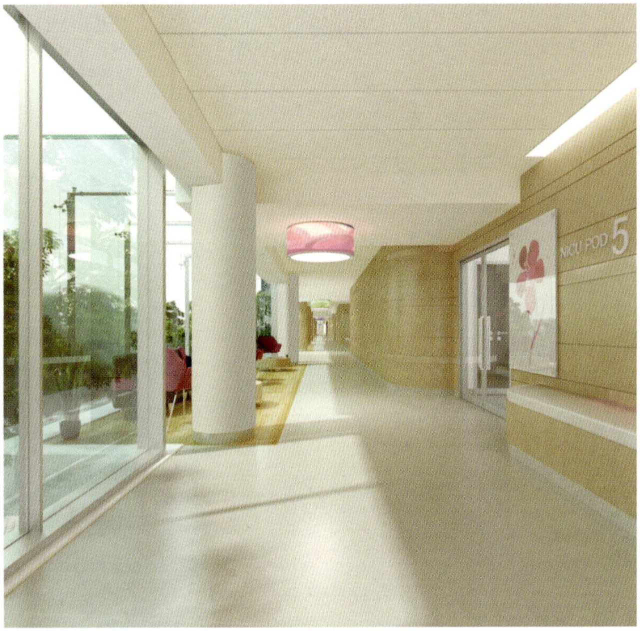

Figure 5.63: *Women and Newborn Hospital, Health Sciences Centre Winnipeg NICU, Winnipeg, Manitoba, Canada (Architects: Parkin Architects Ltd. in association with Smith Carter Architects; Rendering credit: Courtesy of Parkin Architects Ltd.)*

5.4.3 *Staff needs*

While there are a limited number of studies on the anxiety levels and satisfaction of NICU staff, they strongly suggest that working in a NICU is highly stressful (Braithwaite, 2008; Clarke et al., 1984; Dolan, 1987; Oates and Oates, 1995). Overwork or understaffing are among the most critical stress sources (Astbury and Yu, 1982; Clarke et al., 1984; Cusson et al., 2008; Oates and Oates, 1995). Studies that focused on job stress and job dissatisfaction found that job stress was a greater problem (Clarke et al., 1984).

5.4.3.1 Staff stress

Clarke et al. (1984) mailed a five-point-scale job satisfaction questionnaire to neonatologists in the northeastern United States. They found that 34 percent of neonatologists experienced moderately severe stress and 16 percent felt very severe stress. The causes included excessive workload, problems in patient care, and staff disagreements.

Astbury and Yu's study (1982) surveyed the intensity and frequency of stress situations of 22 pediatric consultants and 29 nurses working in NICUs in Australia. More than 70 percent of the consultants rated the following elements as moderately or highly stressful: sudden death/relapse, the conflict between personal life and work, understaffing/overwork; 77.3 percent of consultants highlighted the conflict between personal life and work; and 63.6 percent reported that understaffing/overwork happened often or almost continuously. For the nurses, 75.9 percent chose nurse/doctor conflict and understaffing/overwork, and sudden death/relapse as the most stressful. Nurse/nurse problems, personal life versus work, and nurse/doctor conflict were the top three situations that occurred most frequently or almost continuously among nursing sisters (see Figure 5.64).

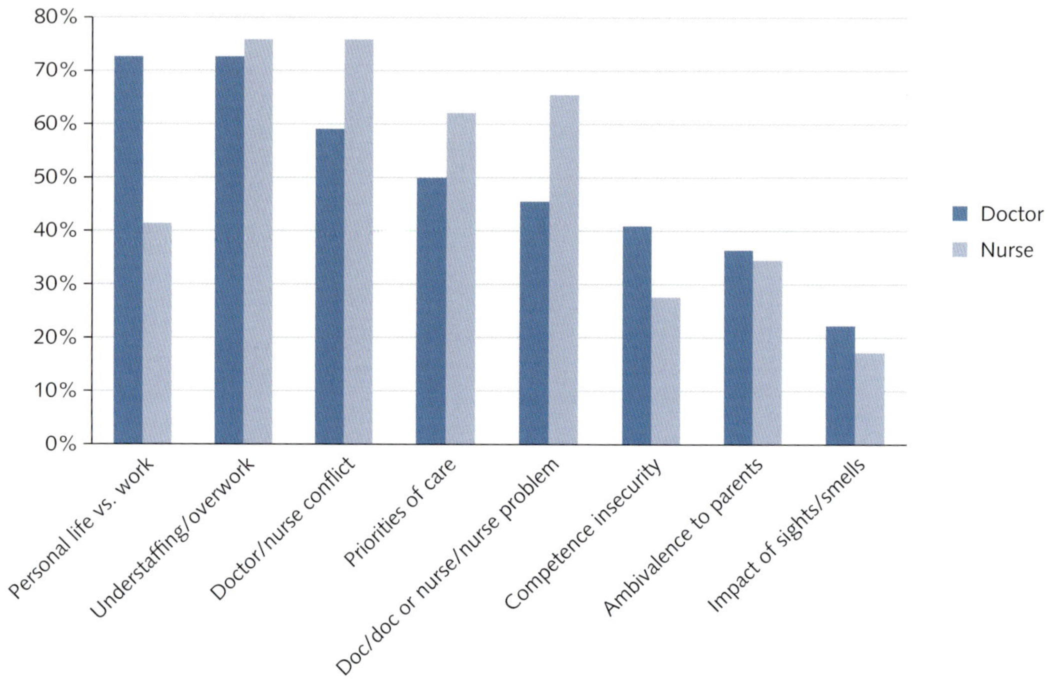

Figure 5.64: *Sources of stress for doctors and nurses (percentage) (Source: Derived from Astbury and Yu, 1982)*

Rosenthal et al. (1989) also studied the frequency and intensity of stress situations, and controllability as well. They categorized eight stressful situations through a literature review: impact of physical environment, concerns about self-competence, demands of infant care, concerns about the family, sudden death/relapse, conflicts with nurses, conflicts with physicians, and ethical issues. In their seven-point Likert scale survey administered to 30 NICU nurses, the overall stress rating was 4.83 (from 0 to 7 was from very little to very much).

Gribbins and Marshall (1984) divided NICU nurse subjects into four groups according to how long they have worked: less than two months, two months to one year, one to three years, and more than three years. They found that the nurses in the first group felt the stress from competence insecurity the most; the other three groups suffered stress from nursing conditions such as understaffing and physician relations; the second and third group also experienced the stress from patients (e.g. death and quality of life) while the third group felt the stress from lack of rewards and job indifference.

Cusson et al. (2008) conducted an internet-based survey of participants of a US neonatal nurse practitioner (NNP) conference. Most of them worked in Level III NICUs. They perceived the responsibility overload and the NNP shortage as the most challenging part as the NNP role.

Shepley et al. (2008) found the NICU staff stress levels lower, staff job satisfaction ratings, and satisfaction with the physical environment higher in the single family room units than in the open-bay units. Tools in this study included the Perception of the Job Satisfaction Scale (Harris et al., 1988), the Nurse Stress Scale (Gray-Toft and Anderson, 1981; French et al., 2000), and the Physical Environment Survey (Fournier, 1999).

5.4.3.2 Staff satisfaction

Staff satisfaction is critical to staff retention. Clarke et al. (1984) found that 17 percent of neonatologists were moderately or very dissatisfied with their work, and the major causes were too much work, lack of resources, too much stress at work, and administrative needs. According to a study by Rosenthal et al. (1989), nurse satisfaction is inversely related to experience and education, and not related to stress. Strategies used by staff for coping involve both problem-solving and emotion-related techniques.

5.4.3.3 Examples of staff spaces in NICUs

Figures 5.65 to 5.75 are examples of staff spaces in NICUs in approximate chronological order. The location, design firm(s), and photo credits are provided. Staff charting, workstations, and meeting areas are shown.

5.5 Facility evaluation

Among the many types of research that can be conducted in PICUs and NICUs are practitioner-focused facility evaluations (PFEs). Evaluation has become particularly critical due to recent paradigm shifts, such as the transition from open-bay to single family room NICUs, as experimental prototypes may be influencing the design of future facilities prior to confirming their appropriateness.

In order to discuss evaluation research, it is helpful to provide a definition of PFEs relative to other types of research. For the purposes of this discussion, PFE research must include three components: an independent variable (the physical environment), a human subject (staff, patient, or family), and an outcome that may be translated into a design solution. Other types of research may not have outcomes that involve persons or are translatable into design solutions. These are still a form of design research but they are not PFEs.

Figure 5.76 gives a list of facility evaluations that have been done in pediatric inpatient settings (both acute and critical care). This list demonstrates that very few evaluations of pediatric and neonatal critical care settings have been published. This is particularly true for PICUs.

5.6 Tools for NICU and PICU research

For those who are interested in conducting design research, one of the first barriers is finding tools to support the research. Having a pre-existing tool enables the researcher in three ways. First, it reduces the time associated with developing and piloting the tool itself; second, the results of the new study may be compared to the results of the previous study that used the tool; and third, the

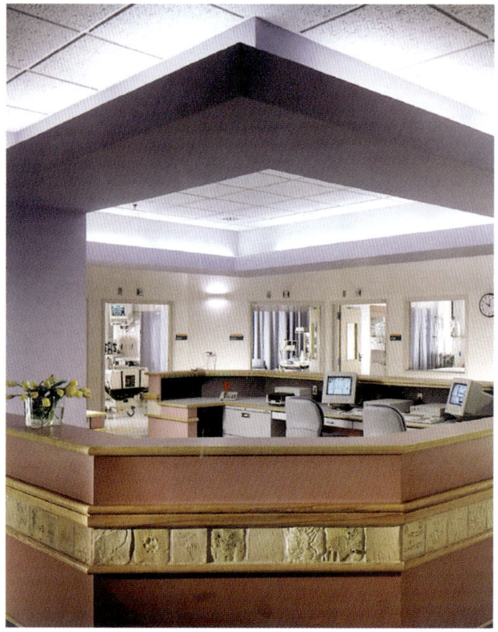

Figure 5.65: *Hasbro Children's Hospital NICU, Providence, RI (Architects: Shepley Bulfinch; Photo credit: Robert Miller)*

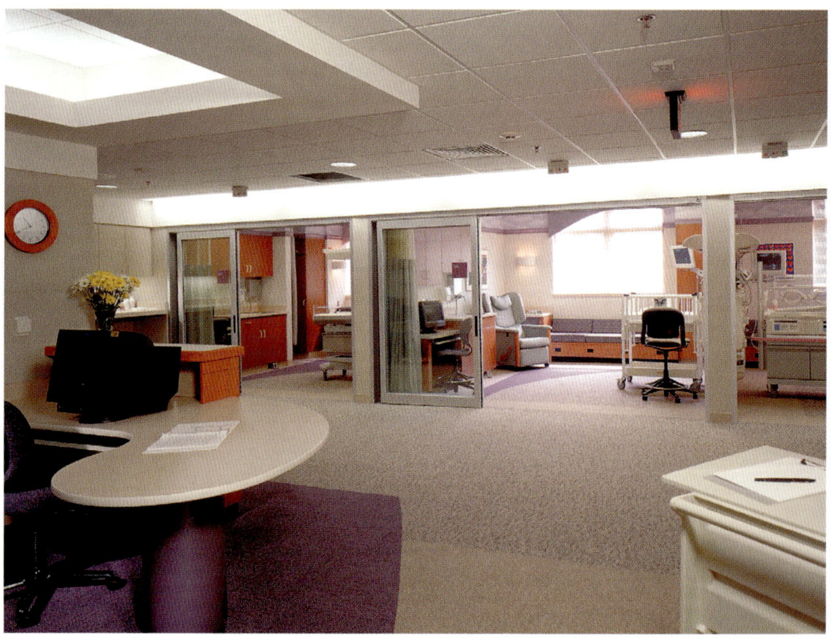

Figure 5.66: *St. Luke's Hospital NICU, Cedar Rapids, IA (Architects: Ellerbe Becket (AECOM); Photo credit: Dana Wheelock/Wheelock Photography)*

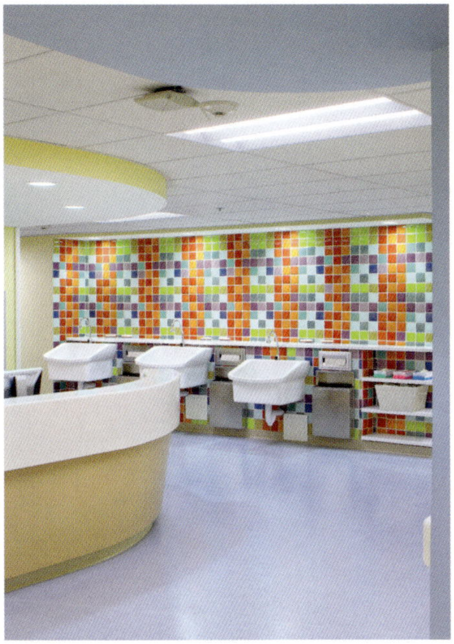

Figure 5.67: *SSM Cardinal Glennon Children's Medical Center NICU, St. Louis, MO (Architects: Christner Inc.; Photo credit: Sam Fentress)*

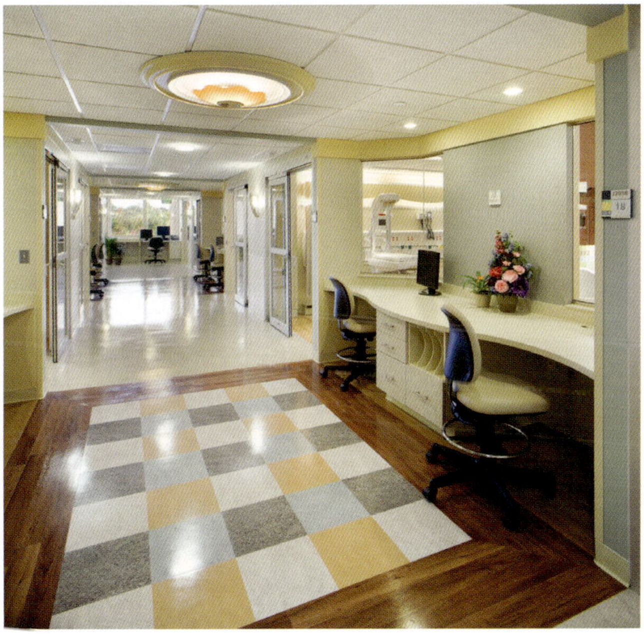

Figure 5.68: *Atlantic Health Systems NICU, Morristown, NJ (Architects: Buckl Architects; Photo credit: Courtesy of www.gregbenson.com)*

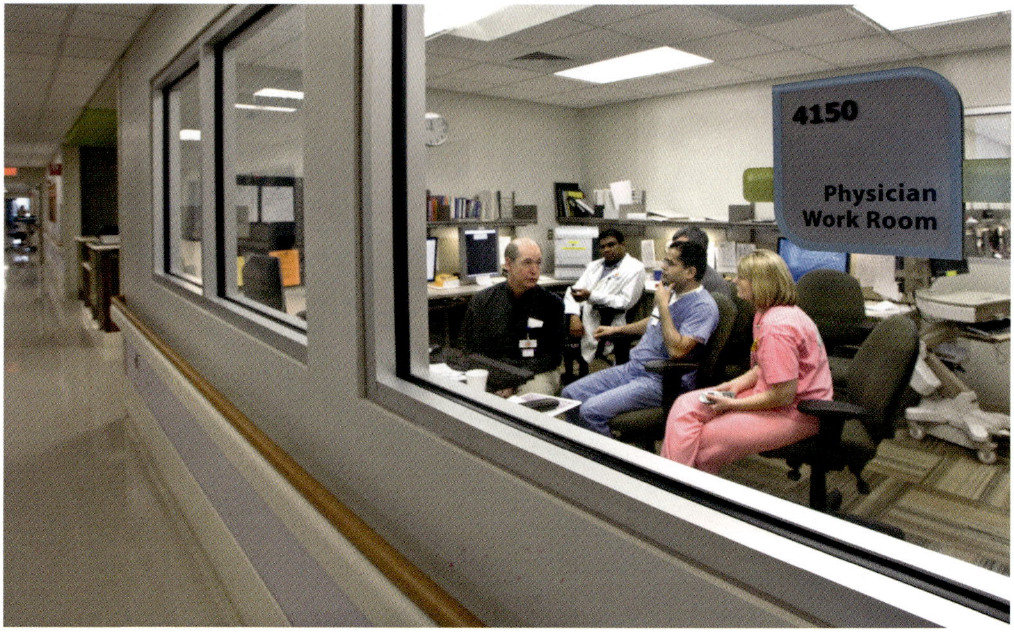

Figure 5.69: *Le Bonheur Children's Hospital NICU, Memphis, TN (Architects: FKP Architects; Photo credit: Courtesy of FKP Architects)*

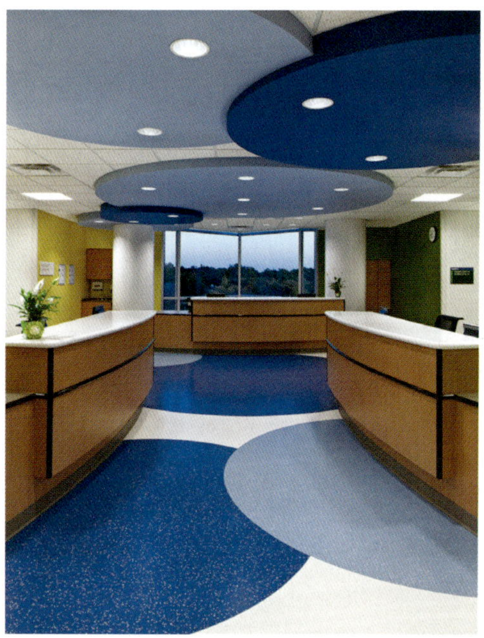

Figure 5.70: *Children's Hospital at St. Francis NICU, Tulsa, OK (Architects: Page Southerland Page, LLP; Photo credit: John W. Davis, DVDesign Group)*

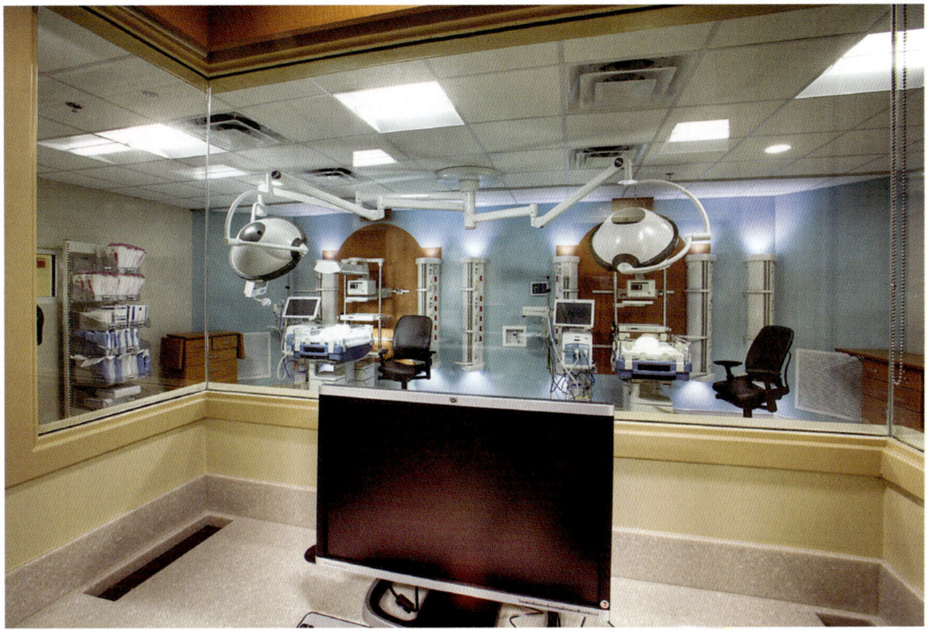

Figure 5.71: *Jennifer Leigh Muma NICU at Tampa General Hospital, Tampa, FL (Architects: Harvard Jolly Architecture; Photo credit: Harvard Jolly Architecture)*

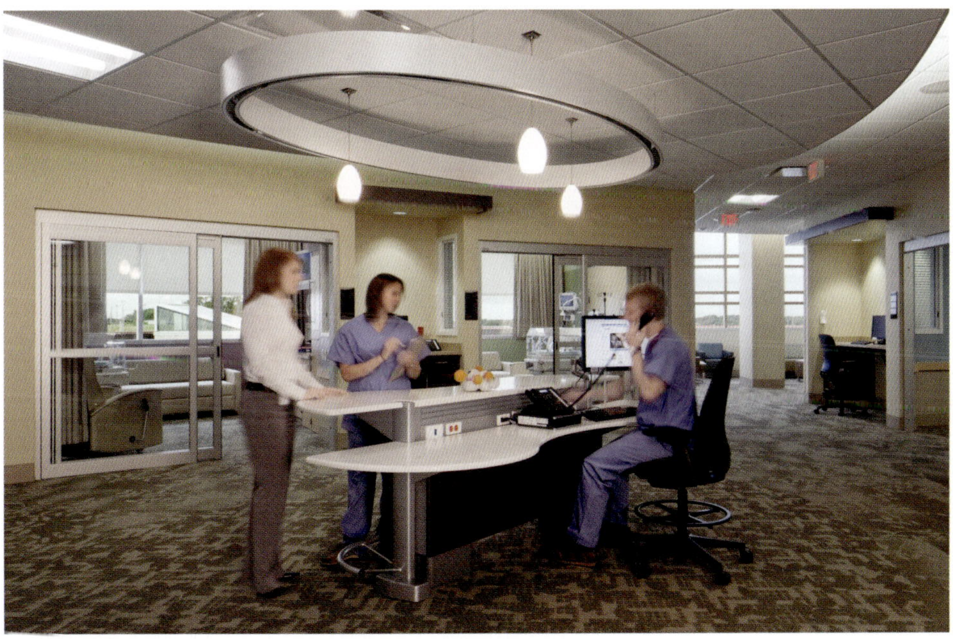

Figure 5.72: *Methodist Women's Hospital NICU, Omaha, NE (Architects: HDR; Photo credit: Ari Burling Photography)*

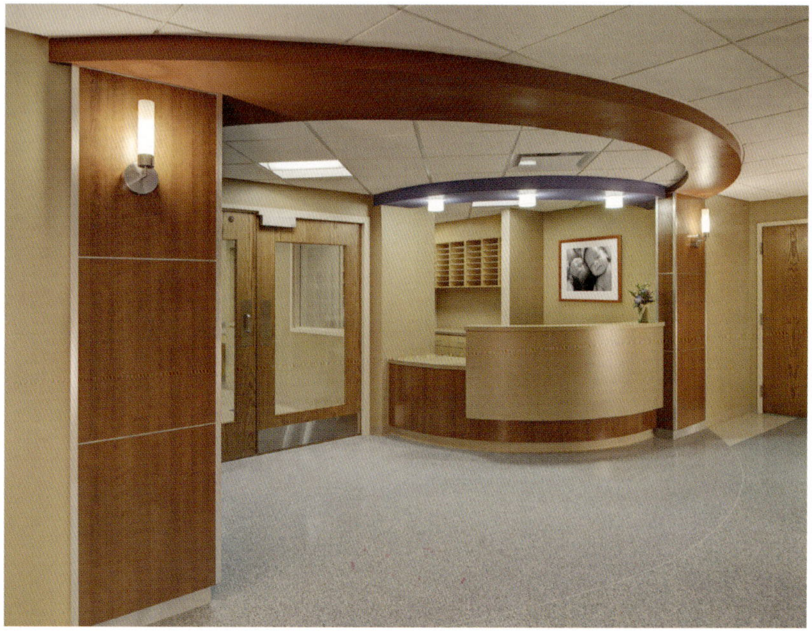

Figure 5.73: *Columbia St. Mary's Hospital NICU, Milwaukee, WI (Architects: Plunkett Raysich Architects, LLP; Photo credit: Tricia Shay Photography)*

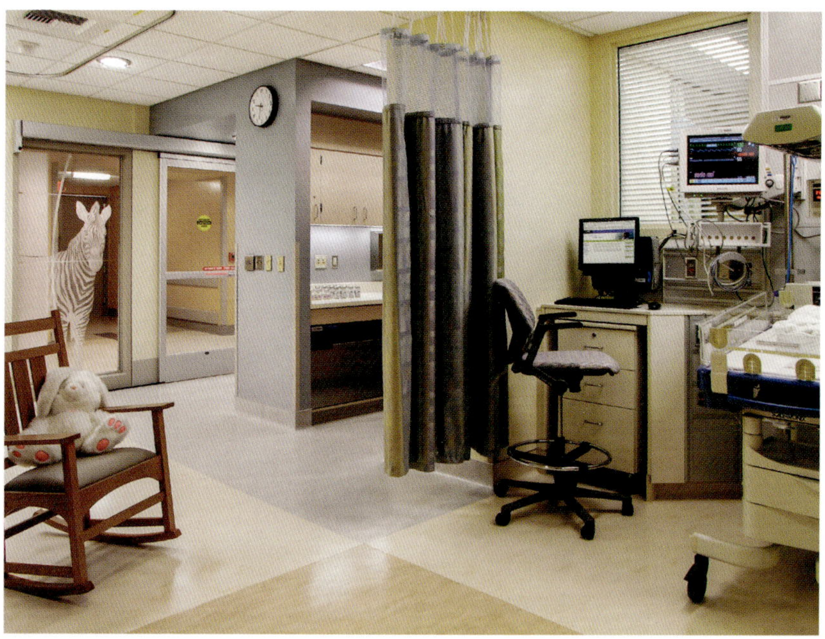

Figure 5.74: *UC Davis Children's Hospital NICU, Sacramento, CA (Architects: Stantec; Photo credit: Dean J. Birinyi, ASMP)*

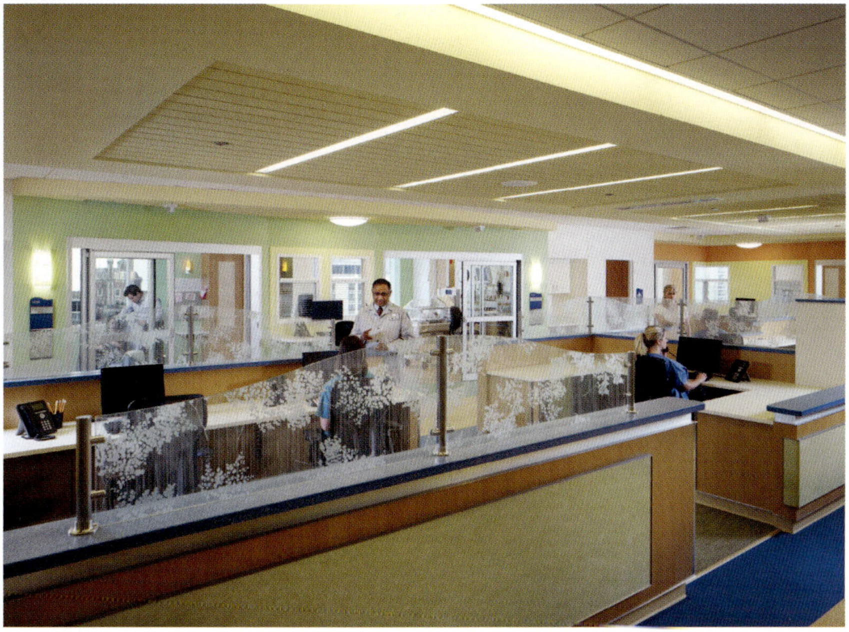

Figure 5.75: *Ann & Robert H. Lurie Children's Hospital of Chicago NICU, Chicago, IL (Architects: ZGF Architects LLP, Solomon Cordwell Buenz, Anderson Mikos Architects, Ltd.; Photo credit: Nick Merrick © Hedrich Blessing)*

authors of the previous study will have had the opportunity to test the reliability and validity of the tool, which will enhance the current research. Sharing similar tools will also support a future meta-analysis of the data.

Among the tools for pediatric design research, several focus specifically on intensive care. The general tools are: the Environmental Assessment Instrument (EAI), the Family Satisfaction with the Physical Environment Survey (FSPES), and the Satisfaction and Perception of the Physical Environment survey (SPPE). The Questionnaire of Stressful Factors in the Intensive Care Unit (QSFICU), the Parental Stressor Scale: Pediatric ICU (PSS: PICU) and the Parental Stressor Scale: Neonatal ICU (PSS: NICU), and the McPherson et al. PICU Parent Satisfaction Survey directly address the ICU. Lastly, James Varni's Pediatric Quality of Life Survey (PedsQL) is a useful tool for assessing parent and child emotional and operational status in children's healthcare settings.

- The EAI was developed to identify child-appropriate features (Curry et al., 1996). The tool includes three parts: minimum standards, accessibility codes, and research-based patient room design recommendations. Responses were provided using yes/no answers; percentages of 90 to 100 percent were considered to be child-oriented. When the tool was used to compare adult and pediatric rooms, Curry et al. found little difference between these units.
- In a comparative study of open-bay and single family-room neonatal intensive care units, to measure degree of satisfaction with the physical environment, Shepley et al. (2008) used the FSPES developed by Fournier (1999), as well as their own instrument, the SPPE. The SPPE has 25 questions addressing physical dimensions of the environment, including overall physical

Figure 5.76: *Facility evaluations in pediatric healthcare environments*

Outcomes (Dependent Variable)	*Environment (Independent Variable)*	*Reference*
Work environment quality Features from guidelines, accessibility standards	Adult and pediatric patient room	Curry, Z.D., Shroyer, J.L., Staton, C.D. & Curry, D.J. (1996). Environmental assessment instrument development and usage for the analysis of adult and pediatric patient room design.
Staff and family behavior	NICU	Harris, D.D., Shepley, M.M., White, R.D., Kolberg, K.J.S., & Harrell, J. W. (2006). The impact of single family room design on patients and caregivers: Executive summary.
Lighting, sound, staff efficiency, family experience, infant sleep time, baby movement	NICU	Marden, V., Grant, D., Abrey, R. & Tooley, M. (2013). Creating a space to grow: Innovative approaches to measuring the impact of a new NICU design on developmental care.
Patient, family, and staff satisfaction and visitation patterns	Pediatric hospital gardens	Pasha, S. (2011). *Usability of outdoor spaces in children's hospitals*.
Safety, length of stay, staffing, family presence	PICU	Poltronieri, L. & Schleien, C.L. (2010). PICU design: Influence on patient outcomes and staff/family satisfaction.
Staff behavior	NICU	Shepley, M.M. (2002). Predesign and postoccupancy analysis of staff behavior in a neonatal intensive care unit.
Satisfaction, family and staff behavior	NICU	Shepley, M.M., Bryant, C., & Frohman, B. (1995). Using a post-occupancy study to validate a building prototype: An evaluation of a new women's medical center.
Patient and family quality of life and satisfaction	Pediatric acute care	Shepley, M.M., Fellows, C., Hintz, R., Johnson, L., & Spohn, J. (2012). Pediatric inpatient room experience.
Staff satisfaction and stress	NICU	Shepley, M.M., Harris, D.D., & White, R. (2008). Open-bay and single-family room neonatal intensive care units: Caregiver satisfaction and stress.
Family behavior	NICU	Shepley, M.M., Harris, D.D., White, R. & Steinberg, F. (2008). Impact of single family NICU rooms on family behavior
Patient and family satisfaction and psychosocial functioning	Oncology inpatient unit	Sherman-Bien, S.A., Malcarne, V.L., Roesch, S., Varni, J.W., & Katz, E.R. (2011). Quantifying the relationship between hospital design, satisfaction, and psychosocial functioning in a pediatric hematology-oncology inpatient unit.
Patient, family, and staff utilization	Pediatric cancer center garden	Sherman, S.A., Varni, J.W., Ulrich, R.S., & Malcarne, V.L. (2005). Post-occupancy evaluation of healing gardens in a pediatric cancer center.
Patient, family, and staff utilization and satisfaction	Pediatric hospital garden	Whitehouse, S., Varni, J.W., Seid, M., Cooper-Marcus, C., Ensberg, M.J., Jacobs, J.R., & Mejlenbeck, R.S. (2001). Evaluating a children's hospital garden environment: Utilization and consumer satisfaction.

environment, window views, natural light, light level, noise level, atmosphere and decor, waiting and resting space, corridors and signage for wayfinding, and places for food and nourishment.

- Huckabay and Jagla (1979) developed the only tool that specifically addresses the ICU. The tool incorporates 32 items and four categories of stressful events in critical care nursing: interpersonal communication difficulties, need for broad knowledge base, environmental problems, and patient care issues. Noise level; physical setup of the unit (e.g. supplies not readily available or not stored in an organized fashion), equipment failure, and physical injury to the nurse are part of the section addressing environmental problems. This subscale has been used by other researchers to examine the relationship between physical features of the workplace and job satisfaction (e.g. Norbeck, 1985).
- McPherson et al. (2000) developed a survey tool specifically for parents of PICU patients. This 23-item survey was developed with the input of parents and tested for validity and reliability. The survey addressed hospital environment (e.g. space around the bed and noise), communication, and patient care.
- The Carter and Miles (1982) Parental Stressor Scale: Pediatric ICU (PSS: PICU) and Miles et al.'s (1993) Parental Stressor Scale: Neonatal ICU (PSS: NICU) have been used in multiple studies to measure parent stress. In addition to psychosocial factors, these tests include items related to the physical environment, such as "sights and sounds," alarms, and surroundings.
- The PedsQL was developed by Dr. James Varni. This tool is a battery of brief surveys that evaluate the quality of life of families and children. It has been used extensively in pediatric healthcare settings and published in more than 840 peer-reviewed journals. Sherman et al. (2006a) used the PedsQL Present Functioning Visual Analogue Scale, which measures in-the-moment emotional status, and the Pediatric Pain Questionnaire to measure anxiety, sadness, anger, worry, fatigue, and pain in parents and children, when they entered a hospital and two hours later, and found a correlation between emotional stress and pain.

Unfortunately, only a handful of studies have been conducted in PICUs. Most of the recent research on NICUs focuses on the issue of shared versus private rooms, although the original emphasis in the literature addressed noise and light levels. These topics and others will be covered.

5.7 Design guidelines from research

In the recently published *Evidence for Innovation* (NACHRI, 2008), the authors generated a list of evidence-based design strategies all for general, NICU, PICU/pediatric, adolescent, staff, and families. This list of strategies is broken down into the categories of pediatric settings and strategies that can be borrowed from adult settings, as well as promising strategies. The latter are not included in this summary, as they are numerous.

Figure 5.77 summarizes conclusions drawn from this report as well as conclusions drawn from the literature discussed in this chapter that include references between 2008 and 2013, not available at the time of the NACHRI publication.

Figure 5.77: *Design strategies suggested by Evidence for Innovation (NAHCRI, 2008) and the literature review in this chapter (EI = Evidence for Innovation; LR = additions based on the preceding literature review)*

	All	*NICU*	*PICU*	*Adol*	*Staff*	*Fam*
Strategies from pediatric settings						
1. Single family rooms		EI	LR			
2. Developmentally appropriate lighting (sometimes circadian)		EI				
3. Noise reduction (in addition to incubators)		EI	LR	LR	LR	
4. Sound-absorbing materials (in addition to ceiling tiles)	EI	LR	LR	LR	LR	
5. Space for families in all patient rooms	EI	LR	LR			
6. Patient and family privacy and environment control		EI	EI	EI		EI
7. Acoustical interventions before/during procedures		EI	EI	EI		
8. Positive distractions to reduce stress				EI		
9. Access to nature through gardens	EI					
10. Age-appropriate play areas				EI		LR
11. Overall ambience and attractiveness	EI	LR	EI			
Applicable strategies from adult settings						
12. Effective way finding systems	EI					
13. Single patient rooms	EI					
14. Hand-washing dispensers and sinks					EI	
15. Access to natural light	EI					
16. Ceiling lifts					EI	
17. Noise audits	EI					
18. Visual access and accessibility to patients	EI					
19. Positive distractions	EI					
20. HEPA filtration for immune-compromised patients		EI	EI			

Reducing noise, providing space for families, supporting patient/family privacy and control, and the use of acoustical interventions are the most frequently discussed objectives in the research literature. In the neonatal literature, recommendations for the use of single family rooms is the most common research topic.

References

Agarwal, S., Classen, D., Larsen, G., Tofil, N.M., Hayes, L.W., Sullivan, J.E., and Sharek, P. (2010). Prevalence of adverse events in pediatric intensive care units in the United States. *Pediatric Critical Care Medicine*, *11*(5), 568–578.

Al-Samsam, R.H., and Cullen, P. (2005). Sleep and adverse environmental factors in sedated mechanically ventilated pediatric intensive care patients. *Pediatric Critical Care Medicine*, 6(5), 562–567.

Archibald, L.K., Manning, M.L., Bell, L.M., Banerjee, S., and Jarvis, W.R. (1997). Patient density, nurse-to-patient ratio and nosocomial infection risk in a pediatric cardiac intensive care unit. *The Pediatric Infectious Disease Journal*, *16*(11), 1045–1048.

Arnon, S., Shapsa, A., Forman, L., Regev, R., Bauer, S., Litmanovits, I., and Dolfin, T. (2006). Live music is beneficial to preterm infants in the neonatal intensive care unit. *Birth, 33*(2), 131–136.

Astbury, J., and Yu, V.Y. (1982). Determinants of stress for staff in a neonatal intensive care unit. *Archives of Disease in Childhood, 57*(2), 108–111.

Bailey, E., and Timmons, S. (2005). Noise levels in PICU: An evaluative study. *Pediatric Nursing, 17*(10), 22–26.

Balluffi, A., Kassam-Adams, N., Kazak, A., Tucker, M., Dominquez, T., and Helfaer, M. (2004). Traumatic stress in parents of children admitted to the pediatric intensive care unit. *Pediatric Critical Care Medicine, 5*(6), 547–553.

Beauchemin, K.M., and Hays, P. (1996). Sunny hospital rooms expedite recovery from severe and refractory depressions. *Journal of Affective Disorders*, *40*(1), 49–51.

Beck, S.A., Weis, J., Greisen, G., Andersen, M., and Zoffmann, V. (2009). Room for family-centered care – A qualitative evaluation of a neonatal intensive care unit remodeling project. *Journal of Neonatal Nursing*, *15*(3), 88–99.

Beeram, M.R. (February 8, 2013). *Medical issues in pediatric care and how they relate to design of children's health facilities*. Presentation at the Architecture-for-Health Spring 2013 Lecture Series. College Station, TX: College of Architecture, Texas A&M University.

Ben Abraham, R., Keller, N., Szold, O., Vardi, A., Weinberg, M., Barzilay, Z., and Paret, G. (2002). Do isolation rooms reduce the rate of nosocomial infections in the pediatric intensive care unit? *Journal of Critical Care*, *17*(3), 176–180.

Benedetti, F., Colombo, C., Barbini, B., Campori, E., and Smeraldi, E. (2001). Morning sunlight reduces length of hospitalization in bipolar depression. *Journal of Affective Disorders*, *62*(3), 221–223.

Berens, R. (1999). Noise in the pediatric intensive care unit. *Journal of Intensive Care Medicine, 14*(3), 118–129.

Bishop, K. (2008). *From their perspectives: Children and young people's experiences in a paediatric hospital environment and its relationship to their feeling of well-being.* Doctoral dissertation retrieved from http://ses.library.usyd.edu.au/bitstream/2123/3962/1/kg-bishop-2008-thesis.pdf

Board, R. (2005). School-age children's perceptions of their PICU hospitalization. *Pediatric Nursing*, *31*(3), 166–175.

Bosch, S., and Bledsoe, T. (March, 2013). Study analyzes staff perceptions of single family rooms in the NICU. *Neonatology Today*, 8–10.

Bosch, S., Bledsoe, T., and Jenzarli, A. (2012). Staff perceptions before and after adding single-family rooms in the NICU. *HERD*, *5*(4), 64–75.

Bowie, B.H., Hall, R.B., Faulkner, J., and Anderson, B. (2003). Single-room infant care: Future trends in special care nursery planning and design. *Neonatal Network, 22*(4), 27–34.

Braithwaite, M. (2008). Nurse burnout and stress in the NICU. *Advances in Neonatal Care, 8*(6), 343–347.

Brandon, D.H., Holditch-Davis, D., and Belyea, M. (2002). Preterm infants born at less than 31 weeks' gestation have improved growth in cycled light compared with continuous near darkness. *Journal of Pediatrics*, *140*, 192–198.

Bratt, M.M., Broome, M., Kelber, S., and Lostocco, L. (2000). Influence of stress and nursing leadership on job satisfaction of pediatric intensive care unit nurses. *American Journal of Critical Care*, *9*(5), 307–317.

Bremmer, P., Byers, J.F., and Kiehl, E. (2003). Noise and the premature infant: Physiological effects and practice implications. *Journal of Obstetric, Gynecologic, and Neonatal Nursing, 32*(4), 447–454.

Brown, P., and Taquino, L.T. (2001). Designing and delivering neonatal care in single rooms. *Journal of Perinatal and Neonatal Nursing, 15*(1), 68–83.

Bruns, D.A., and Klein, S. (2005). An evaluation of family-centered care in a level III NICU. *Infants and Young Children, 18*(3), 222–233.

Buckley, M.S., Erstad, B.L., Kopp, B.J., Theodorou, A.A., and Priestley, G. (2007). Direct observation approach for detecting medication errors and adverse drug events in a pediatric intensive care unit. *Pediatric Critical Care Medicine, 8*(2), 145–152.

Bunker-Hellmich, L.A. (1987). A case study of space use and visiting policy in a neonatal intensive care unit. *Children's Environments Quarterly, 4*(3), 25–32.

Burke, M.A. (2000). *Music Therapy in the NICU: The Personal Journal of a Researcher*. New York: Louis and Lucille Armstrong Music Therapy Program.

Burke, M., Walsh, J., Oehler, J., and Gingras, J. (1995). Music therapy following suctioning: Four case studies. *Neonatal Network, 14*(7), 41–49.

Butt, M.L., and Kisilevsky, B.S. (2000). Music modulates behaviour of premature infants following heel lance. *Canadian Journal of Nursing Research, 31*(4), 17–40.

Byers, J.F., Waugh, W.R., and Lowman, L.B. (2006). Sound level exposure of high-risk infants in different environmental conditions. *Neonatal Network: The Journal of Neonatal Nursing, 25*(1), 25–32.

Cameron, M.A., Schleien, C.L., and Morris, M.C. (2009). Parental presence on pediatric intensive care unit rounds. *The Journal of Pediatrics, 155*(4), 522–528.

Carter, B.S., Carter, A., and Bennett, S. (2008). Families' views upon experiencing change in the neonatal intensive care unit environment: From the "baby barn" to the private room. *Journal of Perinatology, 28*(12), 827–829.

Carter, M.C., and Miles, M.S. (1982). Parental Stressor Scale: Pediatric ICU. *Nursing Research, 31*(2), 121.

Carter, M.C., and Miles, M.S. (1989). The Parental Stressor Scale: Pediatric Intensive Care Unit. *Maternal-Child Nursing Journal, 18*(3), 187–198.

Caskey, M., Stephens, B., Tucker, R., and Vohr, B. (2011). Importance of parent talk on the development of preterm infant vocalizations. *Pediatrics, 128*(5), 910–916.

Cassidy, J.W., and Standley, J.M. (1995). The effect of music listening on physiological responses of premature infants in the NICU. *Journal of Music Therapy, 32(4)*, 208–227.

Clarke, T.A., Maniscalco, W.M., Taylor-Brown, S., Roghmann, K.J., Shapiro, D.L., and Hannon-Johnson, C. (1984). Job satisfaction and stress among neonatologists. *Pediatrics, 74*(1), 52–57.

Colombo, G., and De Bon, G. (2011). Strategies to protect sleep. *Journal of Maternal-Fetal and Neonatal Medicine, 24*(S1), 30–31.

Cooper Marcus, C., and Barnes, M. (1995). *Gardens in Healthcare Facilities: Uses, Therapeutic Benefits, and Design Recommendations*. Martinez, CA: The Center for Health Design.

Curry, Z.D., Shroyer, J.L., Staton, C.D., and Curry, D.J. (1996). Environmental assessment instrument development and usage for the analysis of adult and pediatric patient room design. *Journal of Family and Consumer Sciences, 88*(2), 53–58.

Cusson, R.M., Buus-Frank, M.E., Flanagan, V.A., Miller, S., Zukowsky, K., and Rasmussen, L. (2008). A survey of the current neonatal nurse practitioner workforce. *Journal of Perinatology, 28*(12), 830–836.

Deep, A., Ghildiyal, R., Kandian, S., and Shinkre, N. (2004). Clinical and microbiological profile of nosocomial infections in the pediatric intensive care unit (PICU). *Indian Pediatrics*, *41*(12), 1238–1246.

DiBiasie, A. (2006). Evidence-based review of retinopathy of prematurity prevention in VLBW and ELBW infants. *Neonatal Network: The Journal of Neonatal Nursing*, *25*(6), 393–403.

DiFiore, T., and Schirripa, S. (2013). Effects of NICU design on infection control, patient outcomes and parental satisfaction. *Proceedings from The Physical and Developmental Environment of the High-Risk Infant Conference*. Clearwater, FL: USF Health.

Doheny, L., Hurwitz, S., Insoft, R., Ringer, S., and Lahav, A. (2012). Exposure to biological maternal sounds improves cardiorespiratory regulation in extremely preterm infants. *Journal of Maternal-Fetal and Neonatal Medicine*, *25*(9), 1591–1594.

Dolan, S.N. (1987). The relationship between burnout and job satisfaction in nurses. *Journal of Advanced Nursing, 12*(1), 3–12.

Domanico, R., Davis, D.K., Coleman, F., and Davis, B.O. (2011). Documenting the NICU design dilemma: Comparative patient progress in open-ward and single family room units. *Journal of Perinatology*, *31*(4), 281–288.

Eisen, S.L., Ulrich, R.S., Shepley, M.M., Varni, J.W., and Sherman, S. (2008). The stress-reducing effects of art in pediatric health care: Art preferences of healthy children and hospitalized children. *Journal of Child Health Care, 12*, 173–190.

Ernst, M.E., Messmer, P.R., Franco, M., and Gonzalez, J.L. (2004). Nurses' job satisfaction, stress, and recognition in a pediatric setting. *Pediatric Nursing*, *30*, 219–231.

Farrell, M.F., and Frost, C. (1992). The most important needs of parents of critically ill children: Parents' perceptions. *Intensive and Critical Care Nursing, 8*(3), 130–139.

Fegran, L., Fagermoen, M.S., and Helseth, S. (2008a). Development of parent–nurse relationships in neonatal intensive care units – From closeness to detachment. *Journal of Advanced Nursing*, *64*(4), 363–371.

Fegran, L., Helseth, S., and Fagermoen, M.S. (2008b). A comparison of mothers' and fathers' experiences of the attachment process in a neonatal intensive care unit. *Journal of Clinical Nursing*, *17*(6), 810–816.

Fischer, J.E., Calame, A., Dettling, A.C., Zeier, H., and Fanconi, S. (2000). Experience and endocrine stress responses in neonatal and pediatric critical care nurses and physicians. *Critical Care Medicine*, *28*(9), 3281–3288.

Flynn, E.A., Barker, K.N., Gibson, J.T., Pearson, R.E., Smith, L.A., and Berger, B.A. (1996). Relationships between ambient sounds and the accuracy of pharmacists' prescription-filling performance. *Human Factors: The Journal of the Human Factors and Ergonomics Society*, *38*(4), 614–622.

Flynn, E.A., Barker, K.N., Gibson, J.T., Pearson, R.E., Berger, B.A., and Smith, L.A. (1999). Impact of interruptions and distractions on dispensing errors in an ambulatory care pharmacy. *American Journal of Health System Pharmacy*, *56*, 1319–1325.

Fournier, M.A. (1999). *Impact of a family-centers care approach on the design of neonatal intensivecare units* (Doctoral dissertation). Retrieved from ProQuest Dissertations and Theses (9943483).

Frank, A., Maurer, P., and Shepherd, J. (1991). Light and sound environment. *Physical and Occupational Therapy in Pediatrics*, *11*(2), 27–45.

French, S.E., Lenton, R., Walters, V., and Eyles, J. (2000). An empirical evaluation of an expanded Nursing Stress Scale. *Journal of Nursing Measurement, 8*(2), 161–178.

Gale, G., Franck, L.S., Kools, S., and Lynch, M. (2004). Parents' perceptions of their infant's pain experience in the NICU. *International Journal of Nursing Studies*, *41*(1), 51–58.

Garman, A.N., Garcia, J., and Hargreaves, M. (2004). Patient satisfaction as a predictor of return to provider behavior: Analysis and assessment of financial implications. *Quality Management in Health Care, 13*(1), 75–80.

Giacoia, G.P., Rutledge, D., and West, K. (1985). Factors affecting visitation of sick newborns. *Clinical pediatrics*, *24*(5), 259–262.

Giunta, F., and Rath, J. (1969). Effect of environmental illumination in prevention of hyperbilirubinemia of prematurity. *Pediatrics*, *44*(2), 162–167.

Gold, K.J., Gorenflo, D.W., Schwenk, T.L., and Bratton, S.L. (2006). Physician experience with family presence during cardiopulmonary resuscitation in children. *Pediatric Critical Care Medicine*, *7*(5), 428–433.

Goodfellow, A., Varnam, R., Rees, D., and Shelly, M.P. (1997). Staff stress on the intensive care unit: A comparison of doctors and nurses. *Anaesthesia*, *52*(11), 1037–1041.

Graf, E.R. (2005). Pediatric hospital falls: Development of a predictor model to guide pediatric clinical practice [Abstract]. Paper presented at Sigma Theta Tau International Conference. Retrieved from http://hdl.handle.net/10755/147928

Graham, R.J., Pemstein, D.M., and Curley, M.A. (2009). Experiencing the pediatric intensive care unit: Perspective from parents of children with severe antecedent disabilities. *Critical Care Medicine*, *37*(6), 2064–2070.

Graven, S.N. (2000). Sound and the developing infant in the NICU: Conclusions and recommendations for care. *Journal of Perinatology*, *20*(8; part 2), 88–93.

Graven, S.N. (2004). Early neurosensory visual development of the fetus and newborn. *Clinics in Perinatology*, *31*(2), 199–216.

Gray, L., and Philbin, M.K. (2004). Effects of the neonatal intensive care unit on auditory attention and distraction. *Clinics in Perinatology, 31*, 243–260.

Gray-Toft, P., and Anderson, J. (1981). The Nursing Stress Scale: Development of an instrument. *Journal of Behavioral Assessment, 3*, 11–23.

Greer, B., and Black, A. (2013). I want my own room! The journey from open to private NICU rooms. *Proceedings from The Physical and Developmental Environment of the High-Risk Infant Conference*. Clearwater, FL: USF Health.

Gribbins, R.E., and Marshall, R.E. (1984). Stress and coping strategies of nurse managers in the NICU. *American Journal of Perinatology, 1*(3), 268–271.

Gupta, A., Kapil, A., Lodha, R., Kabra, S.K., Sood, S., Dhawan, B., and Sreenivas, V. (2011). Burden of healthcare-associated infections in a paediatric intensive care unit of a developing country: A single centre experience using active surveillance. *Journal of Hospital Infection*, *78*(4), 323–326.

Guttentag, D.N.W., Albritton, W.L., and Kettner, R.B. (1983). Daytime television viewing by hospitalized children: The effect of alternative programming. *Pediatrics*, *71*(4), 620–625.

Hall, M. (2008). Looking to improve financial results? Start by listening to patients. *Healthcare Financial Management, 62*(10), 76–80.

Hamilton, D.K. (2003). The four levels of evidence based practice. *Healthcare Design*, *3*(4), 18–26.

Harris, D.D., Shepley, M.M., White, R.D., Kolberg, K.J.S., and Harrell, J.W. (2006). The impact of single family room design on patients and caregivers: Executive summary. *Journal of Perinatology*, *26*, S38–S48.

Harris, P.E., Hingley, P., and Cooper, C.L. (1988). *Nurse Stress Index*. Harrogate, North Yorkshire, England: Resource Assessment and Development Ltd.

Heuer, L. (1993). Parental stressors in a pediatric intensive care unit. *Pediatric Nursing*, *19*(2), 128–131.

Huber, D.T. (1998). *Parents' lived-experience with the admission of their newborn into a newborn intensive care unit: A phenomenological study* (Doctoral dissertation). Retrieved from ProQuest Dissertations and Theses. http://search.proquest.com.lib-ezproxy.tamu.edu:2048/docview/304455409/fulltextPDF?accountid=7082

Huckabay, L.M., and Jagla, B. (1979). Nurses' stress factors in the intensive care unit. *The Journal of Nursing Administration, 9*(2), 21–26.

Ireland, S.R., Warren, Y.M., and Herringer, L.G. (1992). Anxiety and color saturation preference. *Perceptual and Motor Skills, 75*(2), 545–546.

Johnson, A.N. (2001). Neonatal response to control of noise inside the incubator. *Pediatric Nursing, 27*(6), 600–605.

Johnson, A.P., Sharland, M., Goodall, C.M., Blackburn, R., Kearns, A.M., Gilbert, R., and Duckworth, G. (2010). Enhanced surveillance of methicillin-resistant Staphylococcus aureus (MRSA) bacteraemia in children in the UK and Ireland. *Archives of Disease in Childhood, 95*(10), 781–785.

Jones, L., Woodhouse, D., and Rowe, J. (2007). Effective nurse–parent communication: A study of parents' perceptions in the NICU environment. *Patient Education and Counseling, 69*, 206–212.

Kaplan, R., and Kaplan, S. (1989). *The Experience of Nature: A Psychological Perspective.* Melborne, AU: Cambridge University Press.

Karande, S., Kelkar, A., and Kulkarni, M. (2005). Recollections of Indian children after discharge from an intensive care unit. *Pediatric Critical Care Medicine*, *6*(3), 303–307.

Kasper, J.W., and Nyamathi, A.M. (1988). Parents of children in the pediatric intensive care unit: What are their needs? *Heart and Lung: The Journal of Critical Care*, *17*(5), 574–581.

Kaushal, R., Bates, D.W., Landrigan, C., McKenna, K.J., Clapp, M.D., Federico, F., and Goldmann, D.A. (2001). Medication errors and adverse drug events in pediatric inpatients. *JAMA: The Journal of the American Medical Association*, *285*(16), 2114–2120.

Kellert, S.R., and Wilson, E.O. (1993). *The Biophilia Hypothesis*. Washington, DC: Island Press.

Kent, W.D., Tan, A.K., Clarke, M.C., and Bardell, T. (2002). Excessive noise levels in the neonatal ICU: Potential effects on auditory system development. *Journal of Otolaryngology, 31*(6), 355–360.

Klassen, J.A., Liang, Y., Tjosvold, L., Klassen, T.P., and Hartling, L. (2008). Music for pain and anxiety in children undergoing medical procedures: A systematic review of randomized controlled trials. *Ambulatory Pediatrics, 8*(2), 117–128.

Larson, E.L., Cimiotti, J., Haas, J., Parides, M., Nesin, M., Della-Latta, P., and Salman, L. (2005). Effect of antiseptic handwashing vs alcohol sanitizer on health care-associated infections in neonatal intensive care units. *Archives of Pediatrics and Adolescent Medicine, 159*(4), 377–383.

Larson, L. (2010) Can you hear me now? *Kentucky Nurse, 58*(3), 10.

Latour, J.M., van Goudoever, J.B., and Hazelzet, J.A. (2008). Parent satisfaction in the pediatric ICU. *Pediatric Clinics of North America*, *55*(3), 779–790.

Latour, J.M., van Goudoever, J.B., Duivenvoorden, H.J., Albers, M.J., van Dam, N.A., Dullaart, E., and Hazelzet, J.A. (2011). Differences in the perceptions of parents and healthcare professionals on pediatric intensive care practices. *Pediatric Critical Care Medicine*, *12*(5), e211–e215.

Lawton, M.P., and Nahemow, L. (1973). Ecology and the aging process. In C. Eisdorfer and M.P. Lawton (eds) *Psychology of Adult Development and Aging* (pp. 657–668). Washington, DC: American Psychological Association.

Lee, S-Y., and Hsu, H-C. (2012). Stress and health-related well-being among mothers with a low birth weight infant: The role of sleep. *Social Science and Medicine*. doi: 10.1016/j.socscimed.2011.12.030

Leske, J. (1991). Internal psychometric properties of the Critical Care Family Needs Inventory. *Heart and Lung, 20*(3), 236–244.

Levy, G.D., Woolston, D.J., and Browne, J.V. (2003). Mean noise amounts in level II vs level III neonatal intensive care units. *Neonatal Network: The Journal of Neonatal Nursing, 22*(2), 33–38.

Lewis, M., Bendersky, M., Koons, A., Hegyi, T., Hiatt, I.M., Ostfeld, B., and Rosenfeld, D. (1991). Visitation to a neonatal intensive care unit. *Pediatrics, 88*(4), 795–800.

Liu, W.F. (2011). Comparing sound measurements in the single-family room with open-unit design neonatal intensive care unit: The impact of equipment noise. *Journal of Perinatology, 32*(5), 368–373.

Marden, V., Grant, D., Abrey, R., and Tooley, M. (2013). Creating a space to grow: Innovative approaches to measuring the impact of a new NICU design on developmental care. *Proceedings from The Physical and Developmental Environment of the High-Risk Infant Conference*. Clearwater, FL: USF Health.

Marks, J. (2009). *A History of Educational Facilities Laboratories (EFL)*. Washington, DC: National Clearinghouse for Educational Facilities.

McGrath, J.M. (2005). Single-room design in the NICU: Making it work for you. *The Journal of Perinatal and Neonatal Nursing, 19*(3), 210–211.

McPherson, M.L., Sachdeva, R.C., and Jefferson, L.S. (2000). Development of a survey to measure parent satisfaction in a pediatric intensive care unit. *Critical Care Medicine, 28*(8), 3009–3013.

Mello, M.J.G.D., Albuquerque, M.D.F.P.M.D., Lacerda, H.R., Souza, W.V.D., Correia, J.B., and Britto, M.C.A.D. (2009). Risk factors for healthcare-associated infection in pediatric intensive care units: A systematic review. *Cadernos de Saúde Pública, 25*, S373–S391.

Miles, M.S., Funk, S.G., and Carlson, J. (1993). Parental Stressor Scale: Neonatal intensive care unit. *Nursing Research, 42*(3), 148–153.

Mirmiran, M., and Ariagno, R.L. (2000). Influence of light in the NICU on the development of circadian rhythms in preterm infants. *Seminars in Perinatology, 24*(4), 247–257.

Mitchell-Dicenso, A., Guyatt, G., Paes, B., Blatz, S., Kirpalani, H., Fryers, M., and Southwell, D. (1996). A new measure of parent satisfaction with medical care provided in the neonatal intensive care unit. *Journal of Clinical Epidemiology, 49*(3), 313–318.

Monroe, K., Wang, D., Vincent, C., Woloshynowych, M., Neale, G., and Inwald, D.P. (2011). Patient safety factors in children dying in a paediatric intensive care unit (PICU): A case notes review study. *BMJ Quality and Safety, 20*(10), 863–868.

Moore, K.A.C., Coker, K., DuBuisson, A.B., Swett, B., and Edwards, W.H. (2003). Implementing potentially better practices for improving family-centered care in neonatal intensive care units: Successes and challenges. *Pediatrics, 111*(Supplement E1), e450–e460.

Mörelius, E., Broström, E.B., Westrup, B., Sarman, I., and Örtenstrand, A. (2012). The Stockholm neonatal family-centered care study: Effects on salivary cortisol in infants and their mothers. *Early Human Development, 88*(7), 575–581.

Morgan, B.E., Horn, A.R., and Bergman, N.J. (2011). Should neonates sleep alone? *Biological Psychiatry, 70*(9), 817–825.

Morgan, H. (2010). Single and shared accommodation for young patients in hospital. *Paediatric Nursing, 22*(8), 20–24.

Morrison, W.E., Haas, E.C., Shaffner, D.H., Garrett, E.S., and Fackler, J.C. (2003). Noise, stress, and annoyance in a pediatric intensive care unit. *Critical Care Medicine, 31*(1), 113–119.

National Association of Children's Hospitals and Related Institutions (NACHRI). (2008). *Evidence for Innovation: Transforming Children's Health through the Physical Environment*. Alexandria, VA: NACHRI.

Needle, J.S., O'Riordan, M., and Smith, P.G. (2009). Parental anxiety and medical comprehension within 24 hrs of a child's admission to the pediatric intensive care unit. *Pediatric Critical Care Medicine*, *10*(6), 668–674.

Norbeck, J.S. (1985). Types and sources of social support for managing job stress in critical care nursing. *Nursing Research, 8*, 252–259.

Oates, R.K., and Oates, P. (1995). Stress and mental health in neonatal intensive care units. *Archives of Disease in Childhood – Fetal and Neonatal Edition, 72*(2), F107–F110.

O'Brien, K., Bracht, M., Macdonell, K., McBride, T., Robson, K., O'Leary, L., and Lee, S.K. (2013). A pilot cohort analytic study of family integrated care in a Canadian neonatal intensive care unit. *BMC Pregnancy and Childbirth, 13*(supplement 1), S12. doi:10.1186/1471-2393-13-S1-S12

Oehler, J.M., and Davidson, M.G. (1992). Job stress and burnout in acute and nonacute pediatric nurses. *American Journal of Critical Care*, *1*(2), 81–90.

Oelrich, T. (2003). Single room NICU: Fad or future. Paper presented at the AIA Academy of Architecture for Health Conference, Denver, CO.

Olds, A. (1995). Nature: The essential healing environment. *Child Health Design, 9*, 3–5.

Olds, A.R., Hall, J.H., and Daniel, P.A. (1987). *Child Health Care Facilities*. Washington, DC: Association for the Care of Children's Health.

Panagiotidis, J., and Lahav, A. (2010). Simulation of prenatal maternal sounds in NICU incubators: A pilot safety and feasibility study. *Journal of Maternal-Fetal and Neonatal Medicine*, *23*(S3), 106–109.

Parsons, R., Tassinary, L.G., Ulrich, R.S., Hebl, M.R., and Grossman-Alexander, M. (1998). The view from the road: Implications for stress recovery and immunization. *Journal of Environmental Psychology*, *18*(2), 113–140.

Pasha, S. (2011). *Usability of outdoor spaces in children's hospitals* (Doctoral dissertation). Abstract retrieved from ProQuest Dissertations and Theses(3471232).

Peng, N.H., Bachman, J., Jenkins, R., Chen, C.H., Chang, Y.C., Chang, Y.S., and Wang, T.M. (2009). Relationships between environmental stressors and stress biobehavioral responses of preterm infants in NICU. *The Journal of Perinatal and Neonatal Nursing*, *23*(4), 363–371.

Pineda, R.G., Neil J., Dierber, D., et al. (2013, in press). Alterations in brain structure and neurodevelopmental outcomes in preterm infants hospitalized in different neonatal intensive care unit environments. *Journal of Psychiatry.*

Playfor, S., Thomas, D., and Choonara, I. (2000). Recollection of children following intensive care. *Archives of Disease in Childhood*, *83*(5), 445–448.

Poltronieri, L., and Schleien, C.L. (2010). PICU design: Influence on patient outcomes and staff/family satisfaction. Paper presented at the annual conference of the National Association of Children's Hospitals and Related Institutions, San Diego, CA.

Poncet, M.C., Toullic, P., Papazian, L., Kentish-Barnes, N., Timsit, J.F., Pochard, F., and Azoulay, E. (2007). Burnout syndrome in critical care nursing staff. *American Journal of Respiratory and Critical Care Medicine*, *175*(7), 698–704.

Razmus, I., Wilson, D., Smith, R., and Newman, E. (2006). Falls in hospitalized children. *Pediatric Nursing*, *32*(6), 568–572.

Reid, T., Bramwell, R., Booth, N., and Weindling, M. (2007). Perceptions of parent–staff communication in Neonatal Intensive Care: The findings from a rating scale. *Journal of Neonatal Nursing*, *13*(2), 64–74.

Rennick, J.E., Lambert, S., Childerhose, J., Campbell-Yeo, M., Filion, F., and Johnston, C.C. (2011). Mothers' experiences of Touch and Talk nursing intervention to optimise pain

management in the PICU: A qualitative descriptive study. *Intensive and Critical Care Nursing, 27*(3), 151–157.
Rice, B.A., and Nelson, C. (2005). Safety in the pediatric ICU: The key to quality outcomes. *Critical Care Nursing Clinics of North America, 17*(4), 431–440.
Rose, P., and Blythe, S. (2008). Use of single rooms on the children's ward: Part I. *Paediatric Nursing, 20*(10), 13–17.
Rosenblum, D. (2005). Single family room care: Before and after data. *Proceedings from The Physical and Developmental Environment of the High-Risk Infant Conference*. Clearwater, FL: USF Health.
Rosenthal, S.L., Schmid, K.D., and Black, M.M. (1989). Stress and coping in a NICU. *Research in Nursing and Health, 12*(4), 257–265.
Routhieaux, R.L., and Tansik, D.A. (1997). The benefits of music in hospital waiting rooms. *Health Care Supervisor, 16*, 31–40.
Sagha Zadeh, R. (2012). *Windows and daylight for healthcare work environments: An evaluation of occupants' performance and wellbeing and building energy use.* Unpublished doctoral dissertation. Texas A&M University, College Station, TX.
Salihoğlu, Ö., Akkuş, C.H., and Hatipoğlu, S. (2011). Recommended standards for the newborn intensive care unit (NICU). *Medical Journal of Bakirköy, 2*(7), 45–51.
Samra, H.A., McGrath, J.M., and Rollins, W. (2011). Patient safety in the NICU: A comprehensive review. *The Journal of Perinatal and Neonatal Nursing, 25*(2), 123–132.
Sargent, A.N. (2009). Predictors of needs in mothers with infants in the neonatal intensive care unit. *Journal of Reproductive and Infant Psychology, 27*(2), 195–205.
Saunders, A.N. (1995). Incubator noise: A method to decrease decibels. *Pediatric Nursing, 21*(3), 265–268.
Saunders, R.P., Abraham, M.R., Crosby, M.J., Thomas, K., and Edwards, W.H. (2003). Evaluation and development of potentially better practices for improving family-centered care in neonatal intensive care units. *Pediatrics, 111*(Supplement E1), e437–e449.
Scott, L.D. (1998). Perceived needs of parents of critically ill children. *Journal for Specialists in Pediatric Nursing, 3*(1), 4–12.
Shepley, M.M. (2002). Predesign and postoccupancy analysis of staff behavior in a neonatal intensive care unit. *Children's Health Care, 31*(3), 237–253.
Shepley, M.M. (2006). The role of positive distraction in neonatal intensive care unit settings. *Journal of Perinatology, 26*, S34–S37.
Shepley, M.M., Bryant, C., and Frohman, B. (1995). Using a post-occupancy study to validate a building prototype: An evaluation of a new women's medical center. *Journal of Interior Design, 21*(2), 19–40.
Shepley, M.M., Fellows, C., Hintz, R., Johnson, L., and Spohn, J. (2012). Pediatric inpatient room experience. *Children, Youth & Environments, 22*(2), 47–65.
Shepley, M.M., Fournier, M.A., and McDougal, K.W. (1998). *Healthcare Environments for Children and their Families*. Dubuque, IO: Kendall/Hunt Publishers.
Shepley, M.M., Harris, D.D., and White, R. (2008). Open-bay and single-family room neonatal intensive care units: Caregiver satisfaction and stress. *Environment and Behavior, 40*(2), 249–268.
Shepley, M.M., Harris, D., White, R., and Steinberg, F. (2008). Impact of single family NICU rooms on family behavior. The AIA Report on University Research, 3. Washington, DC: The American Institute of Architects. Retrieved from www.aia.org/practicing/research/AIAS077439
Sherman, S.A., Eisen, S., Burwinkel, T.M., and Varni, J.W. (2006a). The PedsQL Present

Functioning Visual Analogue Scales: Preliminary reliability and validity. *Health and Quality of Life Outcomes, 41*(1), 75.

Sherman, S.A., Varni, J.W., Ulrich, R.S., and Malcarne, V.L. (2005). Post-occupancy evaluation of healing gardens in a pediatric cancer center. *Landscape and Urban Planning, 73*(2), 167–183.

Sherman, T.I., Greenspan, J.S., St. Clair, N., Touch, S.M., and Shaffer, T.H. (2006b). Optimizing the neonatal thermal environment. *Neonatal Network: The Journal of Neonatal Nursing, 25*(4), 251–260.

Sherman-Bien, S.A., Malcarne, V.L., Roesch, S., Varni, J.W., and Katz, E.R. (2011). Quantifying the relationship between hospital design, satisfaction, and psychosocial functioning in a pediatric hematology-oncology inpatient unit. *Health Environments Research and Design Journal (HERD), 4*(4), 34–59.

Silver, G.H., Kearney, J.A., Kutko, M.C., and Bartell, A.S. (2010). Infant delirium in pediatric critical care settings. *The American Journal of Psychiatry, 167*(10), 1172–1177.

Singh-Naz, N., Sprague, B.M., Patel, K.M., and Pollack, M.M. (2000). Risk assessment and standardized nosocomial infection rate in critically ill children. *Critical Care Medicine, 28*(6), 2069–2075.

Slevin, M., Farrington, N., Duffy, G., Daly, L., and Murphy, J.F.A. (2000). Altering the NICU and measuring infants' responses. *Acta Paediatrica, 89*(5), 577–581.

Smith, A.B., Hefley, G.C., and Anand, K.J.S. (2007). Parent bed spaces in the PICU: Effect on parental stress. *Pediatric Nursing, 33*(3), 215–221.

Smith, T.J., Schoenbeck, K., and Clayton, S. (2009). Staff perceptions of work quality of a neonatal intensive care unit before and after transition from an open bay to a private room design. *Work: A Journal of Prevention, Assessment and Rehabilitation, 33*(2), 211–227.

Smithgall, L.M. (2010). *Perceptions of maternal stress and neonatal patient outcomes in a single private room versus open room Neonatal Intensive Care Unit environment* (Doctoral dissertation). Retrieved from ProQuest Dissertations and Theses (3440888).

Sobo, E.J., Eng, B., and Kassity-Krich, N. (2006). Canine visitation (pet) therapy: Pilot data on decreases in child pain perception. *Journal of Holistic Nursing, 24*(1), 51–57.

Standley, J.M. (1986). Music research in medical/dental treatment: Meta-analysis and clinical applications. *Journal of Music Therapy, 23*(2), 56–122.

Standley, J.M. (2002). A meta-analysis of the efficacy of music therapy for premature infants. *Journal of Pediatric Nursing, 17*(2), 107–113.

Standley, J.M., and Moore, R.S. (1995). Therapeutic effects of music and mother's voice on premature infants. *Pediatric Nursing, 21*(6), 509–512, 574.

Stevens, D.C., Helseth, C.C., Khan, M.A., Munson, D.P., and Smith, T.J. (2010). Neonatal intensive care nursery staff perceive enhanced workplace quality with the single-family room design. *Journal of Perinatology, 30*(5), 352–358.

Stewart, K., and Schneider, S. (2000). The effects of music therapy on the sound environment in the NICU: A pilot study. In J.V. Loewy (ed) *Music Therapy in the Neonatal Intensive Care Unit* (pp. 85–100). New York: Satchnote Press.

Stremler, R., Dhukai, Z., Wong, L., Young, M., and Parshuram, C. (2008). Sleep, sleepiness, fatigue and psychological outcomes in parents with a hospitalized critically ill child. *Sleep, 31*, A312.

Swanson, P.R., Peters, C., and Lee, B.H. (2012). NICU redesign from open ward to private room: A longitudinal study of parent and staff perceptions. *Journal of Perinatology*. Advance online publication, January 3, 2013; doi:10.1038/jp.2012.157

Talmi, A., and Harmon, R.J. (2003). Relationships between preterm infants and their parents: Disruption and development. *Zero to Three, 24*(2), 13–20.

Tansik, D.A., and Routhieaux, R. (1999). Customer stress-relaxation: The impact of music in a hospital waiting room. *International Journal of Service Industry Management*, *10*(1), 68–81.

Thear, G., and Wittmann-Price, R.A. (2006). Project Noise Buster in the NICU: How one facility lowered noise levels when caring for preterm infants. *AJN The American Journal of Nursing*, *106*(5), 64AA–64EE.

Thomas, K.A., Magbalot, A., Shinabarger, K., Mokhnach, L., Anderson, M., Diercks, K., and Berken, M. (2010). Seasonal mapping of NICU temperature study conducted at the University of Washington medical center. *Advances in Neonatal Care: Official Journal of the National Association of Neonatal Nurses*, *10*(2), 83–87.

Thomas, K.A., and Uran, A. (2007). How the NICU environment sounds to a preterm infant: Update. *MCN: The American Journal of Maternal/Child Nursing*, *32*(4), 250–253.

Tsironi, S., Bovaretos, N., Tsoumakas, K., Giannakopoulou, M., and Matziou, V. (2011). Factors affecting parental satisfaction in the neonatal intensive care unit. *Journal of Neonatal Nursing*, *18*(5), 183–192.

Tumulty, G., Jernigan, I.E., and Kohut, G.F. (1994). The impact of perceived work environment on job satisfaction of hospital staff nurses. *Applied Nursing Research*, *7*(2), 84–90.

Turner, M.A., Tomlinson, P.S., and Harbaugh, B.L. (1990). Parental uncertainty in critical care hospitalization of children. *Maternal-Child Nursing Journal*, *90*(1), 45–62.

Ulrich, R. (1984). View through a window may influence recovery from surgery. *Science*, *224*, 420–421.

Ulrich, R., and Lundén, O. (1993). Effects of nature and abstract pictures on patients recovering from heart surgery [Abstract]. Poster presented at the First International Congress of Behavioral Medicine, Uppsala, Sweden.

Ulrich, R.S., Simons, R.F., Losito, B.D., Fiorito, E., Miles, M.A., and Zelson, M. (1991). Stress recovery during exposure to natural and urban environments. *Journal of Environmental Psychology*, *11*(3), 201–230.

Urbanski, B.L., and Lazenby, M. (2012). Distress among hospitalized pediatric cancer patients modified by pet-therapy intervention to improve quality of life. *Journal of Pediatric Oncology*, *29*(5), 272–282.

Vandenberg, K.A. (2007). Individualized developmental care for high risk newborns in the NICU: A practice guideline. *Early Human Development*, *83*(7), 433–442.

Verderber, S. (1986). Dimensions of person–window transactions in the hospital environment. *Environment and Behavior*, *18*(4), 450–466.

Vidyasagar, D. (2005). Stress of admission to pediatric intensive care unit on children. *Pediatric Critical Care Medicine*, *6*(3), 374–376.

Walch, J.M., Rabin, B.S., Day, R., Williams, J.N., Choi, K., and Kang, J.D. (2005). The effect of sunlight on postoperative analgesic medication usage: A prospective study of spinal surgery patients. *Psychosomatic Medicine*, *67*(1), 156–163.

Walsh, W.F., McCullough, K.L., and White, R.D. (2006). Room for improvement: Nurses' perceptions of providing care in a single room newborn intensive care setting. *Advances in Neonatal Care*, *6*(5), 261–270.

Ward-Begnoche, W. (2007). Posttraumatic stress symptoms in the pediatric intensive care unit. *Journal for Specialists in Pediatric Nursing*, *12*(2), 84–92.

White, R.D. (2003). Individual rooms in the NICU – An evolving concept. *Journal of Perinatology*, *23*(Supplement 1), S22–S24.

White, R.D. (2004). Mothers' arms – The past and future locus of neonatal care? *Clinics in Perinatology*, *31*(2), 383–388.

White, R.D. (2011). The newborn intensive care unit environment of care: How we got here, where we're headed, and why. *Seminars in Perinatology, 35*, 2–7.

Whitehouse, S., Varni, J.W., Seid, M., Cooper-Marcus, C., Ensberg, M.J., Jacobs, J.R., and Mejlenbeck, R.S. (2001). Evaluating a children's hospital garden environment: Utilization and consumer satisfaction. *Environmental Psychology, 21*, 201–314.

Wigert, H., Berg, M., and Hellström, A.L. (2010). Parental presence when their child is in neonatal intensive care. *Scandinavian Journal of Caring Sciences*, *24*(1), 139–146.

Wrench, I.J., and Vyas, H.G. (1995). How to equip a paediatric intensive care unit. *Current Paediatrics*, *5*(1), 10–13.

Zuckerman, M., Ulrich, R.S., and McLaughlin, J. (1993). Sensation seeking and reactions to nature paintings. *Personality and Individual Differences, 15*(5), 563–576.

Design Guidelines

6

Several organizations have developed guidelines that address pediatric and neonatal intensive care. This chapter will address some of the documents that focus on the physical environment. The majority of these organizations fully embrace the use of research to support their recommendations. Summaries of guidelines and recommendations from the United States, Abu Dhabi, Australasia, Canada, China, Colombia, Dubai, India, Iran, South Africa, and the United Kingdom are discussed. Lastly, sources of guidelines related to sustainability in healthcare settings will be summarized.

6.1 US Standards

Five of the most commonly used US standards/guidelines will be described in this chapter:

1. *Guidelines for Design and Construction of Healthcare Facilities.*
2. Recommended Standards for the Newborn ICU.
3. Society of Critical Care Medicine guidelines and levels.
4. American Academy of Pediatrics guidelines and levels.
5. US Army Corps of Engineers' *Uniform Facilities Criteria* (Series 4-500) and the *Design Manual of the US Department of Veterans Affairs, Office of Construction and Facilities Management.*

6.1.1 Guidelines for Design and Construction of Healthcare Facilities

The first *General Standards* were published in 1947 in association with the Hill-Burton program (FGI, 2011). In 1974 the title was changed to *Minimum Requirements of Construction and Equipment for Hospital and Medical Facilities* to reinforce the notion that the contents were minimums rather than ideal standards (FGI, 2011). In 1984 the Department of Health and Human Services eliminated the requirement regulations as the associated federal programs had expired, and the title was changed to *Guidelines for Construction and Equipment of Hospital and Medical Facilities* (FGI, 2011). The American Institute of Architects first collaborated with the U.S. Department of Health and Human Services in the revision of the document in 1987 (FGI, 2011). The FGI was founded in 1998 as a not-for-profit corporation, and subsequently Guidelines were produced in 2001, 2006, and 2010. The next edition will be in 2014.

The 2010 *Guidelines for Design and Construction of Healthcare Facilities* (FGI, 2011) contain specific sections on Pediatric Critical Care (2.2–2.9) and Newborn Intensive Care (2.2–2.10), both of which refer back to Section 2.2–2.6.2, Critical Care Patient Rooms and Area, for general requirements.

6.1.2 *Recommended Standards for the Newborn ICU*

In 1991, Ross Products Division of Abbott Laboratories, recognizing that there were no national standards for NICU, convened 25 physicians, nurses, planning officials, developers, consultants, and architects to discuss the influence of the environment on VLBW babies (Harrell and Moon, 2008). This group was transformed into the Committee on Recommended Standards for Newborn Intensive Care. Subsequently the standards were presented to the FGI's *Guidelines for Design and Construction of Healthcare Facilities*, and some elements were incorporated into the 2011 edition of this document.

The Recommended Standards for the Newborn ICU were produced by a volunteer consensus committee starting in 1993 in association with the Physical and Developmental Environment of the High-Risk Infant Project (White, 2007). Various portions of these recommended standards have now been adopted by the FGI and other standards (White, 2007).

6.1.3 *Society of Critical Care Medicine guidelines and levels*

The Society of Critical Care Medicine authored several iterations of guidelines for pediatric intensive care, in 1983, 1993, and 2004 (Committee on Hospital Care and Pediatric Section of the Society of Critical Care Medicine (CHCPSSCCM), 1983, 1993; Rosenberg and Moss, 2004). As the guidelines must be revised within 10 years, the next edition should be available shortly. The contents of these guidelines are discussed in detail in Chapter 2.

6.1.4 *American Academy of Pediatrics guidelines and levels*

The American Academy of Pediatrics has produced documents outlining levels and guidelines in 2004, 2007, and 2012 (American Academy of Pediatrics/American College of Obstetricians and Gynecologists, 2007; Committee on Fetus and Newborn, American Academy of Pediatrics (CoFNAAP), 2004, 2012). These documents are summarized in Chapter 3.

6.1.5 Uniform Facilities Criteria *and the* Design Manual of the Department of Veterans' Affairs

The U.S. Army Corps of Engineers' *Uniform Facilities Criteria* (Series 4-500) address the design of medical military facilities and apply to military departments, defense agencies, and Department of Defense (DoD) field activities (Department of Defense, 2012). The documents are reviewed and updated periodically and administered by the Air Force Civil Engineer Center, the U.S. Army Corps of Engineers, and Naval Facilities Engineering Command (DoD, 2012). The contents address typical construction issues and building systems, as well as sustainable design principles, accessibility, security, and wayfinding.

The U.S. Department of Veterans' Affairs (USDVA), Office of Construction and Facilities Management, provides a variety of design guides for its facilities, which are continuously undergoing upgrades. The guidelines are benchmarked against private sector standards (USDVA, 2011). The guidelines include a section on medical/surgical and intensive care nursing units. While these guidelines are not directed at pediatric and neonatal intensive care, some of the information covered therein is useful to the design process, particularly with regard to PICUs.

6.2 Representative non-US Guidelines

At least one set of guidelines from each of the continents (less Antarctica) – Africa, Asia, Australia, Europe, North America and South America – are included in this overview. While this book made an attempt to incorporate research and design goals from as many international sources as possible, very few examples are available in the literature. The intention of this section is to provide a link to a few of the guidelines that were uncovered via architects located in these countries and representative organizations.

6.2.1 *Abu Dhabi Health Authority Healthcare Facility Design Standards*

The Health Authority – Abu Dhabi (HAAD) created the Healthcare Facility Design Standards for the Emirate of Abu Dhabi in January 2011 (HAAD, 2012). The Standards apply to all healthcare projects in Abu Dhabi. Sections of the Standards include administrative provisions, programming and design, access and occupational health and safety, infection control, and engineering. Requirements for NICUs are found in Section 28, Obstetrics. The model that is described is an open-bay arrangement. Section 21 addresses Intensive Care.

6.2.2 *Australasian Health Facility Guidelines (New South Wales)*

The Australasian Health Facility Guidelines are produced by the Australasian Health Infrastructure Alliance (AHIA) with the intention of supporting planners and designers of healthcare facilities to use common guidelines (AHIA, 2010). Individual jurisdictions provide instructions regarding the particular application of the guidelines to specific capital projects (AHIA, 2010).

The format of the document is similar to those of other guidelines and was likely a predecessor for several of these. The document is subdivided into Introduction, Briefing and Planning, Accessibility and Security, Infection Control, and Building Services. The guidelines include dedicated sections on pediatric/adolescent units and on neonatal/special care nurseries, but PICUs are not addressed. The guidelines reference single family rooms as a reasonable approach to NICU design (AHIA, 2010).

6.2.3 Canadian Health Care Facility Standards CSA Z8000-11

The *CSA Health Care Facility Standards CSA Z8000-11* is the first comprehensive national standard for healthcare facilities for Canada. The document addresses electrical systems, medical gases, plumbing, HVAC, illumination, infection control, area measurement, commissioning, sterilization, and medical devices. Similar to the FGI guidelines, these standards are voluntary and only become implemented once the recommended standards are formally referenced in official regulations (Harvey et al., 2011). The primary objectives include operations, accessibility, safety/security, infection prevention and control, and sustainability. According to CSA Z8000, facilities must identify a structured sustainability program.

6.2.4 Chinese Health Facility Guidelines

The Chinese Ministry of Construction and Ministry of Health (1988) has generated an architectural and design code for general hospitals. The stipulations in this code are mandated by the government. This document lists requirements for pediatric inpatient rooms and infant rooms under the category of Obstetrics. A draft of the 2004 version includes a discussion of intensive care settings, although I was unable to obtain a copy of the most current code. References are made to PICU and NICU care under the code section describing pediatric inpatient care. This same section provides for semi-private isolation rooms. The presence of a baby nursery is accounted for under Obstetrics. In addition, the Chinese Society of Critical Care Medicine (CSCCM) (2006) provides guidelines for the design of intensive care units. The care model suggested is multi-bed rooms with eight to twelve beds per room. Statistics on the status of NICUs and PICUs may be found in Zhang (2011).

6.2.5 Colombian Guidelines

In addition to other health facility components, the Secretaria Distrital de Salud (SDS) in Colombia has a manual dedicated to the design of intensive and intermediate care units. This code is divided into sections focusing on adult ICUs, PICUs, and NICUs, in addition to general requirements, seismic issues (SDS, 2010). Dimensioned floor plans are provided, as well as equipment recommendations. The standards describe open-bay baby stations, but recommend a limit of six to twelve babies in a room at higher levels of care (SDS, 2010).

6.2.6 Dubai Health Facility Guidelines: planning, design, construction and commissioning

The Dubai code adopts the US *Guidelines for Design and Construction of Healthcare Facilities, 2006* (Dubai Health Authority, 2009). Interestingly, the Dubai guidelines include a section (3.3.4) on evidence-based design:

> Architects and Design Consultants are encouraged to use evidence based design strategies to improve patient outcomes in the creation of a healing environment. Evidence indicates improved patient outcomes, staff performance and overall satisfaction where the following principles are incorporated into a design philosophy:
>
> - Build single private room accommodation with external views
> - Reducing noise – refer to section 4.2.4
> - Incorporate nature – glazing with natural lighting and ventilation, internal landscaping
> - Way finding systems – use of color and texture for the visually impaired
> - Improved air quality – minimum standards required – refer to ASHRAE Std 62.1 2004 and Section 4.1.Dubai Design Considerations – Local Factors
> - Encourage hand washing – use of wash hand basins per patient room
> - Adaptability.
>
> (Dubai Health Authority, 2009)

6.2.7 *Indian* Consensus Guidelines for Pediatric Intensive Care Units *and* Toolkit for Setting Up Special Care Newborn Units, Stabilisation Units and Newborn Care Corners

In 2002 the Indian Society of Critical Care Medicine (Pediatric Section) and the Indian Academy of Pediatrics (Intensive Care Chapter) produced the "Consensus Guidelines for Pediatric Intensive Care Units in India." The authors note that while some of the committee members had experience with Western ICUs, care was "taken to adequately develop and adapt the guidelines to be applicable in the Indian context" (Khilnani, 2002, p.43). The guidelines are organized in the following categories:

1. Unit design
   a. Size of PICU: 6–8 beds per unit recommended
   b. Room layout and area: "Patient area in open PICU should be 150 to 200 sq ft. In a cubicle, the minimum area should be 200 to 250 square feet with at least one wash basin for two beds. However, one for each bed is preferred. At least one, preferably two rooms should have an isolation capability with an area of 250 square feet with an ante room ..."
   c. Power supply and temperature control; central HVAC recommended
   d. Beds: maneuverable, railings, emergency call, intercom and bedside patient cart
   e. Crash cart
   f. Receptionist to control visits
   g. Central station with visibility of all patient areas
   h. X-ray viewing
   i. Storage
   j. Clean and dirty utility
   k. Waste disposal
   l. Conference room
   m. Adjacent stat lab
2. Equipment list
3. Organization and staffing
4. Ancillary staffing
5. Levels of PICU care and admission and discharge.

(Khilnani, 2002)

A set of guidelines for neonatal intensive care was also identified. The *Toolkit for Setting up Special Care Newborn Units, Stabilisation Units and Newborn Care Corners* was sponsored by UNICEF and produced in conjunction with the Indian National Neonatology Forum and the WHO Collaborative Center for Training and Research in Newborn Care. This document includes the accreditation committee standards for Level II newborn care and addresses location, space requirements, configuration, electrical and mechanical needs, lighting, temperature, and acoustics (National Neonatology Forum, 2008).

6.2.8 Iranian National Organization for Planning and Budget

The Department of Technology (DoT) of the Office of Technology, Guidelines Production, and Earthquake Hazard Reduction has published a series of volumes addressing healthcare building design. For the purposes of this book, I was only able to identify the guidelines for neonatal intensive care, published in 2005. This detailed document includes a description of the health conditions of the newborns cared for in these units, medical equipment, infection control, safety, architectural design, floor plans, and programming (DoT, 2005).

6.2.9 South Africa Hospital Norms (SAH Norms); National Department of Health

In an effort to represent the African continent, a search was conducted to identify published design standards. While hospital design guidelines certainly exist or are in progress, the research for this book identified one set of guidelines developed in 1980: the South Africa Hospital Norms (SAH Norms) produced by the South African Department of Health (Okpanum and Motanya, 2011). Other African countries may be using guidelines generated by the World Health Organization, such as "Approaches to the Planning and Design of Health Care Facilities in Developing Areas" (Kleczkowski and Pibouleau, 1983), and the Joint Commission International Standards.

6.2.10 United Kingdom Standards

Several references regarding PICU and NICU care standards were identified. Although there are likely to be more updated documents available, the references mentioned help to provide an understanding of the scope and criteria used to evaluate pediatric critical care environments in the United Kingdom (UK).

Health Building Note 57, *Facilities for Critical Care* (NHS Estates, 2003), includes design standards regarding intensive care and high-dependency units and associated locations. Information is provided regarding user requirements, departmental adjacencies, and user views. Subtopics include bed space requirements and number of single rooms, HAIs, privacy, noise reduction, and staff spaces.

A specialized document is available regarding pediatric intensive care – the 4th edition of the *Standards for the Care of Critically Ill Children* (Paediatric Intensive Care Society, 2010) – which, according to the authors, aspires to be based on the available evidence. Concerning neonatology, the recent 2010 version of the *Service Standards for Hospitals Providing Neonatal Care* addresses staffing and operational standards, and the *NHS Toolkit for High Quality Neonatal Services* (Department of Health, 2009) consists of a commissioning framework in support of the strategic development of newborn services. The design of NICUs is addressed by Laing et al. (2004) in *Designing a Neonatal Unit,* a document produced for the British Association of Perinatal Medicine.

6.3 Green Guidelines

Green building means "tailoring a building and its placement on the site to the local climate, site conditions, culture, and community in order to reduce resource consumption, augment resource supply, and enhance the quality and diversity of life" (Adler et al., 2006, p. 3). Adler et al. note that green building is a subset of sustainable development, which enables individuals to achieve their potential and quality of life using methods that maintain the earth's support systems.

Three major guidelines address issues of green design with respect to healthcare facilities. They are the Leadership in Energy and Environmental Design (LEED) guidelines, the Green Guide for Healthcare, and Green Globes. The rating systems are intended to evaluate a whole building or components of a building. As the emphases vary, some buildings may meet the requirements of one system but not another (Wu and Low, 2010). For discussions of the relative merits of these systems see Wu and Low (2010), and Means (2011).

Several design professionals have challenged the effectiveness of the guideline systems on the grounds that some standards limit options with regard to approved materials, or that the processing of the paperwork to achieve certification is too expensive for owners. Few argue, however, that the spirit and goals of these guidelines are not essential to socially responsible design.

6.3.1 Leadership in Energy and Environmental Design (LEED) Guidelines

Of all the whole-building rating systems, LEED is the most commonly used worldwide (Wu and Low, 2010). The pilot for LEED was developed by the U.S. Green Building Council (USGBC), an organization founded in 1993 (USGBC, 2012). The LEED pilot was presented in 1998 (USGBC, 2012), and has been subject to several revisions since. The current version is LEED V.3.

LEED includes six categories (Location and Transportation, Sustainable Sites, Water Efficiency, Energy and Atmosphere, Materials and Resources, and Indoor Environmental Quality), and provides the level designations of certified, silver, gold, and platinum. Dell Children's Hospital in Austin, Texas, which includes a PICU and NICU, was the first platinum LEED hospital. Regarding the cost of LEED projects, a 2008 study of 13 buildings reflected an increase of zero to 5 percent without incentives, and from zero to 3.8 percent with energy incentives (Vittori, 2011).

Apart from LEED for Existing Buildings Operations and Maintenance, LEED categories include Core and Shell, New Construction, Schools, Neighborhood Development, Retail, Homes, Commercial Interiors, and Healthcare. LEED for Healthcare 2009 was made available in 2011, the result of a collaboration with the authors of the Green Guide for Healthcare (GGHC). The GGHC was developed by Healthcare without Harm and the Center for Maximum Potential Building Systems (USGBC, 2012), and is discussed in the following section.

6.3.2 Green Guide for Healthcare

The history of the Green Guide for Healthcare (GGHC) began in 2000 as part of a conference, "Setting Healthcare's Environmental Agenda." Subsequent to this, the American Society of Healthcare Engineering (ASHE) gathered a task force that generated the ASHE Green Healthcare Construction Guidance Statement which addressed health protection at three levels: immediate health of occupants, health of surrounding community, and health of the global community and natural resources (GGHC, 2013a). When LEED for New Construction Version 2.0 was released, it was apparent that standards specifically associated with healthcare were needed, although the tool was several years off from distribution (GGHC, 2013a; Vittori, 2008). In 2004 a pilot tool, 2.0, was released using principles and structure from the ASHE Guidance Statement and LEED for New Construction Version 2.0. An operations section was added in 2005. The Green Guide Version 2.2 Construction was released in 2007 and became the foundation for LEED for Healthcare (GGHC, 2013a). While the point allocations for the Green Guide and LEED differ, the content is largely in common.

The Green Guide is divided into two components: construction and operation. The former addresses new projects, while the latter is a system for measuring ongoing performance. The data is not submitted for third-party verification; rather, guidance is offered for improvement and best practice (GGHC, 2013b). The Green Guide focuses on new and existing hospitals, but could be effectively used on clinics, medical office buildings, and other healthcare facilities.

The Green Guide for Healthcare sunset its operations in December 2011 in response to the successful launch of LEED for Healthcare in April 2011 (G. Vittori, personal communication, March 23, 2013). According to Gail Vittori, co-director, Center for Maximum Potential Building Systems, the Green Guide website

> remains active and holds the body of work that developed over its 10-year history, including the operations-related efforts which, to date, have not been absorbed in the LEED rating system. The final work of GGHC was piloting the operations section and there is a summary report still to be released. We are on hold with further work on the operations section pending feedback from USGBC as to whether they [LEED] may move forward with an Existing Building Operations and Maintenance Supplement to LEED for Healthcare.
>
> (G. Vittori, personal communication, March 23, 2013)

6.3.3 Green Globes for Healthcare

Green Globes, provided by the Green Buildings Initiative (GBI), is an online interactive building assessment and certification program that incorporates an on-site visit by a third-party evaluator (GBI, 2013b). Green Globes was derived from the BRE Environmental Assessment Model (BREEAM) and was introduced into Canada via the BREEAM Green Leaf rating system (Wu and Low, 2010). In 2000 Green Leaf became an online assessment tool as Green Globes for Existing Buildings; in 2002 it was introduced in the UK as the Global Environmental Method (GBI, 2013c). Rights to distribute Green Globes in the US were granted in 2004. Green Globes was the first rating system to be associated with the American National Standard Institute (ANSI) (GBI, 2013c).

Green Globes Continuous Improvement of Existing Buildings Healthcare (CIEB HC) is designed for the specific application to hospitals and extended care facilities with licensed beds. Six areas of assessment are: energy, water, resources, emissions, indoor environment, and environmental management, for which a total of 1,000 points can be received (GBI, 2013a).

6.3.4 Relationship between green design and evidenced-based design

Some professionals question whether sustainable design and evidence-based design (EBD) are compatible. Utilizing a multi-method approach (interviews, focus groups, and questionnaires), we found that there are some areas of conflict. For example, EBD researchers suggest the use of views of water to reduce stress, while sustainable standards attempt to conserve water resources. Likewise, an EBD recommendation to use materials that can be sterilized in order to avoid spreading infection conflicts with the fact that recyclable materials do not do this effectively. However, the majority of experts on EBD and sustainable design find the approaches to be symbiotic (Shepley et al., 2009a, 2009b).

References

Adler, A., Armstrong, J.E., Fuller, S.K., Kalin, M., Karolides, A., Macaluso, J., and Walker, H.A. (2006). *Green Building: Project Planning and Cost Estimating* (2nd edn). Kingston, MA: R.S. Means.

American Academy of Pediatrics/American College of Obstetricians and Gynecologists (AAP/ACOG). (2007). *Guidelines for Perinatal Care* (6th edn). Elk Grove Village, IL/Washington, DC: American Academy of Pediatrics/American College of Obstetricians and Gynecologists.

Australasian Health Infrastructure Alliance (AHIA). (2010). *Australasian Health Facility Guidelines*. Retrieved from http://www.healthfacilityguidelines.com.au/AusHFG_Documents/Guidelines/Archive/AusHFG_v4.pdf

British Association of Perinatal Medicine. (2010). *Standards for Hospitals Providing Neonatal Intensive and High Dependency Care and Categories of Babies Requiring Neonatal Care*. London: British Association of Perinatal Medicine.

Chinese Ministry of Construction and Chinese Ministry of Health. (1988) *Architectural and Design Code for General Hospitals*. Beijing, China: Chinese Ministry of Construction and Chinese Ministry of Health.

Chinese Society of Critical Care Medicine (CSCCM). (2006). *Guidelines for the Construction and Management of Intensive Care Units in China*. Beijing, China: Chinese Society of Critical Care Medicine (CSCCM).

Committee on Fetus and Newborn, American Academy of Pediatrics (COFNAAP). (2004). Levels of neonatal care. *Pediatrics, 114*(5), 1341–1347. doi: 10.1542/peds.2004-1697

Committee on Fetus and Newborn, American Academy of Pediatrics (COFNAAP). (2012). Levels of neonatal care. *Pediatrics, 130*(3), 587–597. doi: 10.1542/peds.2012-1999

Committee on Hospital Care and Pediatric Section of the Society of Critical Care Medicine (CHCPSSCCM). (1983). Guidelines for pediatric intensive care units. *Pediatrics, 72*, 364–371, and *Critical Care Medicine, 11*, 753.

Committee on Hospital Care and Pediatric Section of the Society of Critical Care Medicine (CHCPSSCCM). (1993). Guidelines and levels of care for pediatric intensive care units. *Pediatrics, 92*(1), 166–175.

Department of Defense. (2012). *Unified Facilities Criteria (UFC): Design: Medical Military Facilities*. Washington, DC: U.S. Department of Defense.

Department of Technology, Office of Technology, Guidelines Protection, and Earthquake Hazard Reduction. (2005). *Guidelines for Architectural Programming and Planning for Neonatal Intensive Care Units.* Tehran, Iran: National Organization for Planning and Budget.

Dubai Health Authority. (2009). *Health Facility Guidelines: Planning, design, construction and commissioning.* Dubai, UAE: Dubai Health Authority. Retrieved from http://www.dha.gov.ae/EN/SectorsDirectorates/Directorates/HealthRegulation/Documents/Health%20Facility%20Guidelines.pdf

Facility Guidelines Institute (FGI). (2011). *Guidelines for Design and Construction of Health Care Facilities*. Chicago, IL: ASHE.

Green Buildings Institute (GBI). (2013a). Green building programs. Retrieved from www.thegbi.org/commercial/healthcare

Green Buildings Institute (GBI). (2013b). Green Globes®: A nationally recognized alternative to LEED. Retrieved from http://www.thegbi.org/green-globes/green-globes-leed-green-building-certification.shtml

Green Buildings Institute (GBI). (2013c). History of the Green Globes® system. Retrieved from http://www.thegbi.org/products/green-globes/history.shtml

Green Guide for Healthcare (GGHC). (2013a). Development history. Retrieved from http://www.gghc.org/about.history.php

Green Guide for Healthcare (GGHC). (2013b). Frequently asked questions. Retrieved from http://www.gghc.org/about.faq.php#4

Harrell, J.W., and Moon, R.G. (2008). Designs for the delicate. *Health Facilities Management, 21*(12), 45–48.

Harvey, C., Keen, M., and Snell, R. (2011). *Canadian Health Care Facilities (CSA Z8000-11): The NEW standard for design and construction of Canadian hospitals and health care facility* [Powerpoint slides]. Retrieved from http://www.healthcaredesignmagazine.com/sites/default/files/conference/HCD.11_E33.pdf

Health Authority – Abu Dhabi (HAAD). (2012). *Healthcare Facility Design Standards*. Retrieved from http://www.haad.ae/haad/tabid/1125/Default.aspx

Khilnani, P. (2002). Consensus Guidelines for Pediatric Intensive Care Units in India. *Indian Pediatrics, 39*, 43–50.

Kleczkowski, B.M., and Pibouleau, R. (eds). (1983). *Approaches to Planning and Design of Health Care Facilities in Developing Areas* (Vol. 4). Geneva, Switzerland: World Health Organization.

Laing, I., Ducker, T., Leaf, A., and Newmarch, P. (2004). *Designing a Neonatal Unit for the British Association of Perinatal Medicine*. London: British Association of Perinatal Medicine.

Means, R.S. (2010). *Green Building: Project Planning and Cost Estimating* (Vol. 24). Hoboken, NJ: John Wiley & Sons.

NHS and Department of Health. (2009). *Toolkit for High Quality Neonatal Services*. London: Department of Health.

NHS Estates. (2003). *Facilities for Critical Care*. London: The Stationery Office (TSO).

National Neonatology Forum. (2008). *Toolkit for Setting Up Special Care Newborn Units, Stabilisation Units and Newborn Care Corners.* New Delhi, India: United Nations Children's Fund.

Okpanum, I., and Motanya, J. (2011). Towards flexible and adaptable design of A&E facilities in South Africa: The role of design guidelines. Presentation at Design and Health, 7th World Congress. Boston, MA, July 6–10.

Paediatric Intensive Care Society. (2010). *Standards for the Care of Critically Ill Children*. London: Paediatric Intensive Care Society.

Rosenberg, D.I., Moss, M.M., and the American College of Critical Care Medicine of the Society of Critical Care Medicine. (2004). Guidelines and levels of care for pediatric intensive care units. *Pediatrics, 114*(4), 1114–1125. doi:10.1542/peds.2004-1599

Secretaria Distrital de Salud D.C. (SDS). (2010). *Manual Guia para el Diseño Arquitectonico de Unidades de Cuidados Intensivos e Intermedios.* (*Guide Manual for the Architectural Design of Intensive and Intermediate Care Units*). Bogota, Colombia: Secretaria Distrital de Salud.

Shepley, M.M., Baum, M., Ginsberg, R., and Rostenberg, B. (2009a). Eco-effective design and evidence-based design: Perceived synergy and conflict. *HERD*, *2*(3), 56.

Shepley, M.M., Baum, M., and Rostenberg, B. (2009b). A collaborative research project on evidence-based and eco-effective design. *Enquiry/The ARCC Journal of Architectural Research*, *6*(2), 81–87.

U.S. Department of Veterans Affairs Office of Construction and Facilities Management (USDVA). (2011). *Design Guide: Medical/surgical inpatient units and intensive care nursing units*. Retrieved from http://www.cfm.va.gov/til/dGuide/dgInpatientNU.pdf

U.S. Green Building Council (USGBC). (2012). LEED for Healthcare. Downloaded March 23, 2013 from www.usgbc.org/ShowFile.aspx?DocumentID=8878

Vittori, G. (March 1, 2008). Green Guide for Health Care and LEED: Sorting out the rating systems. Healthcare Design. Downloaded March 23, 2013 from http://www.healthcaredesign-magazine.com/article/green-guide-health-care-and-leed-sorting-out-rating-systems

Vittori, G. (2011). Greening of healthcare: Location and design of facilities are essential mission of health. *Modern Healthcare, Suppl*, 42.

Vittori, G. (2013). Personal communication received March 23, 2013.

White, R.D. (2007). Recommended standards for the newborn ICU. *Journal of Perinatology*, *27*, S4–S19.

Wu, P., and Low, S.P. (2010). Project management and green buildings: Lessons from the rating systems. *Journal of Professional Issues in Engineering Education and Practice,* 136(2), 64–70.

Zhang, Y. (2011). Development of pediatric and neonatal intensive care units: Results of a national survey (2000–2009). *Chung-Hua Erh K'o Tsa Chih* (*Chinese Journal of Pediatrics*), *49*(9), 669–674.

Part Four: The future of design and research

Future of design and design research 7

This chapter is divided into three sections: two separate sections on the future of PICU and NICU design, and a combined section on the future of PICU and NICU design research. Concerning the future of PICU and NICU design, while both settings are influenced by overall trends in critical care, many issues raised in the literature are appropriate to the specific requirements of PICUs and NICUs. Regarding design research, many of the issues and trends are similar; hence, an integrated summary was feasible.

7.1 Future of PICU design

Healthcare futurists rarely make projections about PICU design, although there has been considerable discussion about factors that will impact intensive care units as a group. Due to the functional similarity of pediatric ICUs to adult ICUs, several topics regarding ICUs in general are presented here, as well as PICU-specific information.

7.1.1 Service and programmatic trends

- *Severity of illness*. Several authors have predicted an increase in the number of intensive care patients and, hence, a prolonged length of stay. At least one research team disagrees with this prediction. Namachivayam et al. (2010) reviewed data from three decades of children while they were patients in the PICU and their long-term outcomes. They found that the severity of illness and length of stay in pediatric critical care units has remained the same, and mortality has significantly decreased. However, Namachivayam and colleagues discovered that the percentage of PICU survivors with major and moderate disabilities has increased, and recommend that the health system be aware of the potential impact on services for families and communities over the longer term.
- *Family- and patient-centered care*. A continued emphasis on family- and patient-centered care is expected (Stark, 2004). In addition to space in the patient room for families to sleep, work, and relax, the provision of access to nature, developmentally appropriate art, adequate acoustical control, and appropriate lighting are strong themes (Stark, 2004). The use of the environment as a means of supporting healing objectives is now playing a much more significant role than it has over the past few decades.
- *Lack of critical care physicians and nurses*. Multiple authors predict the forthcoming lack of critical care nurses and doctors (Angus, 2005; Dracup and Bryan-Brown, 2004; Kelley et al., 2004; Robnett, 2006). In response to this situation, the AACN, the American Thoracic Society, the American College of Chest Physicians, and the Society of Critical Care Medicine published "Framing Options for Critical Care in the United States," which recommends regionalizing

resources, standardizing care through the use of practice guidelines, encouraging specialization, and redesigning the work environment (Dracup and Bryan-Brown, 2004; Kelley et al., 2004).

- *Aging population*. Observers of demographic trends predict that there will be a shortage of ICU beds in the future, due to the demands of a large aging patient population (Angus, 2005; Dracup and Bryan-Brown, 2004; Kelley et al., 2004). While PICUs are not directly impacted by the increase in the elderly population, potential critical care staff may be deflected to serve the older adult population. Relatedly, the ICU/PICU workforce is aging, which has an impact on staff needs (Foglia and Milonovich, 2011).
- *Gap between possible and appropriate care*. The gap grows between what is technologically possible and what may be appropriate for health interventions as new medical innovations are brought to the fore (Dracup and Bryan-Brown, 2004). Consideration of treatment choices may cause stress among families, staff, patients, and payers (Dracup and Bryan-Brown, 2004); Foglia and Milonovich (2011) suggest that medically advanced technology and treatment may result in unrealistic expectations on the part of families regarding the healing outcomes of their children.

7.1.2 Technological advances

- *Computer technology developments*. In 2001 Craft suggested that trends in computer technology such as advanced networking, more advanced computer platforms, better computer–human interface, instrumentation changes, increased interoperability among off-the-shelf products, automatic support for mechanistic tasks, more decision-support tools, and just-in-time reference materials would alter the critical care workplace. These fundamental computer interactions continue to evolve. Radio frequency identification devices, such as electronic chips that contain identification/location information, could be used to track assets, medical documents, patients, beds, and blood products (Rashid, 2011). This type of pervasive computing may support the integration of information at the patient's bedside (Rashid, 2011).
- *Tele-ICUs*. Research suggests that ICUs that have intensivists on staff have lower death rates – 15 percent to 60 percent lower than those that do not – and shorter lengths of stay (Gorman, 2011). At the same time the Committee for Manpower for Pulmonary and Critical Care Services predicts a shortfall of 10,000 ICU physicians (Gorman, 2011). Tele-ICUs (also referred to as eICUs) are being introduced to manage patient care in facilities without intensivists physically present (Olff and Clark-Wadkins, 2012). This is a useful approach, particularly in remote parts of the world. eICUS may mitigate the critical care staffing shortage, as intensivists and specialized ICU nursing staff transition into the role of care managers (Jerrard, 2005).
- *Robotics*. Related to eICUs is the use of remote robotics. Robotics technology is a "semi-autonomous, Internet-enabled, real-time, two-way audiovisual telecommunications platform that moves about in a wireless environment" (Reynolds et al., 2012, p. 507). The robots are described as providing a "remote presence" under the control of distant clinicians who can drive the equipment to the bedside, perform a visual exam, coach a local examiner, and analyze the information on monitors, ventilators, and pumps (Reynolds et al., 2012). Research suggests that the presence of this technology supports normal workflow and increases patient/family satisfaction (Reynolds et al., 2012).

- *Health informatics and electronic medical records*. Health informatics has impacted ICU administration, the management of resources, medical records, diagnostics, imaging, and clinical support systems (Rashid, 2011). More pervasive uses of personal digital assistants (PDAs) and bedside computing will permit more immediate access to information (Rashid, 2011). Although electronic medical records have been present in the PICU for more than 20 years, a fully integrated, searchable, accessible, and user-friendly document system is rare (Tegtmeyer, 2009). Advancements in this technology are likely to occur.
- *Patient monitoring*. Portable computed tomographic scanners may eliminate some need to transfer patients to off-unit diagnostic departments (Rashid, 2011), and monitoring devices may gather information suggesting specific trends (Rashid, 2011). Future wireless monitoring equipment systems may travel with the patient to facilitate transport and consistency of information (Rashid, 2011).
- *Infection control*. With regard to infection control, UV-C, high-intensity, broad-spectrum pulsed light has been found to be an effective means of destroying micro-organisms and could be used to treat surfaces (Rashid, 2011).

7.2 Future of NICU design

The following is a list of potential trends that will impact the NICU. The impact of these developments on the NICU population is harder to predict than the likelihood of the evolution of the potential programmatic and technological factors themselves. One potential scenario is that medical advances will save infant lives but may result in longer lengths of stay due to the complex nature of the procedures. On the other hand, medical advances may result in healing babies more quickly, thereby shortening their stays.

7.2.1 *Service and programmatic trends*

- *Trends in premature births*. The March of Dimes and other organizations have made a significant effort to reduce the number of premature births by supporting education programs, research, and prenatal care. There has been a slight downward trend in the number of premature births per capita over the past few years, which may result in a reduced patient census.
- *Importing women's services into children's hospitals*. A few children's hospitals (e.g. Texas Children's Pavilion for Women, Children's Hospital of Philadelphia Center for Fetal Diagnosis and Treatment) have added obstetric or fetal services to their facilities, at least partially, to enhance proximity to neonatal intensive care following high-risk pregnancies. Surgeons associated with NICU settings may be trained in fetal surgery, and other evolving specialties due to advanced knowledge and technology.
- *Couplet care*. Related to rooming-in and family-centered care, couplet care is a system in which mother and child are treated as a pair and not separated after birth. While in vaginal deliveries rooming-in has become standard, separation is more common following a surgical birth. However, organizations that advocate couplet care have successfully implemented specialized co-locational treatment programs for surgical mothers and their infants as well. For example, at the Women's Center at the University Community Hospital in Tampa, Florida, during the

process of redesigning their labor-delivery-recovery rooms and operating suites, a space that had previously been dedicated for surgical holding was redesigned as a couplet room, proximate to staff who were trained for mother/child emergencies (Spradlin, 2009).

- *Single family rooms*. There has been an increase in the United States of the proportion of single family rooms. The research associated with this book made it clear that many organizations that are proposing new, renovated, or expanded facilities are considering single family rooms as an option. In most parts of the world, space and financial constraints will continue to prohibit this possibility, although changes in operational protocols may help to reduce the frequency of infection and achieve the lighting and sound controls sought in the private room settings. In the open units, privacy and family/infant interaction will still be limited, but social interaction among the participants will be common.
- *Family-integrated care*. Highly proactive participation of NICU families in the care of their newborns is demonstrating to have positive outcomes on infants and their families (O'Brien et al., 2013). As poignantly expressed by Dr. Robert White,

  > The developmentally appropriate NICU of the future will not just prepare the baby for home, it will prepare home for the baby. Caregivers will still need technical expertise, but to a far greater extent will be teaching, encouraging, and facilitating family participation in care. The NICU of this future era will have better technology than our current units, yet it will be in the background – tiny, quiet, and efficient – allowing the "feel" of the unit to be closer to that of a multifamily home than of an ICU. After all … the current NICU environment was not the result of evidence that the sights, sounds, and feeling we currently experience are beneficial to babies. … This change is already well under way, and the outlines of the NICU of 2020 are starting to take shape.
  >
  > (White, 2011a, p. 749)

- *Reduction in medical errors*. The inordinately high number of medical errors in NICUs suggests that they will be one of the inpatient settings most significantly impacted by error reduction. With the current healthcare agenda regarding enhanced patient safety and the financial implications of errors, facilities are already experiencing improvements. Reductions in errors are likely to occur as a result of better communication systems, quiet workstations, better task lighting, closer supplies, and more technologies that don't require human intervention (Coull et al., 2011).
- *Education and research*. A shift is predicted that will involve the movement from infant care and tracking of complications to learning about the evolution of disease while caring for the child (Center for Integration of Medicine and Innovative Technology (CIMIT), n.d.).
- *Virtual annex*. The notion of a "virtual annex" to expand expertise to infants from other hospitals and developing countries (CIMIT, n.d.), similar to the concept of tele-ICUs, has been discussed in the context of neonatal critical care.

7.2.2 Technological advances

The number of medical and technological advances that will impact neonatal care is large. The list provided here is not all-inclusive but addresses some of the issues most frequently raised in the literature.

- *The artificial womb*. While in many ways the purpose of the incubator is to serve as an artificial womb, the science of the artificial womb bears a stronger similitude to the actual *in-utero* experience. Tanks filled with a fluid similar to amniotic fluid have brought goat fetuses, which were attached by an artificial umbilical cord that provided oxygen and nutrients, to term (Simonstein, 2006). An artificial womb option might serve to support prematurely born children by allowing them to continue their *in-utero* development outside of the mother's uterus. As the survival rate of extremely low birth weight babies at 23 weeks' gestational age is low – 68 percent in a 2002 study by Wilson-Costello et al. (2007) – this option has the potential of allowing the child to complete the *in-utero* experience and reduce subsequent medical complications. Although the technology may be in the distant future, as one researcher eloquently states, "The history of science tells us that impenetrable barriers are only temporary" (Simonstein, 2006).
- *Fetal surgery*. Significant advances have been made with regard to fetal surgery (Cortes and Farmer, 2004; Upadhyaya and Lander, 2013). Until recently, fetal surgery was limited to fetuses with poor prognoses for survival without the intervention. However, with developments in the imaging technology, endoscopic techniques, and anesthesia, fetal surgery is an option for fetuses for whom the objective is to improve the quality of subsequent life (Upadhyaya and Lander, 2013). Fetal surgery includes *in-utero* procedures (surgery performed while the baby is still in the womb), as well as *exo-utero* procedures (the baby is removed from the mother via surgery while still linked to the umbilical cord while the surgery is performed on the baby). The results of this surgery will generate a patient population with specialized care needs and forge a closer relationship between perinatal and neonatology services (Coull et al., 2011).
- *Genetic medicine*. The discussion of genetic medicine is common in the scientific and popular press. Developments in genetic medicine will impact treatment (Coull et al., 2011). In the 20th century, many physicians perceived genetics as an "esoteric academic specialty," a view that has become outdated (Guttmacher and Collins, 2002). Advancements in neonatal medicine have lowered the survival limits for preterm infants, but several multifactorial diseases (e.g. respiratory distress syndrome and retinopathy of prematurity, a disease of the eye associated with babies receiving intensive care) impact survival and development (Cotten et al., 2006). The recent complete sequencing of the human genome provides opportunities for assessing how genomic and environmental factors influence one another to contribute to disease (Cotton et al., 2006). Related to this, advances in pharmacogenetics (the study of genetic factors and reactions to drugs) will modify the delivery of medicines (Coull et al., 2011).
- *Computer science and engineering technology*. Aschner (2008) suggests that new pathways to discovery will be generated through increased understanding of biological systems and broad access to sensitive, adaptable, and robust technologies and databases. Such technologies include molecular imaging, nanomedicine (an application of nanotechnology, small machines which perform at the scale of molecules to prevent and treat diseases), and bioinformatics and computational biology (the use of computer technology to process biological information).
- *NICU magnetic resource imaging (MRI)*. The presence of MRI technology on the neonatal unit will enhance diagnostics (Coull et al., 2011). A 1.5 T MRI system for infants has been tested on lambs and demonstrated to provide reliable MRI measurements (Tkach et al., 2012). The presence of a neonatal MRI may reduce cost and room requirements, lower noise, improve access to the procedure, and narrow risk (Tkach et al., 2012). The use of MRI technology represents a transition in treatment protocols. The CIMIT (n.d.) predicts that the future NICU

will shift from invasive care, limited to heart and lungs, to real-time non-invasive imaging of multiple organs and comprehension of the disease process.

- *Tools for treatment*. Specific techniques for supporting recovery are in a continuous state of invention and evolution. For example, head cooling (cerebral hypothermia) has been found to be a feasible treatment for neonatal encephalopathy (Gluckman et al., 2005). Neonatal encephalopathy is the presence of nervous system dysfunction typically caused by oxygen deprivation, congenital diseases, or drug reactions.
- *Communication enhancements*. Communication systems, both among staff members and between staff and family, are improving. Regarding staff, silent alarm systems (visual and vibratory), higher quality video monitoring, reduced noise levels, task-specific light levels, and appropriate work areas can increase the effectiveness of communication. Meanwhile, systems such as Baby CareLink, developed by the National Library of Medicine, allow staff and family to remotely monitor babies, at the same time providing access to medical notes, reports, and growth information (Safran, 2003).

7.3 Future of PICU and NICU design research

1. *Performance evaluation*. A critical step in the process of creating built environments is evaluating whether the design has resulted in the intended impact. Methods for conducting pre- and post-evaluations in PICU and NICU settings have been summarized in Chapter 5. These methods include behavioral observation, interviews, questionnaires, physiological indicators, and the analysis of medical record data. Multiple occupancy evaluations have been conducted in NICUs over the past decade; however, few of them involve pre- and post-comparisons. There are very few occupancy evaluations on PICUs. The creation of an information repository for occupancy evaluation research, to allow for the meta-analysis of multiple evaluation case studies, is underway by various organizations such as the Center for Health Design in Concord, CA.
2. *Translational research*. Medical professionals, just like design professionals, indicate that one of the greatest limitations to improvement is delays is translating research into practice (Aschner, 2008). Recognizing this, various organizations are generating materials that mandate the design guidelines suggested by the research. All design research generated by academics (both faculty and researcher students) and practitioners should culminate in recommended guidelines. This approach is currently being practiced by journals, namely *Health Environments Research and Design* (*HERD*), which requires each article to include implications for practice. The concept of practitioner-focused facility evaluation (PFE) (Shepley, 2010) is a critical component of the occupancy evaluation designed to support translational research.
3. *Grounded theory*. Because there is so little research, particularly with regard to PICUs, there is a desperate need for broadly explorative studies to create a framework for subsequent, more focused studies. Grounded theory, described by Glaser and Strauss in 1967, is "a general methodology for developing theory that is grounded in data systematically gathered and analyzed. Theory evolves during actual research, and it does this through continuous interplay between analysis and data collection" (Strauss and Corbin, 1994). This approach will be helpful in determining particular areas of focus and relating various studies to one another. While grounded theory is typically thought of as qualitative research, it may be generated quantitatively as well.

4. *Specific PICU research topics*. It is both difficult and easy to discuss the future of PICU design research. There are only a few studies, and the potential topics are virtually limitless. A few suggestions follow.

   Hilal Ozcan (2006) notes two missing bodies of research regarding PICUs: (1) cross-cultural and transnational comparisons of the physical environment; and (2) sociological and philosophical evaluations of the meaning embedded within the PICU.

   > In the final analysis, 1) positive social interaction and the reduction of anxiety through love, touch, talk, meaningful sharing of experience, transcendence of prejudices, relaxation and rejuvenation, and provision of an equal and democratic practice of caring, 2) a psychological sense of belonging to a local and cultural environment (sense of place and community), and 3) spiritual transformation or self-transcendence … inform the functional, psychological and phenomenological requirements of healing ICU design.
   >
   > (Ozcan, 2006, p. 279)

   Most topics appropriate to adult units would serve to support PICUs, including studies on the impact of centralized versus decentralized nursing, but there are several areas of interest that pertain specifically to pediatrics. One of the most controversial is the use of private rooms for all pediatric inpatient settings. Several studies have reflected on the isolation of pediatric patients when families and caregivers are not present, but most agree that there are huge benefits regarding noise, light, family privacy, and infection control. PICU patients in particular are in need of private rooms, but studies should examine ways of mitigating isolation. Another discussion revolves around creating environments that are suitable for children of all ages. Little work has been done on specific dimensions (light, sound, color) for PICUs, although initial data has been gathered on preference for art. A few studies have addressed the impact of integrating family in the caregiving process, but this topic needs to be researched in more detail.

5. *Specific NICU research topics*. Although NICUs have been among the most studied healthcare environments, the number of topics that still need to be addressed or reaffirmed is significant. When choosing a topic, there are multiple possible approaches: (1) study prototypes and innovations, such as facilities with couplet care recovery rooms, as these projects may be emulated in other facilities when there are shortcomings that have not been identified and shared; (2) address pressing debates, such as the presence of windows to the outdoors as opposed to mere access to natural light in single family rooms; or (3) select research projects that focus on the most frail infants and their families, such as extremely low birth weight children. Developmental care has been promoted for many years; however, with the advent of single family rooms, studies should be carried out confirming the most effective protocols and room designs for achieving this care. Lastly, (4) consider addressing the social and human issues through both qualitative and quantitative research. As noted by Robert White,

   > We have nearly come full circle, from eons when infants spent most of their time in direct human contact, through a period where human contact was rare and usually unpleasant in our early NICUs. We are now approaching a day when the best medical care and nurturing are not mutually exclusive concepts, and where the mother's arms are considered the optimal locus of care. The goal of NICU design has evolved from efficient provision of optimal medical technology to providing the best environment of care for babies, families and caregivers alike. State-of-the-art technology and design are necessary but not sufficient

to reach this goal. Optimizing brain growth and development in the preterm infant and mental health in families and caregivers requires collaboration and a nurturing environment for all to thrive.

(White, 2011b, p. 6)

References

Aschner, J. (2008). *Future of NICU Care* [PowerPoint slides]. Retrieved from http://www2.aap.org/sections/perinatal/presentations/FutureofNICUCare_Aschner4-2008.pdf

Angus, D. (2005). The future of critical care. *Critical Care Clinics, 21*, 163–169.

Center for Integration of Medicine and Innovative Technology. (n.d.). Shaping the future of healthcare: Clinical systems innovation [PDF document]. Retrieved from http://www.cimit.org/images/media_center/ShapingTheFutureOfHealthcare.pdf Powerpoint presentation. www.cimit.org

Cortes, R.A., and Farmer, D.L. (2004). Recent advances in fetal surgery. *Seminars in Perinatology, 28*(3), 199–211.

Cotten, C.M., Ginsburg, G.S., Goldberg, R.N., and Speer, M.C. (2006). Genomic analyses: A neonatology perspective. *Journal of Pediatrics*, *148*(6), 720–726.

Coull, A., Mare, G., and Henson, M.M. (2011). Healthcare 201: Patient unit – neonatal intensive care unit and pediatric intensive care unit. Retrieved from http://www.aia.org/aiaucmp/groups/aia/documents/presentation/aiab087097.pdf

Craft, R.L. (2001). Trends in technology and the future intensive care unit. *Critical Care Medicine*, *29*(8), N151–N158.

Dracup, K., and Bryan-Brown, C.W. (2004). Navigating the future of critical care. *American Journal of Critical Care*, *13*(3), 187–188.

Foglia, D.C., and Milonovich, L.M. (2011). The evolution of pediatric critical care nursing: Past, present, and future. *Critical Care Nursing Clinics of North America*, *23*(2), 239–253.

Glaser, B.G., and Strauss, A.L. (1967). *The Discovery of Grounded Theory: Strategies for Qualitative Research*. New Brunswick, NJ, and London: Aldine Transaction.

Gluckman, P.D., Wyatt, J.S., Azzopardi, D., Ballard, R., Edwards, A.D., Ferriero, D.M., and Gunn, A.J. (2005). Selective head cooling with mild systemic hypothermia after neonatal encephalopathy: Multicentre randomised trial. *The Lancet*, *365*(9460), 663–670.

Gorman, M.J. (June 30, 2011). The future of tele-ICUs: An insider's perspective. Retrieved from http://www.medgadget.com/2011/06/the-future-of-tele-icus-an-insiders-perspective.html

Guttmacher, A.E., and Collins, F.S. (2002). Genomic medicine – a primer. *New England Journal of Medicine*, *347*(19), 1512–1520.

Jerrard, J. (November, 2005). The future of critical care. *The Hospitalist*. Retrieved from http://www.the-hospitalist.org/details/article/255801/The_Future_of_Critical_Care.html

Kelley, M.A., Angus, D., Chalfin, D.B., Crandall, E.D., Ingbar, D., Johanson, W., and Vender, J.S. (2004). The critical care crisis in the United States: A report from the profession. *Chest Journal*, *125*(4), 1514–1517.

Namachivayam, P., Shann, F., Shekerdemian, L., Taylor, A., van Sloten, I., Delzoppo, C., and Butt, W. (2010). Three decades of pediatric intensive care: Who was admitted, what happened in intensive care, and what happened afterward. *Pediatric Critical Care Medicine*, *11*(5), 549–555.

O'Brien, K., Bracht, M., Macdonell, K., McBride, T., Robson, K., O'Leary, L., and Lee, S.K. (2013).

A pilot cohort analytic study of family integrated care in a Canadian neonatal intensive care unit. *BMC Pregnancy and Childbirth, 13*(Supplement 1), S12. doi:10.1186/1471-2393-13-S1-S12
Olff, C., and Clark-Wadkins, C. (2012). Tele-ICU partners enhance evidence-based practice: Ventilator weaning initiative, *AACN Advanced Critical Care, 23*(3), 312–322.
Ozcan, H. (2006). *Healing design: A holistic approach to social interaction in pediatric intensive care units in the United States and Turkey* (Doctoral dissertation). Retrieved from ProQuest Dissertations and Theses (3202268).
Rashid, M. (2011). Technology and the future of intensive care unit design. *Critical Care Nursing Quarterly, 34*(4), 332–360.
Reynolds, E.M., Grujovski, A., Wright, T., Foster, M., and Reynolds, H.N. (2012). Utilization of robotic "remote presence" technology within North American intensive care units. *Telemedicine and e-Health, 18*(7), 507–515.
Robnett, M. (2006). Critical care nursing: Workforce issues and potential solutions. *Critical Care Medicine, 35*(3), S25–S31.
Safran, C. (2003). The collaborative edge: Patient empowerment for vulnerable populations. *International Journal of Medical Informatics*, *69*(2), 185–190.
Shepley, M. (2010). *Health Facility Evaluation for Design Practitioners*. Myersville, MD: Asclepion Publishing.
Simonstein, F. (2006). Artificial reproduction technologies (RTs) – all the way to the artificial womb? *Medicine, Health Care and Philosophy*, *9*(3), 359–365.
Spradlin, L.R. (2009). Implementation of a couplet care program for families after a cesarean birth. *AORN*, *89*(3), 553–562.
Stark, A. (May, 2004). Innovation in the design of the ICU: New trends that incorporate patient- and family-centered design. *Minnesota Physician*, 32–34.
Strauss, A., and Corbin, J. (1994). Grounded theory methodology: An overview. In N.K. Denzin and Y.S. Lincoln (eds) *Handbook of Qualitative Research* (pp. 273–285). Thousand Oaks, CA: Sage.
Tegtmeyer, K. (2009). The pediatric intensive care unit of the future: Technological advances in pediatric critical care medicine. In D.S. Wheeler, H.R. Wong, and T.P. Shanley (eds) *Science and Practice of Pediatric Critical Care Medicine* (pp. 105–111). London: Springer.
Tkach, J.A., Hillman, N.H., Jobe, A.H., Loew, W., Pratt, R.G., Daniels, B.R., and Dumoulin, C.L. (2012). An MRI system for imaging neonates in the NICU: Initial feasibility study. *Pediatric Radiology*, *42*(11), 1347–1356.
Upadhyaya, M., and Lander, A. (2013). Advances in fetal surgery. *Surgery*, *31*(3), 114–118.
White, R. (2011a). Design environment for developmental care. *Clinics in Perinatology, 38*(4), 745–749.
White, R. (2011b). The newborn intensive care unit environment of care: How we got here, where we're headed and why. *Seminars in Perinatology, 35*(1), 2–7.
Wilson-Costello, D., Friedman, H., Minich, N., Siner, B., Taylor, G., Schluchter, M., and Hack, M. (2007). Improved neurodevelopmental outcomes for extremely low birth weight infants in 2000–2002. *Pediatrics*, *119*(1), 37–45.

Conclusion

As mentioned in the introduction, *Design for Pediatric and Neonatal Critical Care* was formulated to supplement *Design for Critical Care* (2009). A compendium of works focusing on other specific healthcare environments and addressing similar topics would make a welcome addition to this series and contributions from future authors are welcome.

While thousands of resources were consulted in the process of generating these two publications, in some ways we have only scratched the surface of the subject of intensive care unit design. For example, supplemental material could be gleaned by examining specialized critical care units (e.g. cardiac), or step-down and transitional inpatient facilities. The issue of the impact of technology on critical care has been raised, but this inspiring topic deserves even more attention. Examining the role of embedded memory in spatial experiences and personal experiences in critical care settings would make for engaging expeditions. Lastly, a vast body of research from associated disciplines, such as sociology, psychology, engineering, and aesthetics, could be explored and would make an excellent foundation for future research on healthcare design.

In this book I have addressed the history of pediatric and neonatal care, design issues, design research topics, guidelines, and future directions. In Chapters 2 and 3 on the history of pediatric and neonatal care, I found that these fields, while supported by a sizable entourage of dedicated medical professions, are relatively new and still establishing their foothold. In terms of design issues, discussions in Chapter 4 revealed consensus around multiple topics, ranging from the developmental needs of children to the role of families, to factors that support staff efficacy. The summary of research, in Chapter 5, is wide-ranging in the disciplines that are addressed (e.g. sociology, psychology), as a result of the need to turn to other fields when information was not available that specifically addressed the physical environment. Chapter 6 allows us to put our feet back on the ground and consider in-the-trenches design practice regarding standards and recommendations. The codes and standards included in this book permit firms to pursue international practice, and give a sense of the approaches used in regions outside of North America. Chapter 7 encourages a release from the constraints of the present and engagement in conjecture about the future.

Constructing a manuscript like this is a learning process for the writer, and I welcome comments and reinterpretations from the readership. However, I can draw some pertinent conclusions from the experience. The exploration of the literature and consultation with practitioners led me to the following: (1) pediatric and neonatal care will remain specialized services and continue to evolve with the changing needs of the population; (2) some design goals for critical care environments are broadly agreed upon (e.g. the role of family-centered care), while others are still the subject of debate (e.g. the prevalent use of single family rooms); (3) while progress is being made regarding research on neonatal intensive care unit environments, research on pediatric intensive care is very limited; (4) a variety of countries provide guidelines/standards for neonatal intensive care, but few have guidelines specific to pediatric critical care; and (5) a prediction regarding the impact of future technology on care delivery is at best guesswork; transitions are occurring so rapidly that major impacts cannot be foreseen.

There is no higher calling for an architect or designer than to serve the most frail among our society. For this reason, addressing design and research in support of patients, families, and staff in pediatric and neonatal intensive care units feeds an important need to make a contribution and allows us to meet our social responsibility. Of course, we need help to meet this responsibility. Engagement by the entire cast of design team participants in the process of creating a new project, be they members of the healthcare community for the project that is being undertaken or adjunct experts, makes an incalculable difference in the success of a new project. The only way to excel in developing the most appropriate healing environments is to enlist the contributions of champions from all groups of stakeholders.

As architects and researchers, our purpose is to create environments that provide a supportive and minimally stress-inducing experience for staff. Our purpose is to design environments that best afford the opportunity for parents to bond with and care for their children. Our purpose is to provide intensive care environments that enable children to be soothed and healed.

Index

Note: Page numbers in *italics* indicate Figures.